The
Pandemic
Century

The Pandemic Century

A History of Global Contagion from the Spanish Flu to Covid-19

Mark Honigsbaum

WH ALLEN

3 5 7 9 10 8 6 4 2

WH Allen, an imprint of Ebury Publishing,
20 Vauxhall Bridge Road,
London SW1V 2SA

WH Allen is part of the Penguin Random House group of companies
whose addresses can be found at global.penguinrandomhouse.com

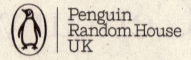

Penguin Random House UK

Copyright © Mark Honigsbaum 2019
Chapter 10 and epilogue copyright © Mark Honigsbaum 2020

Mark Honigsbaum has asserted his right to be identified as the author of this
Work in accordance with the Copyright, Designs and Patents Act 1988

First published by C. Hurst & Co. in 2019
This edition with new chapter and epilogue published by WH Allen in 2020

www.penguin.co.uk

A CIP catalogue record for this book is available from the British Library

ISBN 9780753558287

The epigraph taken from Albert Camus's *La Peste*, or *The Plague*, is reproduced
with kind permission of Editions Gallimard © Editions Gallimard, Paris, 1947.
All rights reserved.

The epigraph taken from René Dubos' 'Despairing Optimist' is reproduced
with kind permission of *The American Scholar* (Vol. 48, No. 2, Spring 1949).
© The Phi Beta Kappa Society, 1949.

Printed and bound in Great Britain by Clays Ltd, Elcograf S.p.A.

Penguin Random House is committed to a sustainable future
for our business, our readers and our planet. This book is made
from Forest Stewardship Council® certified paper.

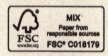

For Mary-Lee

"Everyone knows that pestilences have a way of recurring in the world; yet somehow we find it hard to believe in ones that crash down on our heads from a blue sky. There have been as many plagues as wars in history; yet always plagues and wars take people equally by surprise."

Albert Camus, *The Plague*, 1947.

CONTENTS

PROLOGUE

SHARKS AND OTHER PREDATORS

Sharks never attack bathers in the temperate waters of the North Atlantic. Nor can a shark sever a swimmer's leg with a single bite. That's what most shark experts thought in the blisteringly hot summer of 1916 as New Yorkers and Philadelphians flocked to the beaches of northern New Jersey in search of relief from the sweltering inland temperatures. That same summer the East Coast had been gripped by a polio epidemic, leading to the posting of warnings about the risk of catching "infantile paralysis" at municipal pools. The Jersey shore was considered a predator-free zone, however.

"The danger of being attacked by a shark," declared Frederic Lucas, director of the American Museum of Natural History, in July 1916, "is infinitely less than that of being struck by lightning and ... there is practically *no* danger of an attack from a shark about our coasts." As proof, Lucas pointed to the reward of $500 that had been offered by the millionaire banker Hermann Oerlichs "for an authenticated case of a man having being attacked by a shark in temperate waters [in the United States, north of Cape Hatteras, North Carolina]"—a sum that had gone unclaimed since Oerlichs had posted the challenge in the *New York Sun* in 1891.[1]

But Oerlichs and Lucas were wrong, and so were Dr Henry Fowler and Dr Henry Skinner, the curators of Philadelphia's Academy of Natural Science who had categorically stated, also in 1916, that a shark lacked the power to sever a man's leg. The first exception to these *known* facts had come on the evening of 1 July 1916, when Charles Epting Vansant, a wealthy young broker holidaying in New Jersey with his wife and family, decided to go for a pre-dinner swim near his hotel at Beach Haven. A graduate of the University of Pennsylvania's class of 1914, Vansant, or "Van" to his chums, was a scion of one of the oldest families in the country—Dutch immigrants who had settled in the United States in 1647—and famed for his athleticism. If he had any concerns about entering the cool Atlantic waters that evening, they would have been offset by the familiar sight of the beach lifeguard, Alexander Ott, a member of the American Olympic swimming team, and a friendly Chesapeake Bay retriever that ran up to him as he slid into the surf. In the fashion of young Edwardian men of the time, Vansant swam straight out beyond the lifelines, before turning to tread water and call to the dog. By now his father, Dr Vansant, and his sister, Louise, had arrived on the beach and were admiring his form from the lifeguard station. Much to their amusement, the hound refused to follow. Moments later, the reason became apparent—a black fin appeared in the water, bearing down on Vansant from the east. Frantically, his father waved for his son to swim to shore, but Vansant spotted the danger too late and when he was fifty yards from the beach he felt a sudden tug and an agonizing pain. As the sea around him turned the colour of wine, Vansant reached down to discover that his left leg was gone, severed neatly at the thigh bone.

By now Ott was at his side and dragging him through the water to the safety of the Engelside Hotel where his father desperately tried to stem the bleeding. But it was no use—the wound was too deep—and to his father and young wife's horror Vansant died then and there, the first known victim of a shark attack in the North Atlantic. From that moment on, neither would be able to look at Jersey's Atlantic seaboard without imagining the jaws lurking beneath the surface.

They were not alone. Within fourteen days, four more bathers would also be attacked on the Jersey shore and three would be killed, sparking an obsessive fear of "man-eating" sharks* that persists to this day.[2] It makes little difference that sightings of great whites and other large sharks in the North Atlantic are rare and attacks on swimmers rarer still. Beachgoers now *know* better than to swim too far from shore, and should they become blasé about the risks and dismissive of the menace, there is always a rerun of *Jaws* or an episode of the Discovery channel's *Shark Week* to set them straight. The result is that many children and a fair number of adults are now terrified of playing in the surf, and even those brave enough to venture beyond the breakers *know* to keep a wary eye on the horizon for the tell-tale sight of a dorsal fin.

* * *

At first glance, the New Jersey shark attacks would seem to have little to do with the Ebola epidemic that engulfed West Africa in 2014 or the Zika

---

* The species of shark or sharks responsible for the attacks has never been identified. Some experts believe they were the work of a juvenile great white, *Carcharodon carcharias*; others that they are consistent with the feeding pattern of bull sharks, which are known to favour shallow coastal waters.

epidemic that broke out in Brazil the following year, but they do, for just as in the summer of 1916 most naturalists could not conceive of a shark attack in the cool waters of the North Atlantic, so in the summer of 2014 most infectious disease experts could not imagine that Ebola, a virus previously confined to remote forested regions of Central Africa, might spark an epidemic in a major city in Sierra Leone or Liberia, much less cross the Atlantic to threaten citizens of Europe or the United States. But that is precisely what happened when, shortly before January 2014, Ebola emerged from an unknown animal reservoir and infected a two-year-old boy in the village of Meliandou, in south-eastern Guinea, from whence the virus travelled by road to Conakry, Freetown, and Monrovia, and onward by air to Brussels, London, Madrid, New York and Dallas.

And something very similar happened in 1997 when a hitherto obscure strain of avian influenza, known as H5N1, which had previously circulated in ducks and other wild waterfowl, suddenly began killing large numbers of poultry in Hong Kong, triggering a worldwide panic about bird flu. The great bird flu scare, of course, was followed by the panic about Severe Acute Respiratory Syndrome (SARS) in 2003, which was followed, in turn, by the 2009 swine flu—an outbreak that began in Mexico and set off an alarm about the threat of a global influenza pandemic that saw the drawdown of stockpiles of antiviral drugs and the production of billions of dollars' worth of vaccines.

Swine flu did not turn into a man-eater—the pandemic killed fewer people globally than common or garden strains of flu have in the United States and the United Kingdom most years—but in the spring of 2009 no one knew that would be the case. Indeed, with disease experts focused on the re-emergence of bird flu in Southeast Asia, no one had anticipated the emergence of a novel swine flu virus in Mexico, let alone one with a genetic profile similar to that of the virus of the 1918 "Spanish flu"—a pandemic that is estimated to have killed at least 50 million people worldwide and is considered a byword for viral Armageddon.[*]

* * *

---

[*] An epidemic is the rapid spread of infectious disease to a large number of people in a given population within a short period of time. By contrast, a pandemic is an epidemic that has spread across a large region, for instance, multiple countries and continents. This spread may be rapid or may take many months or years. The World Health Organization defines a pandemic simply as the "worldwide spread of a new disease."

PROLOGUE

In the nineteenth century, medical experts thought that better knowledge of the social and environmental conditions that bred infectious disease would enable them to predict epidemics and, as the Victorian epidemiologist and sanitarian William Farr put it in 1847, "banish panic." But as advances in bacteriology led to the development of vaccines against typhoid, cholera, and plague, and fear of the great epidemic scourges of the past gradually receded, so other diseases became more visible and new fears developed. A good example is polio. The month before sharks began attacking bathers on the Jersey shore, a polio epidemic had broken out near the waterfront in South Brooklyn. Investigators from New York's Board of Health immediately blamed the outbreak on recent Italian immigrants from Naples living in crowded, unsanitary tenements in a district known as "Pigtown." As cases of polio multiplied and the papers filled with heart-breaking accounts of dead or paralyzed infants, the publicity prompted hysteria and the flight of wealthy residents (many New Yorkers headed for the Jersey shore). Within weeks, the panic had spread to neighbouring states along the eastern seaboard, leading to quarantines, travel bans, and enforced hospitalizations.[3] These hysterical responses partly reflected the then-prevalent medical conviction that polio was a respiratory disease spread by coughs and sneezes and by flies breeding in rubbish.*

In his history of poliomyelitis, the epidemiologist John R. Paul describes the epidemic of 1916 as "the high-water mark in attempts at enforcement of isolation and quarantine measures." By the time the epidemic petered out with the cooler weather in December 1916, 27,000 cases and 6,000 deaths had been recorded in twenty-six states, making it the world's then-largest polio outbreak. In New York alone there had been 8,900 cases and 2,400 deaths, a mortality rate of around one child in four.[4]

The scale of the outbreak made polio appear a peculiarly American problem. But what most Americans did not realize is that a similarly devastating outbreak had visited Sweden five years earlier. During that outbreak, Swedish scientists had repeatedly recovered polio virus from the small intestine of victims—an important step in explicating the true aetiology and pathology of the disease. The Swedes also succeeded in culturing the virus in monkeys who had been exposed to secretions from asymptomatic human cases, fuelling suspicion about the role of "healthy carriers" in the preservation of the virus between epidemics. However, these insights were ignored by leading

---

* In fact, polio is spread principally via the oral-faecal route and nonparalytic polio had been endemic to the United States for several decades prior to 1916.

polio experts. The result is that it was not until 1938 that researchers at Yale University would take up the Swedish studies and confirm that asymptomatic carriers frequently excreted the polio virus in their stools and that the virus could survive for up to ten weeks in untreated sewage.

Today, it is recognized that in an era before polio vaccines, the best hope of avoiding the crippling effects of the virus was to contract an immunizing infection in early childhood when polio is less likely to cause severe complications. In this respect, dirt was a mother's friend and exposing babies to water and food contaminated with polio could be considered a rational strategy. By the turn of the nineteenth century, most children from poor immigrant neighbourhoods had become immunized in exactly this way. It was children from pristine, middle-class homes that were at the greatest risk of developing the paralytic form of the disease—people like Franklin Delano Roosevelt, the thirty-second president of the United States, who escaped polio as a teen only to contract the disease in 1921 at the age of thirty-nine while holidaying at Campobello Island, New Brunswick.

* * *

This is a book about the way that advances in the scientific knowledge of viruses and other infectious pathogens can blind medical researchers to these ecological and immunological insights and the epidemic lurking just around the corner. Ever since the German bacteriologist Robert Koch and his French counterpart, Louis Pasteur, inaugurated the "germ theory" of disease in the 1880s by showing that tuberculosis was a bacterial infection and manufacturing vaccines against anthrax, cholera and rabies, scientists—and the public health officials who depend on their technologies—have dreamed of defeating the microbes of infectious disease. However, while medical microbiology and the allied sciences of epidemiology, parasitology, zoology, and, more recently, molecular biology, provide new ways of understanding the transmission and spread of novel pathogens and making them visible to clinicians, all too often these sciences and technologies have been found wanting. This is not simply because, as is sometimes argued, microbes are constantly mutating and evolving, outstripping our ability to keep pace with their shifting genetics and transmission patterns. It is also because of the tendency of medical researchers to become prisoners of particular paradigms and theories of disease causation, blinding them to the threats posed by pathogens both known and unknown.

Take influenza, the subject of the first chapter. When the so-called "Spanish flu" emerged in the summer of 1918, during the closing stages of World War

I, most physicians assumed it would behave in a similar way to previous flu epidemics and dismissed it as a nuisance. Few thought the pathogen might pose a mortal threat to young adults, much less to soldiers en route to the Allied lines in northern France. This was partly because they had been informed by no less an authority than Koch's protégé, Richard Pfeiffer, that flu was transmitted by a tiny Gram-negative bacterium, and that it would only be a matter of time before bacteriologists trained in German laboratory methods had manufactured a vaccine against the influenza bacillus, just as they had against cholera, diphtheria, and typhoid. But Pfeiffer and those who put their faith in his experimental methods were wrong: influenza is not a bacterium but a virus that is too small to be seen through the lens of an ordinary optical microscope. Moreover, the virus passed straight through the porcelain filters then used to isolate bacteria commonly found in the nose and throat of influenza sufferers. Although some British and American researchers had begun to suspect that flu might be a "filter-passer," it would be many years before Pfeiffer's misconception would be corrected and influenza's viral aetiology divined. In the meantime, many research hours were wasted and millions of young people perished.

However, it would be a mistake to think that simply knowing the identity of a pathogen and the aetiology of a disease is sufficient to bring an epidemic under control, for though the presence of an infectious microbe may be a necessary condition for ill health, it is rarely sufficient. Microbes interact with our immune systems in various ways, and a pathogen that causes disease in one person may leave another unaffected or only mildly inconvenienced. Indeed, many bacterial and viral infections can lie dormant in tissue and cells for decades before being reactivated by some extrinsic event or process, whether it be coinfection with another microbe, a sudden shock to the system due to an external stress, or the waning of immunity with old age. More importantly, by taking specific microbial predators as our focus we risk missing the bigger picture. For instance, the Ebola virus may be one of the deadliest pathogens known to humankind, but it is only when tropical rain forests are degraded by clear-cutting, dislodging from their roosts the bats in which the virus is presumed to reside between epidemics, or when people hunt chimpanzees infected with the virus and butcher them for the table, that Ebola risks spilling over into humans. And it is only when the blood-borne infection is amplified by poor hospital hygiene practices that it is likely to spread to the wider community and have a chance of reaching urban areas. In such circumstances, it is worth keeping in mind the view expressed by George Bernard Shaw in *The Doctor's Dilemma*, namely that "The characteristic microbe of a disease might be a symptom instead of a cause." Indeed, updating Shaw's axiom for the present day, we might say that infectious diseases nearly always have wider environmental and social causes. Unless and until we take account of the ecological, immunological, and behavioural factors that govern the emergence and spread of novel pathogens, our knowledge of such microbes and their connection to disease is bound to be partial and incomplete.

In fairness, there have always been medical researchers prepared to take a more nuanced view of our complex interactions with microbes. For instance, in 1959 at the height of the antibiotics revolution, the Rockefeller researcher René Dubos railed against short-term technological fixes for medical problems. At a time when most of his colleagues took the conquest of infectious disease for granted and assumed that the eradication of the common bacterial causes of infections was just around the corner, Dubos, who had isolated the first commercial antibiotic in 1939 and knew what he was talking about, sounded a note of caution against the prevailing medical hubris. Comparing man to the "sorcerer's apprentice," he argued that medical science had set in motion "potentially destructive forces" that might one day usurp the dreams of a medical utopia. "Modern man believes that he has achieved almost completely mastery over the natural forces which molded his evolution in the past and that he can now control his own biological and cultural destiny," wrote Dubos. "But this may be an illusion. Like all other living things, he is part of an immensely complex ecological system and is bound to all its components by innumerable links." Instead, Dubos argued that complete freedom from disease was a "mirage" and that "at some unpredictable time and in some unforeseeable manner nature will strike back."[5]

Yet for all that Dubos's writings were hugely popular with the American public in the 1960s, his warnings of a coming disease Armageddon were largely ignored by his scientific colleagues. The result was that when, shortly after Dubos's death in 1982, the Centers for Disease Control and Prevention (CDC) coined the acronym AIDS, to describe an unusual autoimmune condition that had suddenly appeared in the homosexual community in Los Angeles and was now spreading to other segments of the population, it took the medical world by surprise. But really the CDC shouldn't have been surprised because something very similar had happened just eight years earlier when an outbreak of atypical pneumonia among a group of war veterans who had attended an American Legion convention at a luxury hotel in Philadelphia sparked widespread hysteria as epidemiologists scrambled to identify the "Philly Killer" (the outbreak initially flummoxed the CDC's disease detectives and it took a microbiologist to identify the pathogen, *Legionella pneumophila*, a tiny bacterium that thrives in aquatic environments, including the cooling towers of hotels). That year, 1976, saw not only a panic over Legionnaires' disease, but a panic over the sudden emergence of a new strain of swine flu at a US Army base in New Jersey—an emergence event for which the CDC and public health officials were likewise unprepared and that would eventually result in the needless vaccination of millions of Americans. And something very similar happened again in 2003 when an elderly Chinese professor of nephrology checked into the Metropole Hotel in Hong Kong, igniting cross-border outbreaks of a severe respiratory illness that was initially blamed on the H5N1 avian influenza virus but which we now know to have been due to a novel coronavirus* associated with SARS. In that case, a pandemic was averted by some nifty microbiological detective work and unprecedented cooperation between networks of scientists sharing information, but it was a close call, and since then we have seen several more unanticipated—and initially misdiagnosed—emergence events.

This is a book about these events and processes, and the reasons why, despite our best efforts to predict and prepare for them, they continue to take us by surprise. Some of these epidemic histories, such as the panic over the 2014–16 Ebola epidemic or the hysteria over AIDS in the 1980s, will be familiar to readers; others, such as the pneumonic plague outbreak that erupted in the Mexican quarter of Los Angeles in 1924, or the great "parrot fever" panic that swept the United States a few months after the Wall Street Crash, less so. Whether familiar or not, however, each of these epidemics illustrates how quickly the received medical wisdom can be overturned by the emergence of new pathogens and how, in the absence of laboratory knowledge and effective vaccines and treatment drugs, such epidemics have an unusual power to provoke panic, hysteria, and dread.

Far from banishing panic, better medical knowledge and surveillance of infectious disease can also sow new fears, making people hyperaware of epidemic threats of which they had previously been ignorant. The result is that just as lifeguards now scan the sea for dorsal fins in the hope of forewarning bathers, so the World Health Organization (WHO) routinely scans the internet for reports of unusual disease outbreaks and tests for mutations that might signal the emergence of the next pandemic virus. To some extent this hypervigilance makes sense. But the price we pay is a permanent state of anxiety

---

* Coronaviruses primarily infect the respiratory and gastrointestinal tracts of mammals and are thought to be the cause of up to one-third of common colds.

about the next Big One. It's not a question of *if* the Apocalypse will occur, we're repeatedly told, but *when*. In this febrile atmosphere it is not surprising that public health experts sometimes get it wrong and press the panic button when, in reality, no panic is warranted. Or, as in the case of the West African Ebola epidemic, misread the threat entirely.

To be sure, the media plays its part in these processes—after all, nothing sells like fear—but while 24/7 cable news channels and social media help to fuel the panic, hysteria, and stigma associated with infectious disease outbreaks, journalists and bloggers are, for the most part, merely messengers. I argue that by alerting us to new sources of infection and framing particular behaviours as "risky," it is medical science—and the science of epidemiology in particular—that is the ultimate source of these irrational and often prejudicial judgments. No one would wish to deny that better knowledge of the epidemiology and causes of infectious diseases has led to huge advances in preparedness for epidemics, or that technological advances in medicine have brought about immense improvements in health and well-being; nevertheless, we should recognize that this knowledge is constantly giving birth to new fears and anxieties.

Each epidemic canvassed in this book illustrates a different aspect of this process, showing how in each case the outbreak undermined confidence in the dominant medical and scientific paradigm, highlighting the dangers of overreliance on particular technologies at the expense of wider ecological insights into disease causation. Drawing on sociological and philosophical insights into the construction of scientific knowledge, I argue that what was "known" before the emergence event—that water towers and air conditioning systems *don't* present a risk to hotel guests and the occupants of hospitals, that Ebola *doesn't* circulate in West Africa and *can't* reach a major city, that Zika is a relatively harmless mosquito-borne illness—was shown to be false; and I explain how, in each case, the epidemics would spark much retrospective soul-searching about "known knowns" and "unknown unknowns"* and what scientists and public health experts should do to avoid such epistemological blind spots in the future.[6]

The epidemics canvassed in this book also underline the key role played by environmental, social, and cultural factors in changing patterns of disease

---

* The concepts of "known knowns" and "unknown unknowns" were infamously introduced into public discourse by the former US secretary of defense Donald Rumsfeld at a Pentagon news conference in 2002 (see endnotes for further discussion).

prevalence and emergence. Recalling Dubos's insights into the ecology of pathogens, I argue that most cases of disease emergence can be traced to the disturbance of ecological equilibriums or alterations to the environments in which pathogens habitually reside. This is especially true of animal origin or zoonotic viruses such as Ebola, but it is also true of commensal bacteria such as streptococci, the main cause of community-acquired pneumonias. The natural host of Ebola is thought to be a fruit bat. However, though antibodies to Ebola have been found in various species of bats indigenous to Africa, live virus has never been recovered from any of them. The reason, most likely, is that as with other viruses that are adapted to their hosts as a result of long evolutionary association, the Ebola virus is quickly cleared from the bloodstream by the bat's immune system, but not before, presumably, it has been transmitted to another bat. The result is that the virus circulates continually in bat populations, without leading to the destruction of either. A similar process occurs with pathogens that have evolved so as to infect only humans, such as measles and polio, with a first infection in childhood usually resulting in a mild illness, after which the subject recovers and enjoys lifelong immunity. However, every now and again these states of immunological balance are disrupted. This may occur naturally if, for instance, sufficient numbers of children escape infection in childhood to cause herd immunity to wane, or if the virus suddenly mutates, as occurs frequently with influenza, leading to the circulation of a new strain against which people have little or no immunity. But it can also occur when we accidentally interpose ourselves between the virus and its natural host. This is presumably what happened with Ebola in 2014 when children in Meliandou began taunting long-tailed bats roosting in a tree stump in the middle of their village. And it is thought that something very similar may have prompted the spillover* of the HIV progenitor virus from chimpanzees to humans in the Congo in the 1950s. Tracing the precise genesis of these epidemics is the subject of ongoing research. In the case of AIDS, there is little doubt that the inauguration of steamship travel on the Congo River at the turn of the twentieth century and the construction of new roads and railways in the colonial period were important contributing factors, as was the greed of loggers and timber companies. However, social and cultural factors also played a part: were it not for the practice of consuming bushmeat and widespread prostitution near the camps supplying labour to the

---

* A term popularized by David Quammen's 2012 book *Spillover: Animal Infections and the Next Human Pandemic*. See further discussion in Chapter 6.

rail and timber companies, the virus would probably not have spread so widely or been amplified so rapidly. Similarly, were it not for entrenched cultural beliefs and customs in West Africa—in particular, people's adherence to traditional burial rituals and their distrust of scientific medicine—it is unlikely that Ebola would have morphed into a major regional epidemic, let alone a global health crisis.

However, perhaps the most important insight medical history can bring is the long association between epidemics and war. Ever since Pericles ordered Athenians to sit out the Spartan siege of their harbour city in 430 BC, wars have been seen as progenitors of deadly outbreaks of infectious disease (this was certainly the case in West Africa in 2014, where decades of civil war and armed conflict had left Liberia and Sierra Leone with weak and under-resourced health systems). Though the pathogen responsible for the plague of Athens has never been identified and perhaps never will be (candidates include anthrax, smallpox, typhus, and malaria), there is little doubt that the decisive factor was the crowding of upwards of 300,000 Athenians and refugees from Attica behind the Long Walls of the Greek city. That confinement created the ideal conditions for the amplification of the virus—if virus it was—turning Athens into a charnel house (as Thucydides informs us, as there were no houses to receive the refugees from the countryside "they had to be lodged at the hot season of the year in stifling cabins, where the mortality raged without restraint"). The result was that by the third wave of the disease in 426 BC, Athens's population had been reduced by between one-quarter and one-third.[7]

In the case of the Athenian plague, for reasons that are unclear, the disease does not appear to have affected the Spartans, or spread far beyond the borders of Attica. But 2,000 years ago, towns and cities were more isolated and there was far less passage of people and pathogens between countries and continents. Unfortunately, this is not the case today. Thanks to global trade and travel, novel viruses and their vectors are continually crossing borders and international time zones, and in each place they encounter a different mix of ecological and immunological conditions. This was nowhere more true than during World War I, when the congregation of tens of thousands of young American recruits in training camps on the eastern seaboard of the United States and their subsequent passage to and from Europe provided the ideal conditions for the deadliest outbreak of pandemic disease in history.

1

THE BLUE DEATH

It was an unassuming village, much like any you would have encountered on a rural tour of New England in 1917. Blink and you might have missed it. Set in drab scrubland thirty-five miles northwest of Boston, Ayer comprised fewer than three hundred cottage-like dwellings, plus a church and a couple of stores. Indeed, were it not for the fact that the village sat at the junction of the Boston and Maine and Worcester and Nashua railroads and boasted two stations, there would have been little to recommend it. But in the spring of 1917, as America prepared to go to war and military planners began looking for suitable sites to train thousands of men responding to the draft, those railroad stations and empty fields marked Ayer out as special, unusual even. Perhaps that is why in May 1917 someone in Washington, DC stuck a pin with a red flag in a map of Lowell County, Massachusetts, and designated Ayer as the site of the cantonment of the new Seventy-Sixth Division of the US Army.

In early June leases were signed with owners of some 9,000 acres of tree-less "sprout" land adjacent to the Nashua River, and two weeks later engineers arrived to transform the site into a camp fit for Major General John Pershing's doughboys. In the space of just ten weeks, engineers constructed 1,400 build-ings, installed 2,200 shower baths, and laid sixty miles of heating pipes. Measuring seven miles by two, the cantonment contained its own restaurant, bakery, theatre, and fourteen huts for reading and fraternizing, plus a post and telegraph office. Arriving from Ayer—a short half-mile walk that led across the tracks of the Fitchburg railroad—the first sight to greet newly drafted men was the huge YMCA auditorium and the barracks of the 301st engineers.

To the right lay the barracks of the 301st, 302nd, and 303rd infantry divisions, and nearby, those for the field artillery, depot brigade, and machine-gun brigade. Beyond that lay fields for practicing drill and bayoneting skills, and an eight-hundred-bed hospital, also run by the YMCA. In all, the cantonment was capable of housing 30,000 men. But over the next few weeks, as raw recruits arrived from Maine, Rhode Island, Connecticut, New York, Minnesota, and as far south as Florida, the rough wooden barracks would be filled with in excess of 40,000 men, forcing engineers to erect tents for the overflow. In recognition of its importance to the north-eastern military command, the cantonment was named Camp Devens in honour of General Charles Devens, a Boston lawyer turned Civil War commander whose Union troops were the first to occupy Richmond after its fall in 1865. As Roger Batchelder, a propagandist for the War Department, put it, admiring Camp Devens from a hill outside Ayer in December 1917, the cantonment resembled nothing so much as a "huge city of soldiers."[1] What the observer did not say was that Devens also represented an unprecedented immunological experiment. Never before had so many men from so many different walks of life—factory workers and farmhands, machinists and college graduates—been brought together in such numbers and forced to live cheek by jowl.

Camp Devens was not the only camp to be hastily constructed that summer, nor was it the biggest. In all, draftees destined for the American Expeditionary Force would be sent for training to forty large camps across the United States. Some, such as Camp Funston, built on the site of a former cavalry station at Fort Riley, Kansas, accommodated as many as 55,000 men. Meanwhile, on the opposite side of the Atlantic at Étaples in northern France, the British had constructed an even larger facility. Built on low-lying meadows adjoining the railway line from Boulogne to Paris, Étaples had bunks for up to 100,000 British and Imperial troops and hospital beds for 22,000. In the course of the war, it is estimated that one million soldiers passed through Étaples en route to the Somme and other battlegrounds.

Nor were the facilities at many of these camps always as good as war supporters suggested. Indeed, in many cases mobilization had been so swift that engineers had been unable to complete the construction of hospitals and other medical facilities in time, and barracks were often so drafty that men were forced to huddle around stoves in the evening to keep warm and to sleep in extra layers of clothing at night. Some, such as Batchelder, saw this as a way of toughening recruits and preparing them for the hardships of trench warfare in northern France. "At Ayer it is cold, but … the cold weather is exhilarating; it inures the men who have always lived in hot houses to the out-door life."[2] However, others criticized the War Department for selecting a site so far north, saying it would have been better if Devens had been located in the South where the weather was more hospitable.

In truth, the principal danger was not the cold so much as the overcrowding. By bringing together men from so many different immunological backgrounds and forcing them to live at close quarters for weeks on end, the mobilization greatly increased the risk of communicable diseases being spread from one to another. Wars have always been incubators of disease, of course. What was different in 1917 was the scale of the call-up and the intermixing of men raised in very different ecological settings. In urban areas, where populations are denser, the chances of being exposed to measles or common respiratory pathogens, such as *Streptococcus pneumoniae* and *Staphylococcus aureus*, is far higher and usually occurs in childhood. By contrast, in an era before cars and buses, when children raised in rural areas tended to be educated at primary schools close to their homes, many avoided exposure to measles. Nor would many have been exposed to *Streptococcus pyrogenes* and other haemolyticus bacteria that cause "strep throat." The result was that as the US Army grew from 378,000 in April 1917 to a force of 1.5 million by the turn of 1918 (by the war's end, in November 1918, the combined strength of the US Army and Navy would be 4.7 million), epidemics of measles and pneumonia erupted at camps all along the eastern seaboard, as well as in several southern states.[3]

Prior to the introduction of antibiotics, pneumonia accounted for roughly one-quarter of all deaths in the United States. These pneumonias could be triggered by bacteria, viruses, fungi, or parasites, but by far the largest source of community-acquired outbreaks were pneumococcal bacteria (*Streptococcus pneumoniae*). Under the microscope these pneumococcal bacteria resemble any other streptococcus. However, one of *S. pneumoniae*'s unusual features is that it possesses a polysaccharide (sugar) capsule that protects it from drying out in air or being ingested by phagocytes, one of the immune system's principal cellular defences. Indeed, in moist sputum in a darkened room, pneumococci can survive on surfaces for up to ten days

Worldwide, there are more than eighty subtypes of pneumococcal bacteria, each one differing from the others in terms of the constitution of its capsule. For the most part, these bacteria reside in the nose and throat without causing illness, but if a person's immune system is impaired or compromised by another disease, such as measles or influenza, the bacteria can get the upper hand, triggering potentially fatal lung infections. Typically, such infections begin as an inflammation of the alveoli, the microscopic sacs that

3

absorb oxygen in the lungs. As the bacteria invade the alveoli, they are pursued by leukocytes and other immune cells, as well as fluids containing proteins and enzymes. As the air sacs fill they become "consolidated" with material, making it harder for them to transfer oxygen to the blood. Usually, this consolidation appears in patches surrounding the bronchi—the passages which branch from the bronchus, the tube that carries air from the trachea into the right and left lungs. When this consolidation is localized it is known as bronchopneumonia. However, in more severe infections, this consolidation can spread across entire lobes (the right lung has three, the left two) turning the lungs into a solid, liverlike mass. The effect on lung tissue is dramatic. A healthy lung is spongy and porous and a good conductor of sound. When a doctor listens to the breathing of a healthy patient through a stethoscope he or she should hear very little. By contrast, a congested lung conducts breathing sounds to the wall of the chest, resulting in rattling or cracking sounds known as rales.

In the late Victorian and Edwardian period, pneumonia was perhaps the most feared disease after tuberculosis and nearly always fatal, particularly in the elderly or those whose immune systems were compromised by other diseases. Prominent victims included the ninth president of the United States, William Henry Harrison, who died one month after his inauguration in 1841, and the Confederate general Thomas Jonathan "Stonewall" Jackson, who died of complications of pneumonia eight days after being wounded at the Battle of Chancellorsville in 1863. Another victim was Queen Victoria's grandson, the Duke of Clarence, who suffered a fatal case of double lobar pneumonia after contracting "Russian influenza" at Sandringham in the winter of 1892. Little wonder then that Sir William Osler, the so-called father of modern medicine, dubbed pneumonia the "Captain of the Men of Death."[4]

When contracted in childhood measles usually results in a rash and high fever accompanied by a violent cough and sensitivity to light, but in the case of the camp-acquired measles cases the symptoms were far more severe. The outbreaks produced the highest infection rates the army had seen in ninety-seven years and were often accompanied by an aggressive bronchopneumonia. The result was that between September 1917 and March 1918, more than 30,000 American troops were hospitalized with pneumonia, nearly all as a result of complications of measles, and some 5,700 died. The extent of the outbreaks astonished even battle-hardened doctors, such as Victor Vaughan, the dean of the University of Michigan's School of Medicine and a veteran of the Spanish-American War. "Not a troop train came into Camp Wheeler (near Macon, Georgia) in the fall of 1917 without bringing one to six cases of measles already in the eruptive stage," he wrote. "These men had brought the infection from their homes and had distributed its seed at the state encampment and on the train. No power on earth could stop the spread of measles through a camp under these conditions. Cases developed, from one hundred to five hundred a day, and the infection continued as long as there was susceptible material in the camp."[5]

By the spring of 1918 the War Department was being lambasted by Congress for shipping recruits to training camps before facilities were fully ready and under conditions that failed to meet basic standards of public health, and by July the department had appointed a pneumonia commission to investigate the unusual prevalence of the disease in the large cantonments. The commission read like a future who's who of American medicine, and included Eugenie L. Opie, the future dean of Washington University School of Medicine; Francis G. Blake, who would go on to become professor of internal medicine at Yale University; and Thomas Rivers, who would become one of the world's leading virologists and director of the Rockefeller University hospital in New York. Assisting them in the surgeon general's office with the rank of commanders were Victor Vaughan and William H. Welch, the dean of the Johns Hopkins School of Medicine and then the most famous pathologist and bacteriologist in America, and Rufus Cole, the first director of the Rockefeller University Hospital and a specialist in pneumococcal disease. Together with his assistant Oswald Avery, Cole would direct laboratory investigations of the pneumonia outbreaks and train medical officers in the correct techniques for culturing the bacteria and making serums and vaccines. Meanwhile, keeping a watch over their endeavours would be Simon Flexner, the head of the Rockefeller Institute and a former student and protégé of Welch.

* * *

While American physicians were worrying about camp-acquired measles and pneumonia cases, medics in the British Army were becoming concerned about another respiratory disease. Labelled "purulent bronchitis" for want of a better term, the disease had broken out at Étaples in the bitterly cold winter of 1917, and by February 156 soldiers were dead. The initial stages resembled ordinary lobar pneumonia—a high fever and the expectoration of blood-streaked sputum. But these symptoms soon gave way to a racing pulse accompanied by the discharge of thick pale yellow dollops of pus, suggesting bronchitis. In half of these cases death from "lung block" followed soon after.

Another striking feature was cyanosis. This condition occurs when a patient becomes breathless because the lungs can no longer transfer oxygen efficiently to the blood and is characterized by a dusky purple-blue discolouration of the face, lips, and ears (it is oxygen that turns blood in the arteries red). However, in the case of the Étaples patients, their breathlessness was so acute that they tore off their bedclothes in distress. At autopsy, the pathologist, William Rolland, was shocked to find a thick, yellowish pus blocking the bronchi. In the larger bronchi, the pus was mixed with air, but when he cut a section through the smaller tubes he wrote, "the pus exudes spontaneously ... with little or no admixture of air."[6] This explained why the attempt to relieve patients' symptoms by giving them piped oxygen had been of little use. Étaples was not the only army camp where this peculiar disease appeared. In March 1917 a similar outbreak had occurred at Aldershot, "The Home of the British Army," in southern England. Once again the disease proved fatal to half to those it infected, the signature feature being the exudation of a yellowish pus followed by breathlessness and cyanosis. Of the cyanosed patients, physicians noted, "no treatment that we have been able to devise appears to do any good." To some, the short shallow breathing recalled the "effects of gas poisoning,"[7] but later the bacteriologists and pathologists who examined the Aldershot and Étaples cases became convinced it had been a type of influenza.[8] Flu had long been recognized as a trigger for bronchial infections. During influenza epidemics and the seasonal outbreaks of the disease which occurred every fall and winter, epidemiologists were accustomed to seeing a spike in respiratory deaths, particularly among the very young or elderly sections of the population. But for young adults and those below the age of seventy, flu was considered more of a nuisance than a mortal threat to life, and convalescents were frequently viewed with suspicion.

* * *

We may never know whether the outbreaks at Étaples and Aldershot were flu, but in March 1918 another unusual respiratory outbreak visited a large army camp—this time at Camp Funston in Kansas. Initially, physicians thought they were seeing another wave of camp-acquired pneumonias, but they soon revised their opinion.

The first casualty was supposedly the camp cook. On 4 March, he woke with a splitting headache and aches in his neck and back and reported to the base hospital. Soon, one hundred other members of the 164th Depot Brigade had joined him, and by the third week in March more than 1,200 men were on the sick list, forcing Fort Riley's chief medical officer to requisition a hangar adjacent to the hospital for the overflow. The illness resembled classic influenza: chills followed by high fever, sore throat, headache, and abdominal pains. However, many patients were so incapacitated that they found it impossible to stand up; hence the malady's nickname, "knock-me-down fever." Most of the men recovered within three to five days, but, disturbingly, several went on to develop severe pneumonias. Unlike the pneumonias after measles, which tended to localize in the bronchi, these post-influenzal pneumonias frequently extended to the entire lobe of a lung. In all, such lobar pneumonias had developed in 237 men, roughly one-fifth of those hospitalized, and by May there had been 75 deaths. As Opie and Rivers discovered the following July when the pneumonia commission eventually arrived to conduct an investigation, there were other disturbing features, too: after the initial epidemic had petered out in March there had been further outbreaks in April and May, each one corresponding to the arrival of a new group of draftees.[9] Not only that, but men transferred to camps in the East appeared to carry the disease with them, and when many of these same men joined the American Expeditionary Force and mingled freely with soldiers sailing for Europe, they sparked further outbreaks on board Atlantic troopships. The pattern continued when the transports arrived at Brest, the main disembarkation point for American troops, and disgorged their cargo. "Epidemic of acute infectious fever, nature unknown," reported a medical officer at a US Army hospital in Bordeaux on 15 April. By May, "grippe" had broken out in the French lines and scores of British soldiers at Étaples were sick with PUO—"pyrexia of unknown origin." As at Funston, the initial cases were mild but by June thousands of Allied troops were being hospitalized, and by August alarm was mounting. "These successive outbreaks tended to be progressively more severe both in character and extent, which would speak for an increasing virulence of the causative agent," observed Alan M. Chesney, a medical officer at an AEF artillery training camp in Valdahon.[10]

Chesney's was a rare example of concern. In the summer of 1918 no one had experienced a pandemic of influenza for twenty-eight years. Compared to typhus, a deadly blood-borne disease spread by lice that lived in soldiers' clothing, or the septicaemia that bred in gunshot and shrapnel wounds, influenza was a trifling infection from the point of view of army medical officers. Civilian physicians regarded flu with similar disdain, particularly the British, who had long considered influenza a suspect Italian word for a bad cold or catarrh.*

---

* *Influenza* derives from the Latinate Italian phrase *influenza coeli*, meaning "influence of the heavens."

Besides, after nearly five years of brutal trench warfare which had already claimed the lives of tens of thousands of Europeans, and with two million Allied troops now dug in in northern France and Flanders, officers had more pressing issues on their minds. "Quite 1/3 of the Batt. and about 30 officers are smitten with the Spanish Flu," the poet Wilfred Owen informed his mother, Susan, disdainfully in a letter from a British Army camp in Scarborough, North Yorkshire, in June. "The thing is much too common for me to take part in. I have quite decided not to! Imagine the work that falls on unaffected officers."[11]

Owen was wrong to be so complacent. Between the summer of 1918 and the spring of 1919, tens of thousands of soldiers and millions of civilians would be mown down by Spanish flu (so-called because Spain was the only country not to censor reports of the spreading epidemic) as the disease ricocheted between America and northern Europe before engulfing the entire globe. In the United States alone, some 675,000 Americans would perish in the successive waves of flu; in France, perhaps as many as 400,000; in Britain, 228,000. Worldwide, the death toll from the Spanish flu pandemic has been estimated at 50 million—five times as many as died in the fighting in World War One and 10 million more than AIDS has killed in thirty years.

One reason Owen and others were so relaxed about influenza was that in 1918 medical scientists were confident that they knew how the disease was transmitted. After all, in 1892 Richard Pfeiffer, the son-in-law of Robert Koch, the German "father" of bacteriology, had announced that he had identified the disease's "exciting cause," a tiny Gram-negative bacterium he dubbed *Bacillus influenzae*. Pfeiffer's "discovery" came at the height of the so-called Russian influenza pandemic and made headline news around the world, fuelling expectations that it would only be a matter of time before scientists trained in German laboratory techniques had produced a vaccine. Never mind that other researchers were not always able to isolate "Pfeiffer's bacillus," as the bacterium was popularly known, from the throat washings and bronchial expectorations of influenza patients. Or that it was notoriously difficult to cultivate the bacteria on artificial media and it often took several attempts to grow colonies of sufficient size that the small, spherical, and colourless bodies could be visualized through a microscope using special dyes. Or that despite inoculating monkeys with the bacillus, Pfeiffer and his Berlin colleague, Shibashuro Kitasato, had so far been unable to transfer the disease, thereby failing the test of Koch's fourth postulate.[12] As far as most medical authorities were concerned, Pfeiffer's bacillus *was* the aetiological agent of influenza and that was that. Rare was the man of science who dared to challenge the authority of Koch and his disciples by expressing unease at the failure to find the bacillus in each and every case of influenza.

Perhaps that explains why, on arriving at Camp Funston in July, Opie, Blake, and Rivers had ignored the fact that researchers had failed to find *Bacillus influenzae* in 77 per cent of the pneumonia cases, or that the bacillus had also been isolated from the mouths of one-third of the healthy men, i.e., those who had *not* shown any signs or symptoms of influenza.* Instead, they tried to make sense of the higher pneumonia attack rates observed among African American draftees from Louisiana and Mississippi, an incidence they attributed to racial differences between white and "coloured" troops. This was despite observing that the units that had suffered most severely from post-influenzal pneumonias were the ones that were new to the camp and had only been at Fort Riley for three to six months, and that a greater proportion of the African American draftees came from rural areas.[13] For the most part, the survey was dull, repetitive work and Blake soon found himself longing for a change of scene. As he complained to his wife on 9 August, "No letter from my beloved for two days. No cool days, no cool nights, no drinks, no movies, no dances, no club, no pretty women, no shower bath, no poker, no people, no fun, no joy, no nothing save heat and blistering sun and scorching winds and sweat and dust and thirst and long and stifling nights and working all hours and lonesomeness and general hell—that's Fort Riley, Kansas."[14]

Very soon Opie, Blake, and Rivers would get orders to leave Kansas, only to be thrust into a far worse hell when they found themselves in the midst of a raging epidemic of influenza and pneumonia at Camp Pike, Arkansas. They were spared the worst hell of all, however.

* * *

In August 1918, Clifton Skillings, a 23-year-old farmer from Ripley, Maine, boarded a southbound Boston train. Like thousands of other American men of fighting age, Skillings had received his draft papers a few weeks earlier and had now been ordered to report for duty to Camp Devens. Alighting at Ayer, he fell into step with other draftees dressed in their Sunday best and began striding toward the camp, with a trooper on horseback leading the way. To the eyes of the Boston men, Ayer was a "hick town."[15] Whether Skillings thought it so he does not say, but to judge by his letters and his postcards he did not

---

* Today the bacillus is referred to as *Haemophilus influenzae*.

care particularly for the food. "We have your beans at noon but they are not like the beans you get at home," he complained to his family on 24 August. "It makes me think of mixing up dog food." Skillings immediately fell in with a group from Skowhegan, Maine, but was amazed to learn that the camp included men from midwestern states such as Minnesota. "There is a good many thousand men in this campground. It seems awful funny to see nothing but men ... I wish you folks could come in & look around." Four weeks later the size of the camp and the quality of food is the least of his concerns, however. "Lots of the boys are sick and in the hospital," he wrote home on 23 September. "It is a disease. Some [thing] like the Gripp ... I don't think I will get it."[16]

It's not known where the fall wave of influenza originated. It could have been incubating in America over the summer, but more likely it was introduced by troops returning from Europe. From an ecological point of view, northern France was a vast biological experiment—a place where large masses of men from two continents converged and mingled freely with men from a host of other nations, including Indian soldiers from the Punjab, African regiments from Nigeria and Sierra Leone, Chinese "coolies," and Indochinese labourers from Vietnam, Laos, and Cambodia. One theory is that the second wave began with an outbreak at a coaling station in Sierra Leone at the end of August, from whence it spread rapidly to other West African countries and to Europe via British naval vessels.[17] Another is that the bug was already in Europe, hence the pre-pandemic waves recorded in Copenhagen and other northern European cities in July.[18]

In the United States, the second wave had first announced itself toward the end of August at Commonwealth Pier in Boston, one of the main entry points for returning AEF troops, when several sailors were suddenly taken ill. By 29 August, fifty had been transferred to the Chelsea Naval Hospital, where they came under the care of Lieutenant Commander Milton Rosenau, a former director of the US Public Health Service's Hygienic Laboratory and a member of Harvard Medical School. Rosenau isolated the sailors in an effort to contain the outbreak, but by early September US naval stations in Newport, Rhode Island, and New London, Connecticut, were also reporting significant numbers of flu cases.[19] At around the same time, Devens saw an increase in pneumonia cases. Then, on 7 September, a soldier from Company B, 42nd infantry, was admitted to the base hospital with "epidemic meningitis." In fact, his symptoms—runny nose, sore throat, and inflammation of the nasal passages—were consistent with influenza, and when the following day twelve more men from the same company fell ill with similar symptoms, doctors had no hesitation in labelling it a "mild" form of Spanish influenza.[20] It would not remain mild for long.

When a parasitic organism meets a susceptible host for the first time, it triggers an arms race between the pathogen and the host's immune system. Having never encountered the pathogen before, the immune system is initially blindsided and takes time to mobilize its defences and launch a counterattack. With nothing to stop it, the pathogen tears through the host's tissue, invading cells and multiplying at will. At this stage, the parasite resembles a child having a tantrum. With no one and nothing to discipline it, its tantrum can easily escalate and its behaviour can become increasingly virulent. Eventually, in the most extreme cases of all, its rage may become all-consuming. This is usually bad news for the host. From a Darwinian point of view, however, the parasite does not want to kill its host; its primary objective is to survive long enough to escape and infect a new susceptible. In other words, the death of the host is a bad strategy for a parasite, an "accident" of biology if you will. A far better survival strategy over the long term is to evolve in the other direction, toward avirulence, resulting in an infection that is mild or barely detectable in the host. But in order for that to happen, the immune system must first find a way of taming the parasite.

It did not take long for the infection to spread from the 42nd infantry to adjacent barracks, and when it did, the flu was nothing like the "mild" spring wave. It was explosive. By 10 September more than five hundred men had been admitted to the base hospital at Devens. Within four days, those numbers had tripled, and on 15 September a further 705 were admitted. The next three days were the worst, however. On 16 September medical orderlies had to find beds for a further 1,189 men and the following day beds for 2,200 more. The pneumonia cases began to mount soon afterward, but they were nothing like the bronchopneumonias associated with measles. Instead, they resembled more severe versions of the lobar pneumonias that had developed in some of the flu cases at Camp Funston in the spring. "These men start with what appears to be an ordinary attack of *La Grippe* or Influenza, and when brought to the Hosp. they very rapidly develop the most vicious type of Pneumonia that has ever been seen," recalled a Scottish physician named Roy, who was present when pneumonia ripped through the wards. "Two hours after admission they have the Mahogany spots over the cheek bones, and a few hours later you can begin to see the Cyanosis extending from their ears and spreading all over the face, until it is hard to distinguish the coloured men from the white.... One could stand it to see, one, two or twenty men die, but to see these poor devils dropping like flies ... is horrible."[21]

As the writer John Barry noted in his book *The Great Influenza*, in 1918 these cyanoses were so extreme that victims' entire bodies would take on a dark purple hue, sparking "rumours that the disease was not influenza, but the Black Death."[22] British Army medical officers, many, like Welch and Vaughan, experienced civilian physicians and pathologists who had taken military commissions at the outset of war, were similarly impressed by these cyanotic cases and, struck by the resemblance to the cyanoses seen at Étaples and Aldershot in the winter of 1917, commissioned an artist from the Royal Academy to paint patients in the last throes of illness. The artist labelled the final stage "heliotrope cyanosis" after the deep blue flowers of the same name beloved by English gardeners.[23]

As concerns about measles and pneumonia had grown over the summer, the surgeon general's office in Washington had kept Welch, Vaughan and Cole busy. They were sent to make an inspection of Camp Wheeler, near Macon, Georgia, and other camps in the South. On leaving Macon in early September, Welch had suggested they stop at the Mountain Meadows Inn, a fashionable retreat in Asheville, North Carolina. A portly man famous for his love of cigars and gourmet dining, Welch was now in his late sixties and, except for a strip of white around the ears, almost completely bald. To offset the absence of hair on top, he sported a fashionable goatee and moustache, which were also white. To some this gave him the appearance of an elder statesmen—an impression underscored by his reputation for being an aloof and distracted teacher. But that was the older Welch. In his youth his imagination had been fired by reports from Germany of the advances being made in the understanding of disease processes using the microscope and new laboratory methods, and in 1876 he had set sail for Leipzig to work with Carl Ludwig, then the foremost experimental pathologist in the world. From Ludwig, Welch learned that "the most important lesson for a microscopist [was] not to be satisfied with loose thinking and half proofs ... but to observe closely and carefully facts." The experience made an indelible impression and, on his return to the United States, Welch set about conveying the principles and techniques he had acquired in Europe to a new generation of American medical students, first at Bellevue Medical College, New York, and later at Johns Hopkins, the university that, more than any other American institution, is credited with creating a new paradigm for medical education in the United States.[24] There, to contemporaries such as William Osler and William Steward Halstead, Welch was considered a bon vivant whose favourite pastimes were swimming, carnival rides, and five-dessert dinners in Atlantic City. But for all that they might tease the confirmed bachelor by referring to him as "Popsy," they also recognized that few could equal Welch's skills as an anatomist. When Welch cared to, he could also awe his students with his intellect and knowledge of art and culture. As Simon Flexner, who went on to write a biography of his former teacher, recalled, Welch's technique was initially to ignore his students and leave them to their own devices in the laboratory. But on rare evenings when he invited promising students to dine with him, "a spell fell over the room as the quiet voice talked on, and the young men, some of them already a little round-shouldered from too much peering into the microscope ... resolved to go to art galleries, to hear music, to read the masterpieces of literature about which Welch discoursed so excitingly."[25]

Welch and his colleagues used their stay in North Carolina to go over what they had learned during their tour of the South. The consensus was that a better understanding of the immunity of newly drafted men held the key to understanding the measles and pneumonia outbreaks. The Meadows Inn "is a delightful, restful, quiet place," Welch observed on 19 September. It would be the last respite the group would enjoy for some time.

Two days later they were back in Washington, DC, but no sooner had they alighted at Union Station than they were informed that Devens had been struck by Spanish influenza and they were to proceed immediately to Ayer. The scene that confronted them there was shocking and difficult to comprehend. By now the base hospital was overflowing with patients and care was almost non-existent. More than 6,000 men were crammed into the 800-bed facility, with cots installed in every nook, crevice, and cranny. Nurses and doctors had so exhausted themselves caring for the sick that many also now lay ill or dying, having failed, as one observer put it, to "buck the game."[26] Everywhere Welch and Vaughan looked there were men coughing up blood. In many instances, crimson fluids poured from nostrils and ears. Even eight years later the images were still etched in Vaughan's memory. "I see hundreds of young, stalwart men in the uniform of their country coming into the wards of the hospital in groups of ten or more," he wrote in 1926. "They are placed on the cots until every bed is full and yet others crowd in. The faces soon wear a bluish cast; a distressing cough brings up the bloodstained sputum. In the morning the dead bodies are stacked about the morgue like cord wood ... such are the grewsome [sic] pictures exhibited by the revolving memory cylinders in the brain of an old epidemiologist."[27]

The scene that greeted them in the autopsy room, once they had stepped over the cadavers blocking the entrance, was possibly even more gruesome. Before them, on the autopsy table, lay the corpse of a young man. According to Cole, when they tried to move him, bloody fluids poured from his nose.

Nevertheless, Welch decided it was imperative to take a closer look at his lungs. What he saw astonished the veteran pathologist. As Cole recalled: "When the chest was opened and the blue swollen lungs were removed and opened, and Dr Welch saw the wet, foamy surfaces with real consolidation, he turned and said, 'This must be some new kind of infection or plague' ... it shocked me to find that the situation, momentarily at least, was too much even for Dr Welch."[28]

By the end of October one-third of the camp's population, some 15,000 soldiers, had contracted influenza and 787 had died of the pneumonic complications of the disease. Two-thirds of these pneumonias were of the lobar variety.[29] Such pneumonias tended to have a very rapid onset and terminated in either massive pulmonary haemorrhage or pulmonary edema. The devastation was far more extensive than is usually seen in lobar pneumonias, with damage to the epithelial cells that line the respiratory tract but little evidence of bacterial action. The other type was more akin to an acute aggressive bronchopneumonia and was characterized by more localized changes, from which pathogenic bacteria could usually be cultured at autopsy.[30]

The first kind of pneumonia was unlike anything pathologists had observed before in either lobar or bronchopneumonias, fully justifying Welch's description of it as some new kind of plague. But while Welch's intuition may have been correct, he was not yet ready to abandon old certainties. Perhaps it was the fault of his formative years in Leipzig, followed by his battles to get the American medical profession to embrace the new German laboratory methods, that made him reluctant to challenge the conclusions reached by Pfeiffer as to the aetiological role of his bacillus, even when his gut instincts as a pathologist told him that this was something both new and terrifying. Or perhaps it was the fact that by now American scientists trained in the same bacteriological techniques were finding *B. influenzae* in influenza patients with similarly gruesome lung pathologies. Foremost among these scientists was William H. Park, the chief of the laboratory division of the New York City Health Department, and his deputy Anna Williams, both highly respected medical researchers. Mindful of the importance of observing "closely and carefully" and "not to be satisfied with ... half proofs," Welch approached Burt Wolbach, the chief pathologist of Brigham Hospital, Boston, and asked him to conduct further autopsies to see if all cases of this influenza shared the same peculiar lung pathology he had seen at Devens. Next he called the surgeon general's office to give a detailed description of the disease and urge that "immediate provision be made in every camp for the rapid expansion of hospital space."[31] The third person he approached was Oswald Avery at the Rockefeller Institute.

A methodical medical researcher, famous for his austere lifestyle, Avery lived for the laboratory. Working with Cole, he had already perfected techniques for identifying the four main subtypes of pneumococcus responsible for lobar pneumonia using specific serums. Next he had gone on to study how efficiently each type killed mice and in what dosages—experiments that led him to conclude that virulence was a function of the ability of the polysaccharide capsule of the pneumococcus to resist ingestion by white blood cells, the immune system's first line of defence against invasive bacteria.

One of the challenges of culturing *Bacillus influenzae* is that it is a fastidious organism that grows only within a very narrow temperature range and which depends heavily on oxygen, meaning it is usually found only on the surface of culture mediums. Because it tends to grow singly or in pairs, and its colonies are translucent and lacking in structure, it is also very easy to miss when looking through the field of an optical microscope. Pfeiffer had realized that a substrate of haemoglobin greatly facilitated growth of the bacillus and promoted his blood agar culture as necessary for establishing it (Pfeiffer recommended pigeon's blood; other researchers used rabbit's blood). Once a bacteriologist had obtained colonies of the bacillus, the next step was to stain it with an appropriate dye, wash it with alcohol, then stain it again with a contrasting dye (Gram-positive bacteria retain crystal violet stains, whereas *B. influenzae* and other Gram-negative bacteria, such as mycobacteria, require red counterstains).[32] Such stains could also be applied directly to slides smeared with sputum from influenza cases. However, a more precise and conclusive method was to prepare pure cultures of the bacillus by inoculating mice with sputum from flu patients and then growing the bacteria from fluids taken from the mice and reintroduced to the blood agar media.

Like other researchers, Avery at first found it difficult to grow Pfeiffer's bacillus from the sputum and bronchial expectorations of flu victims, so, to increase his chances, he refined his methods, adding acids to his agar culture medium and substituting defibrinated blood for untreated blood (other researchers heated the blood or filtered and dried it to separate the haemoglobin from the fibrin). Gradually, as Avery perfected his techniques, he was able to find the bacillus more and more frequently, until he was able to tell Welch it was present in twenty-two of thirty dead soldiers examined at Devens. Wolbach's results were even more definitive: he had found the bacillus in every case he examined at Brigham Hospital. That was enough for Welch, Cole, and Vaughan. "It is established that the influenza at Camp Devens is caused by the bacillus of Pfeiffer," they wired the surgeon general on 27 September.[33]

* * *

In fact, influenza is a viral infection. *B. influenzae* is merely a fellow traveller. Like other bacteria commonly found in the mouths, throats, and lungs of influenza patients, it is not the primary cause of the disease, though it may play a role in secondary infections.[34] However, in the fall of 1918 no one knew this, though some researchers had begun to suspect it. Instead, failure to cultivate *B. influenzae* reflected badly on researchers, not the theory of bacterial causation. Indeed, so dominant was the scientific view that influenza was a bacterial infection that, rather than doubt Pfeiffer's claim, scientists chose to doubt their instruments and methods. If the bacillus could not be cultivated on the first attempt, they needed to improve their culture medium, refine their dyes, and try again.

Anomalies are a common occurrence in science. No two experiments are ever exactly alike, but by refining methods and sharing tools and technologies, scientists are broadly able to reproduce each other's observations and findings, thereby arriving at a consensus that this or that interpretation of the world is correct. That is how knowledge emerges and a particular paradigm comes to be adopted. However, there is no such thing as absolute certainty in science. Paradigms are constantly being refined by new observations and, if enough anomalies are found, faith in the paradigm may be undermined and a new one may come to supplant it. Indeed, the best scientists welcome anomalies and uncertainty as this is the way scientific knowledge advances.

When Pfeiffer first put forward his claim for the aetiological role of his bacillus, the science of bacteriology and the germ-theory paradigm (one germ, one disease) was in the ascendancy. With the invention of improved achromatic lenses and better culture-staining techniques, by the late 1880s Robert Koch and Louis Pasteur had brought a series of hitherto hard-to-detect germs into view. These included not only such landmark bacteria as the bacilli of fowl cholera and tuberculosis, but streptococcus and staphylococcus. In short order, their discoveries paved the way for the development of serums and bacterial vaccines against diseases such as cholera, typhoid and plague, and by the eve of World War I, Avery and Cole were using the same methods to develop vaccines for pneumococcal pneumonias.

When Pfeiffer made his announcement in 1892, it raised hopes that it would not be long before bacteriology had also delivered a vaccine for influenza. But from the beginning, Pfeiffer's claim was dogged by doubts and anomalous observations. The first problem was that Pfeiffer had failed to find *B. influenzae* in the majority of clinical cases he had examined in Berlin during the Russian influenza epidemic. Second, as noted previously, he had been unable to reproduce the disease in monkeys inoculated with pure cultures of the bacillus (Pfeiffer does not specify what type of monkey he used, but his failure may have been because many monkeys are a poor refractory species for human influenzas).[35] Soon afterwards, Edward Klein, a Vienna-trained histologist and author of the leading British textbook on bacteriology, succeeded in isolating the bacillus from a series of patients admitted to hospitals in London during the same epidemic of Russian flu. However, Klein also noted finding "crowds" of other bacteria in sputum cultures and observed that as the condition of influenza patients improved, it became progressively more difficult to find Pfeiffer's bacillus in the colonies on the agar plating medium used to grow bacteria. Finally, Klein noted that *B. influenzae* had also been isolated from patients suffering diseases *other than* influenza.

After 1892, the Russian influenza epidemic abated and it was no longer possible to conduct bacteriological exams of influenza patients. Now and then there would be a resurgence of Russian flu, however, and investigators would attempt to culture the bacillus from the sputum and lung secretions of convalescents. Sometimes these efforts succeeded, but just as often they did not. For instance, in 1906 David J. Davis, from the Memorial Institute for Infectious Disease in Chicago, reported being able to isolate the bacillus in only three of seventeen cases of influenza. By contrast he had found the bacillus in all but five of sixty-one cases of whooping cough. The following year, W. D'Este Emery, clinical pathologist at King's College London, noted that *B. influenzae* grew more readily in culture in the presence of other respiratory bacteria and seemed to be more virulent for animals in the presence of killed streptococci, leading him to speculate that Pfeiffer's bacillus might, for the most part, be a "harmless saprophyte" and that it required other respiratory pathogens to make it pathogenic.[36]

With the emergence of Spanish flu in 1918, researchers were able to resume their investigations. Again, the results were mixed, and again the anomalies cast doubt on Pfeiffer's claim. By the summer, concerns had reached such a pitch that a special meeting was convened at the Munich Medical Union. Summarizing the debate, *The Lancet* wrote that "Pfeiffer's bacillus has been found but exceptionally," and that if any bacteria had a claim to be the cause of influenza it should be the far more common streptococci and pneumococci.[37] Britain's Royal College of Physicians concurred, arguing that there was "insufficient evidence" for Pfeiffer's claim, though it was happy to allow that the bacillus played an important secondary role in fatal respiratory complications of influenza.[38] In other words, the aetiological role of *B. influenzae* might be open to question, but the bacterial paradigm was not. However, this paradigm was now facing a serious challenge from another quarter.

If Koch was the German father of bacteriology, then Louis Pasteur was its French parent or, as one writer puts it, microbiology's "lynchpin."[39] In his first biological paper, published in 1857 at the age of 35, Pasteur, then a relatively unknown French chemist working in Lille, boldly formulated what he called the germ theory of fermentation—namely, that each particular type of fermentation is caused by a specific kind of microbe. In the same paper he suggested that this theory could be generalized into a specific microbial aetiology of disease and, later, a general biological principle captured by his phrase, "Life is the germ, and the germ is life." However, in his own lifetime Pasteur's fame rested on a famous set of public experiments conducted two decades later, in which he isolated the bacteria of anthrax and chicken cholera and, using basic chemical techniques (heat or exposure to oxygen), weakened the microbes to the point where they lost their virulence. Next, he demonstrated that these weakened strains could confer protection to animals challenged with fully virulent versions of the same bacteria. In so doing, Pasteur opened up a whole new branch of microbiology: the study of immunology. Pasteur realized that weak or attenuated microbes stimulated the host (sheep in the case of anthrax; chickens in the case of cholera) to produce substances (antibodies) that protected them against challenge with more virulent, disease-causing microbes. Eight years later, in 1885, Pasteur conducted an even more astounding microbiological experiment by applying the same principles to the rabies virus. Taking the spinal cord from a rabid dog, he injected the diseased material into a rabbit, and, when the rabbit fell ill, repeated the procedure with another rabbit. By passaging the virus in rabbits every few days, he was able to heighten its virulence for rabbits, but reduce its virulence for dogs. Next, he went a stage further and removed the spinal cord of a dead rabbit and dried it for fourteen days. This new attenuated virus no longer caused disease in dogs at all. Instead, it immunized them against challenge with fully virulent rabies. Next, Pasteur staged a daring public demonstration by administering his vaccine to a nine-year-old boy, Joseph Meister, who had been bitten in fourteen places by a rabid dog. Meister made a rapid recovery, prompting banner headlines. Other than smallpox, this was the first successful immunization with a virus vaccine, and within a few months Pasteur was inundated with requests from victims of rabid animal attacks from Smolensk to Seville. However, perhaps the most remarkable aspect of Pasteur's breakthrough in retrospect is that he developed the vaccine without being able to see the rabies virus or having much idea what a virus was. The reason is that rabies, like other viruses, is too small to be seen through an optical microscope (it measures 150 nanometres, or 0.15 micrometres, and requires magnifications ten thousand times greater than were available in Pasteur's day). But although Pasteur could not visualize the virus or cultivate it in the laboratory, he could intuit its existence by excluding microbes that he *could* grow and see, i.e., bacteria. Indeed, in 1892, the same year that Pfeiffer had claimed that a bacillus was the cause of influenza, the Russian botanist Dmitry Ivanovski had shown that tobacco mosaic disease was caused by an unseen agent that passed through porcelain filters with pores too small to admit bacteria. By the turn of the century, these filters, known as Chamberland filters after their inventor Charles Chamberland, were being manufactured and used in research laboratories in Europe and elsewhere, leading to the identification of a variety of "filter passing" agents, including the agents of foot and mouth disease of cattle, bovine pleuropneumonia, rabbit myxomatosis and African horse sickness. Then, in 1902, a commission headed by US Army Surgeon Walter Reed identified the first filter-passing human disease, yellow fever.[40] At the Pasteur Institute in Paris, these agents were referred to as "*virus filtrants*"—"filter-passing viruses."

After his death in 1885, Pasteur's disciples, such as Emile Roux and Roux's star pupil Charles Nicolle, continued these investigations. Dividing his time between biomedical research and administrative duties—it was Roux who created the Pasteur Institute—by 1902 Roux had identified ten diseases that he believed were due to filter-passing viruses. The same year, he persuaded Nicolle to join the Pasteur Institute in Tunis. Though greatly attracted by literature, Nicolle had bowed to the wish of his physician father and studied medicine, but while practicing in Rouen had suffered a hearing loss that prevented him from effectively using a stethoscope—an accident that may have persuaded him to concentrate on bacteriology instead and accept the position in North Africa. Nicolle quickly showed himself worthy of Roux's faith, and on arriving in Tunis launched a study of epidemic typhus. At the time, most doctors thought typhus, which tended to decimate armies at times of war and was a particular problem in prisons and other closed institutions, was a disease of filth and squalor. No one realized typhus was actually transmitted by the body louse (*Pediculus humanis corporis*), which infested unlaundered clothing, or that the agent was a tiny intracellular organism belonging to the *Rickettsia* family—the same family responsible for the tick-borne disease Rocky Mountain spotted fever. Nicolle began by injecting guinea pigs with blood from patients with typhus, showing that, although they did not develop the disease, the inoculations resulted in transient fevers—evidence that they were sub-clinically or, as Nicole put it, "inapparently" infected by something in the blood. However, the crucial observation came when he was observing typhus patients entering the Sadiki Hospital in Tunis and realized that they ceased to be infectious as soon as their clothing was removed and they were bathed and dressed in hospital uniforms. Suspecting that lice, not dirt, was the cause, Nicolle requested a chimpanzee from Roux and injected the chimp with blood from a typhus patient. When the chimp developed fever and skin eruptions, he injected its blood into a macaque monkey, and when the macaque also fell ill he allowed lice to feed on it. In this way, he was able to transfer the infection to other macaques and, eventually, a chimp. In September 1909, he communicated his finding that lice were the carriers of typhus to the French Academy of Sciences—a discovery for which in 1928 he was awarded the Nobel Prize.[41]

Although Nicolle's efforts to develop a vaccine for typhus would be unsuccessful (this would be left to others), it was only natural that when the influenza epidemic struck he would want to study it using similar methods. There is no evidence that Nicolle had worked on influenza before or had tried to culture its putative bacillus, but by the summer of 1918 French bacteriologists raised in the Pastorian tradition were finding it increasingly difficult to isolate Pfeiffer's organism and were becoming increasingly sceptical of the German's claims. Instead, Nicolle and his assistant, Charles Lebailly, began to suspect that, like the microbe of yellow fever, influenza might be a filter-passer.

By late August the flu had reached Tunis and there were signs of *la grippe* everywhere. Whether this was an extension of the same flu that had visited Europe in the spring and early part of the summer or a different strain, such as the more virulent strain seen at Devens in the autumn of 1918, is difficult to say. The point is that rather than trying to cultivate the bacillus, Nicolle decided to use the same method he had used with typhus. Accordingly, in late August he and Lebailly requested more test animals and began monitoring patients with flu. Chimpanzees were now impossible to obtain, so once again Nicolle settled on macaques, a fortunate choice as it turned out. Nicolle and Lebailly then looked for a household afflicted by the epidemic to be sure that they were examining a definitive case of *la grippe*, and not some other disease. The patient they selected was a 44-year-old man, identified only as "M.M.," who had fallen ill on 24 August, together with his daughters. Six days later, M.M. was displaying classic symptoms of influenza—nasopharyngitis, a violent headache, and fever—and Nicolle and Lebailly drew some blood. The following day, 1 September, they also collected bronchial expectorations. At this point, Nicolle and Lebailly had no idea if it was possible to transmit flu to a monkey or if the organism responsible for the disease was to be found in human blood, sputum, or other bodily fluids. However, while noting that

M.M.'s sputum contained "diverse" bacteria, including *B. influenzae*, they observed that the bacillus was present in "minimal" amounts and did not attempt to prepare pure cultures of the bacillus. Instead, they removed *B. influenzae* and other bacteria from M.M.'s bronchial expectorations using a Chamberland filter and injected the filtrate directly into the eyes and nose of a Chinese bonnet monkey (*Macacus sinicus*). At the same time, they administered the filtrate to two human volunteers, a 22-year-old who was inoculated under the skin, and a 30-year-old who received the filtrate intravenously. Six days later, both the macaque and the first volunteer came down with symptoms highly suggestive of flu—the monkey developed a fever and marked depression with loss of appetite, while the 22-year-old experienced rapid onset of fever, accompanied by a runny nose, headache and generalized body aches. As no one else in the first volunteer's living quarters developed influenza at the same time, Nicolle and Lebailly reasoned that the person had contracted flu from the filtrate. However, the second volunteer showed no signs of illness, even after fifteen days. Nicolle and Lebailly also attempted to infect other macaques by inoculating them with blood from M.M., but without success (the injections were given in either the monkeys' peritoneal cavities or their brains). Using blood from the macaque, they also inoculated a third volunteer who developed apparent symptoms of influenza, but this also proved unsuccessful. Finally, on 15 September they repeated the first experiment with a long-tailed macaque (*Macacus cynomolgus*) and a fourth volunteer. This time the filtered expectorations resulted in only a slight rise in temperature in the monkey and induced mild symptoms of flu in the volunteer.

By today's standards the experiments were hardly ideal—for instance, Nicolle and Lebailly did not use other monkeys or humans as controls (presumably because macaques were in short supply), nor do they appear to have been "blinded" from their subjects, as would be required today. Moreover, they did not investigate the pathogenic effect of filtered sputum from *non-influenza* cases, nor were they able to conduct passage experiments, as Pasteur had done with rabies in rabbits, to manipulate the virulence of the organism and reproduce the disease through several generations. Nevertheless, Nicolle and Lebailly concluded that the bronchial expectorations of influenza patients were virulent and that both the bonnet monkey and the long-tailed macaque were susceptible to subcutaneous inoculation with the filtered fluids. Flu therefore was an "*organisme filtrant*"—a filtered organism. They further concluded that the filtered virus had "reproduced the disease" in the two people inoculated subcutaneously.[42]

Nicolle and Lebailly's paper detailing their findings was read by Roux before the French Academy of Sciences in Paris on 21 September—the day before Welch arrived at Devens and witnessed the carnage sweeping the camp. Ordinarily, such an announcement before a respected scientific body would make other researchers around the world sit up and take notice. But the world was in the midst of war and Welch and his colleagues had more pressing concerns. Besides, even if reports of Nicolle and Lebailly's study had reached the surgeon general's office in Washington, DC in time and the news had been communicated to Welch—and there is no evidence that at this stage it was—it is unlikely that he would have given it particular credence. After all, Nicolle and Lebailly's investigations could hardly be considered conclusive. Moreover, before accepting their findings, Welch would have wanted other researchers—preferably American ones—to duplicate their experiments. The ideal place to do this was at the Rockefeller Institute, now an auxiliary laboratory of the US Army, or at nearby naval research laboratories in Boston and Rhode Island. The bacteriological paradigm of influenza could not be overturned on the basis of a just a few experiments conducted in North Africa thousands of miles from the main theatres of war and the world's preeminent medical research institutions.

Today, we know that Nicolle and Lebailly's supposition was correct. Influenza *is* a virus. To be precise, it is composed of eight slender strands of ribonucleic acid (RNA)—by contrast the building blocks of human and other mammalian cells are comprised of double-stranded helix spirals of deoxyribonucleic acid (DNA). However, Nicolle and Lebailly were almost certainly not justified in reaching that conclusion based on their experiments. First, while it is possible they could have infected the human volunteers with influenza if they had dripped the filtrate directly into their noses, it is extremely unlikely they could have done so by injecting the filtrate under the skin. That is not to say that the volunteers did not have influenza, only that they probably did not get it the way that Nicolle and Lebailly thought they did. Second, although it is possible to infect a range of Old-World monkeys with human flus (squirrel monkeys are particularly susceptible), macaques are a poor refractory species for human influenza and rarely develop visible respiratory symptoms or lung damage. It is also very difficult to get them to "take" the disease by dripping filtrate into their noses or by exposing them to aerosols containing the virus—indeed, in studies conducted in monkeys since 1918 researchers have reported far greater success with intravenous inoculations of the virus, somewhat ironic given Nicolle and Lebailly's reported failure in this respect.[43]

To be fair, in the absence of a reliable animal model for human influenza and a means of propagating the virus in living cells, in 1918 no researcher stood much chance of demonstrating that influenza was a virus. That only became possible after 1933, when a team of British researchers studying canine distemper demonstrated that ferrets were highly sensitive to influenza and could be inoculated simply by introducing filtered sputum into their nasal passages. When, soon after, one of the ferrets sneezed on a scientist who was handling it and the scientist went on to develop flu, the viral aetiology of flu was considered proven. This was followed in 1934 by the discovery that influenza viruses could be cultivated in chick egg embryos, freeing researchers from the need to collect samples from patients during an outbreak or to abandon their research when epidemics ended and the supply of flu patients dried up.[44] With chick embryo cultivation, the virus could now be propagated continuously in the laboratory, and scientists could be sure that they were performing experiments with the same strain of virus, something that had not been possible in 1918. By passaging flu viruses through embryonated hen's eggs, scientists could also attenuate the viruses and manufacture vaccines, thereby providing protection against whichever type of flu happened to be circulating that season.[*]

* * *

Unlike AIDS and smallpox, influenza is not a particularly disfiguring disease; for the most part, it does not leave visible marks or scars on the body. Nor does it cause victims to retch black fluids from their stomachs as yellow fever does, or induce uncontrollable diarrhoea as cholera does. But for those who witnessed the gruesome cyanotic end stages of the disease, when victims' lungs were compromised by pneumonia and their cheeks and lips turned blue then dark purple, Spanish flu was shocking to behold. This was not only the case at Devens and other US Army camps, but on the transatlantic troopships that conveyed American soldiers to Europe. On the *Leviathan*, a massive transport that set sail from New York at the end of September, eyewitnesses described having to step through "pools of blood from severe nasal haemorrhages." At first men were confined to steel cabins below deck in the hope of containing the infection, but within days of leaving New York so many were ill and the stench below decks was so overpowering that they were brought

_____

* Chick egg embryo cultivation is still the principal means of making flu vaccines.

on deck to breathe the sea air. In an era before antibiotics, and with no vaccine, doctors were powerless to heal the afflicted. Instead, they distributed fresh fruit and water. Sadly, like the bloody discharges, these also soon ended up on the floor, so that the decks became "wet and slippery, [with the] groans and cries of the terrified added to the confusion of the applicants clamoring for treatment." By the time the *Leviathan* arrived at Brest on 8 October, some 2,000 soldiers were ill and eighty had died, the majority of their bodies having been disposed of at sea.[45]

New Yorkers were unaware of the dreadful scenes on the *Leviathan*. When the vessel set sail, most New Yorkers still thought of Spanish influenza as an exotic foreign disease. Public health officials, keen to contribute to the war effort, colluded in the deception, downplaying the flu's impact on American servicemen even as they talked up the toll it was exacting on German troops. "You haven't heard of our doughboys getting it, have you?," queried New York's Commissioner of Health Royal S. Copeland. "You bet you haven't, and you won't."[46] Slowly but surely, however, the virus was swimming closer to shore, conveyed in the bodies of the passengers and crew of returning troopships and commercial liners. And all the while, as it passaged through more and more bodies, it was growing in virulence. The result was that when it made landfall on the eastern seaboard of the United States soldiers would not be the only casualties.

It is difficult to say how and where the second wave broke. Perhaps the fall outbreak began at Commonwealth Pier, in Boston, before spreading to Ayer and other towns in Massachusetts. Or perhaps there were several simultaneous introductions of the virus. New York, for instance, saw a marked increase in influenza deaths, particularly in middle age groups, in February–April 1918, though the first cases in the second wave were associated with passengers alighting from a Norwegian steamer in the middle of August. By the end of September, cases in New York were running at eight hundred a day, and Copeland took the unusual step of ordering quarantines (wealthy patients were allowed to remain in their homes, but those living in boarding houses or tenements were removed to city hospitals where they were kept under strict observation). Quarantines were something new and unprecedented for influenza—before the war, flu had not even been a notifiable disease—and New Yorkers could not help but be reminded of the polio epidemic two years earlier. Then, officials had gone door-to-door rounding up children with symptoms of "infantile paralysis," spreading terror in neighbourhoods like Brooklyn where recent Italian immigrants were suspected of harbouring the disease. However, the Spanish flu was as likely to visit a Park Avenue brownstone as a Brooklyn tenement, and as each day brought new reports of sickness, the city grew increasingly uneasy. Copeland tried to reassure New Yorkers by explaining that influenza was only communicable "in the coughing and sneezing of one who actually has influenza," not from someone living in the same household as someone stricken with flu but who did not show symptoms.[47] He also insisted that a vaccine was imminent.[48] He was referring to the efforts by scientists like Park and Williams at the New York Public Health Laboratory who were experimenting with vaccines using mixed strains of *B. influenzae*. By the middle of October, Park was reporting that animals immunized with a heat-killed vaccine made from these bacterial cocktails showed specific antibodies against the bacillus. Scientists at Tufts Medical School in Boston and the University of Pittsburgh's medical school were reporting similar progress with their own version of heat-killed bacterial vaccines. But while Park was having more success culturing *B. influenzae* and getting it to agglutinate to antibodies in serum, privately he was beginning to worry that the results might be a reflection of improved culture techniques rather than proof of the bacillus's aetiological role. "There is of course the possibility that some unknown filterable virus may be the starting point," he wired a colleague.[49] In spite of these misgivings, Park's vaccine was eventually released to the military. It was also used to immunize 275,000 employees of the US Steel Company.[50] There is no evidence that these primitive vaccines and serums had any effect on influenza whatsoever.

By 6 October more than 2,000 people a day in New York were being quarantined and the panic was palpable. From several districts came reports that patients were holding nurses captive in their homes because they were so frightened. Then nurses and doctors also started falling sick. By now the flu had reached San Francisco and was also raging in cities in the Midwest and South. The flu erupted in Chicago in mid-September, most likely introduced by sailors from the nearby Great Lakes Naval Station. With a capacity for 45,000 men, the station was the largest naval training facility in the world, and, like Devens, a breeding ground for respiratory disease. As flu and pneumonia gripped Chicago, citizens were advised to avoid crowds and other public gatherings and to cover their mouths when sneezing. The most visible signs of the contagion were the gauze face masks worn by policemen and tram attendants. The trend quickly caught on, prompting a prominent Illinois physician to warn that homemade masks were inadequate because they were "made from gauze with meshes too large to catch and strain out the bacilli from the fine spray issuing from the mouths of victims." This was of special concern in hospitals and other confined spaces as the spray was thought to be infectious at distances of up to twenty feet. Instead, he persuaded the *Chicago Herald Examiner* to publish a cut-out-and-keep guide on its front page for the proper procedure for making a gauze mask with a narrow mesh.[51] Unfortunately, these masks made little difference as influenza virus particles are many times smaller than the smallest bacteria, and by mid-October Chicago was already reporting 40,000 cases. The city hit hardest of all, however, was Philadelphia.

By 1918 Philadelphia had grown considerably since its Quaker beginnings as the capital of the Pennsylvania colony and the place where the founding fathers signed the Declaration of Independence. Ringed by steel mills and with its huge shipyards overlooking the Delaware River, Philadelphia was an industrial powerhouse. The needs of war (naval vessels, aircraft, munitions) brought tens of thousands of additional workers flocking to the city, and as its population swelled to nearly two million, so living conditions in Philadelphia became increasingly intolerable. In cramped rooming houses and over-crowded tenements, the virus found ample fodder and steadily increased in virulence, killing people rapidly and indiscriminately. At a time when authorities in other cities were advising people to avoid large public gatherings, the epidemic was almost certainly exacerbated by the decision of Philadelphia's mayor to proceed with a Liberty Loan Drive on 28 September. The drive brought thousands of people crowding into the downtown area, and within two weeks Philadelphia had recorded more than 2,600 flu deaths. By the third week of October deaths had soared to over 4,500. As bodies piled up in morgues for lack of undertakers, the stench became overpowering and the city resorted to digging mass graves—something that had not been seen since the yellow fever epidemics of the late eighteenth century. The sight of rotting bodies became so commonplace that adults made little effort to shield children from the horrors. The fear of influenza was now palpable, and with fear came panic. But this panic was not the fault of the press. "Panic is the worst thing that can happen to an individual or a community," warned the *Philadelphia Inquirer* in an editorial at the height of the fall wave. "Panic is exaggerated fear and fear is the most deadly word in any language." The remedy, it suggested, was to expel fearful thoughts by an act of will. "Do not dwell on the influenza. Do not even discuss it. ... Terror is a big ally of the influenza."[52] But once seen, the sight of a cyanotic, influenza-ridden body was not easily forgotten, either in Philadelphia or other places the flu visited, including London where by October deaths were running at 1,500 a week. The sight of "big strong men, heliotrope blue and breathing 50 to the minute" was unforgettable, observed Dr Herbert French, a pathologist based at Guy's

Hospital in London and a physician to Her Majesty's Household. But the worst case by far was the type that became "totally unconscious hours or even days before the end, restless in his coma, with head thrown back, mouth half open, a ghastly sallow pallor of the cyanosed face, purple lips and ears." It was "a dreadful sight," he concluded.[53]

* * *

The 1918 influenza pandemic was a shot heard around the world. The scenes described by French were not confined only to London and other large European and American cities but were the same everywhere. In Cape Town, observed one eyewitness, the autumn wave "made orphans of between two to three thousand children."[54] One such orphan who was co-opted into burial duties reported: "I carry the coffin, holding my nose ... no longer were church bells tolling for the dead ... there was no sexton to ring the bells."[55] It was the same in Bombay (Mumbai), where the disease arrived courtesy of a container ship in May. Deaths peaked in the first week of October, the same time as Boston. By the end of the year, the flu had killed an estimated one million people in this populous Indian city. All told, the pandemic claimed the lives of 18.5 million people across the Indian subcontinent, according to the latest estimates, and perhaps as many as 100 million worldwide. With the exception of Australia, where strict maritime quarantines delayed the onset of flu until the winter of 1919, virtually the entire globe suffered the pandemic at the same time. Only American Samoa, St. Helena, and a handful of islands in the South Atlantic escaped the plague. It was truly a shared global disaster.

It is difficult to imagine deaths of this order of magnitude, much less process them. The scale is too vast. "When one has fought a war, one hardly knows any more what a dead person is," remarks Camus. "And if a dead man has no significance unless one has seen him dead, a hundred million bodies spread through history are just a mist drifting through the imagination."[56] However, if there is little point in trying to imagine death on this scale, there is much to be gained from examining variations in mortality rates observed in different geographical locations and ecological and immunological settings. When influenza reached New Zealand, for instance, the local Maori population died at seven times the rate of British settlers. Similarly wide variations in mortality rates were observed between indigenous and European-descended peoples in Fiji and other South Pacific islands (one of the most striking discrepancies was observed in Guam, where the pandemic killed 5%

of the local population but just one sailor at the US naval base on the island). While the case fatality rate for "white" South Africans was 2.6%, for "blacks, Indians, and Coloureds" it was nearly 6%. For those who toiled underground in the Kimberley diamond mines the mortality rate was even worse—22%. Similar variations were observed at Devens and other large army training camps, with recent arrivals suffering far worse clinical outcomes than men of a similar age who had been at the camps for four months or longer. On the AEF transports, sailors permanently assigned to the ships fared far better than soldiers who had just embarked, even though both were attacked by influenza in more or less equal numbers.[57]

But perhaps the most striking aspect of the Spanish flu pandemic was the mortality pattern observed in young adults. In a normal flu season, curves of mortality by age at death are typically U-shaped, reflecting high mortality in the very young (children under three) and the elderly (seventy-five and over), with low mortality at all ages in between. This is because infants and the aged tend to be those with the weakest immune systems. By contrast, the 1918–19 pandemic and the succeeding winter recurrences in 1919 and 1920 produced a W-shaped curve, with a third mortality peak in adults aged 20–40 years. Moreover, adults in these age ranges accounted for half the total influenza deaths, including the majority of excess respiratory deaths.[58] This abnormal mortality pattern was observed both in cities and rural areas, in major European metropolises and distant outposts of empire. In other words, it was the same everywhere.

Why this should have been the case has never been satisfactorily explained. Nor, despite the advances in influenza virology and immunology and a better understanding of the pathophysiology of flu, are scientists today in a much better position to say whether the Spanish flu pandemic was a one-off occurrence—a never-to-be-repeated epidemiological disaster—or whether it could happen again. By reviewing what has been learned about the 1918 virus, and the likely identity of previous pandemic viruses, it is possible to rule out some hypotheses and rule others in. However, perhaps the biggest clue to the epidemiological patterns and unusual lung pathologies observed in 1918 comes from the ecology of large army camps and the contemporary accounts of medics who observed the ravages wrought by influenza in them at first hand.

* * *

Influenza, we now know, is a member of the family *Orthomyxoviridae*, and comes in three types—A, B, and C—named in the order of their discovery.

Type C rarely causes disease in humans. Type B can cause epidemics, but the course of infection is milder and the spread of the virus tends to be slower. By contrast, type A is associated with explosive spread and high rates of morbidity and mortality, making it the leading cause of epidemics and pandemics. Like all influenza viruses, type A influenzas are RNA viruses and must infect a living cell in order to replicate. Generally, they do this by attacking the epithelial cells that line the respiratory tract from the nose and through the windpipe to the lungs.

Although in 1933 scientists had demonstrated that influenza was a virus that could be transferred from ferrets to man (the breakthrough was made by a team headed by Sir Patrick Laidlaw at the Farm Laboratory, in Mill Hill, north London, part of the UK's National Institute for Medical Research), it was not until the 1940s and the invention of the electron microscope that researchers were able to see the influenza virion for the first time. It measured approximately 100 nanometres (0.10 micrometres), making it slightly smaller than the rabies virus but larger than rhinovirus, the cause of the common cold. Magnified, it resembled nothing so much as the surface of a dandelion bristling with tiny spikes and mushroom-like spines. The spikes are made of a protein called haemagglutinin (HA) that derives its name from its ability to agglutinate to red blood cells. When a person inhales an air droplet containing the virus, it is these spikes that stick to the receptors on the surface of the epithelial cells in the respiratory tract, much as a prickly seed case catches on the fibres of clothing in tall grass. The square-headed mushroom-like protrusions, fewer in number, consist of a powerful enzyme, neuraminidase (NA). It is the combination of these proteins and enzymes that enables the virus to invade epithelial cells and evade the body's immune defences. These permutations of proteins and enzymes give each virus a signature shape, making for easy classification. In all, scientists have identified sixteen types of haemagglutinin and nine types of neuraminidase in mammals and birds (beside ferrets, type A flu viruses commonly infect pigs, whales, seals, horses and wild waterfowl), but to date only influenza viruses of the H1, H2 and H3 types have caused pandemics.

Unlike DNA, RNA does not possess an accurate proofreading mechanism. During replication, when the virus invades and colonizes animal cells, the RNA makes small copying errors, resulting in genetic mutations to the H and N molecules on its surface. In the Darwinian world of the virus, some of these copies can confer a competitive advantage, allowing the viruses to escape the antibodies designed to neutralize them and enabling them to spread more efficiently via coughs and sneezes to the wider environment, ready to infect the next person. This process of gradual mutation is known as "antigenic drift." Type A viruses can also spontaneously "swap" or exchange genetic material. This process is typically thought to occur in intermediary hosts such as pigs, which can be infected with swine and human type A strains simultaneously, and is known as "antigenic shift."[59] In this case, the result is the emergence of a completely new subtype that codes for proteins that may be new to the immune system and for which human populations may possess few or no antibodies. It is these strains that historically have been the cause of pandemics. However, it is thought that the virus responsible for the 1918 pandemic may have emerged in yet another way.

In the 1990s, scientists at the Armed Forces Institute of Pathology in Bethesda, Maryland, led by molecular biologist Jeffery Taubenberger, succeeded in retrieving fragments of the Spanish flu virus from lung autopsy specimens stored in the institute's archives. Further genetic viral material came from a woman who had died of influenza in 1918 in Alaska and had been buried in permafrost, which preserved her lungs from decay. Using this material, Taubenberger's group was eventually able to sequence the virus's entire genome. Published in 2005, the results came as something of a surprise because none of the eight genes came from a strain that had previously infected humans, as one would have expected if the Spanish flu had been the result of antigenic shift. Furthermore, large portions of the genetic code matched sequences only found in wild birds. This suggested that the virus may have begun as a bird-adapted strain that, with just a handful of mutations, made the leap to humans.[60] Alternatively, the pandemic strain may have begun life as an H1 which re-assorted with an avian virus shortly before 1918.[61] By 2005, it was recognized that mallards and teals were an important reservoir of avian influenza viruses in the wild, and the idea that birds might be the source of novel genes in pandemic viruses was gaining currency. Taubenberger's sequencing studies also coincided with growing concern about an avian virus that was then infecting chicken flocks across Southeast Asia. The virus, known as H5N1, had first emerged in Hong Kong in 1997, where it infected eighteen people and caused six deaths, before re-emerging for a second time in 2002. Since then the virus had spread from Asia to Europe and Africa, sparking hundreds of human cases and forcing authorities to cull millions of chickens. Alarmingly, the H5N1 virus was able to replicate in the human respiratory tract, and the mortality rate averaged 60 per cent. However, it did not transmit easily from person to person. Nevertheless, its emergence demonstrated that people could be directly infected with a wholly avian influenza virus, meaning it was no longer necessary to invoke pigs as intermediary hosts in the generation of pandemic strains. Theoretically, such reassortments, or mixing, of avian and mammalian flu strains could also occur in humans. The question was, could something like this have happened in 1918? The short answer is that no one knows, but the possibility cannot be ruled out.[62]

The precise genetic identities of pandemic strains prior to 1900 are lost to history, but in the twentieth century there have been three major shifts. The first was the H1N1 Spanish flu virus that emerged in 1918, or possibly a little earlier (by comparing older and more recent strains of the virus and running molecular clocks backward in time, evolutionary biologists suggest the virus may have acquired its avian genes somewhere between 1913 and 1917).[63] This was the prevailing strain until 1957, when it was replaced by a new viral strain, typed H2N2. Known as the "Asian flu," the H2N2 seems to have been generated by a reassortment of descendants of the 1918 virus with an avian influenza strain derived from Eurasian wild waterfowl. It spread rapidly around the globe, displacing descendants of H1N1 Spanish flu and killing an estimated two million people. In 1968 there was a third shift, when an H3N2 suddenly emerged in Hong Kong, also apparently as a result of the acquisition of novel proteins from Eurasian wild waterfowl. Known, unsurprisingly, as the "Hong Kong" flu, this virus is estimated to have killed one million people globally, and at the time of writing remains the leading cause of morbidity and mortality from influenza.

To complete the picture of pandemic viruses in the modern period, we also need to include the Russian flu. Like the 1918 Spanish flu, this was a true worldwide pandemic. Originating in the Eurasian "steppes"—a vast expanse of grassland that encompassed parts of Russia plus Tsarist-controlled Uzbekistan and Kazakhstan—it spread rapidly along international rail and shipping routes and is conservatively thought to have killed one million in the period between 1889 and 1892.[64] Unfortunately, scientists have been unable to recover fragments of the virus, so its precise genetic identity is unknown. However, serology tests on elderly people who were examined for antibodies at the time of the 1968 Hong Kong flu suggest that, like that virus, it was caused by an H3. This may be an important clue, as those most at risk of dying in 1918 were born in or around 1890, meaning they belonged to a birth cohort whose first exposure to a flu virus would almost certainly have been to the Russian flu. We will return to this in a moment, but first it is necessary to consider the nature of the pneumonias that killed people in 1918.

As noted earlier, broadly speaking these pneumonias can be divided into two types—lobar and bronchial. However, it is also important to note that in a pre-virological era, these distinctions rested on clinical observations and histological examinations of lung tissue and that the two types were often closely related, with the clinical-pathological syndromes sometimes overlapping. The most common type by far appears to have been an acute aggressive bronchopneumonia. In this type, pathological changes were most obvious in the bronchi, and pathogenic bacteria could usually be cultured at autopsy from different parts of the lung. Close to 90 per cent of the pneumonias fell into this category. In the second type, the outstanding features were pulmonary haemorrhage and edema with extensive damage to one or more of the lobes, and pathogenic bacteria were less frequently or rarely recovered. In this type, the infection appears to have triggered an acute inflammation of the pulmonary alveoli resulting in cell death (necrosis) and the deposit of damaged cells and fluids in the alveolar air spaces—the microscopic sacs that absorb oxygen in the lung.[65] These features were found whenever victims died within a few days of the onset of illness, as well as in 70 per cent of cases in which pneumonia developed after influenza. And they were nearly always found in deaths involving healthy young soldiers or civilians.[66] However, it must be reiterated that this type accounted for only a small percentage of deaths overall. The later-onset bronchopneumonias and mixed infections, in which bacteria could be readily cultured after death, were the ones encountered most frequently. Indeed, it is these bacterial fellow travellers of flu—or what pathologists at the time called "secondary invaders"—that many experts believe best explain the majority of deaths seen at camps like Devens and the variations in mortality observed between recruits of the same age from rural and urban areas.

It is perhaps also worth remarking that as doubts about the aetiological role of *B. influenzae* grew, so pathologists took care to distinguish between lung lesions attributable to commensal bacteria and those due to the presumed, though as yet unproven, virus of the epidemic. By the mid-1920s, this was a view that Welch was also coming to endorse. Addressing a meeting of public health officials in Boston in 1926, Welch said that the idea that influenza was due to an "unknown virus" had much to recommend it, and he now thought that "when there was a lesion of the lung ... it was attributable to the virus, the real influenza virus, not general respiratory manifestations." He had also been struck by the "crowding together" of soldiers at the base hospital at Devens, an occurrence that he thought increased patients' risk of exposure to other organisms and was "largely responsible for the enormous extent of the disease."[67]

Unlike in 1918, today it is possible to study the virus in the laboratory using a process called reverse genetics. Beginning in 2005, this is exactly what scientists have done, re-assembling the virus in Biosafety Level Four facilities and then challenging mice and other test animals. The resurrected virus kills mice in three to five days and causes a severe lung inflammation reminiscent of the lesions reported by doctors in 1918. It also replicates very efficiently in bronchial epithelial cells.[68] Indeed, so striking is the virulence of the 1918 virus in laboratory animal studies that some virologists argue that infection with the virus alone could have triggered the rapid onset pneumonias and symptoms of cyanosis described by pathologists in 1918 and that it is unnecessary to invoke secondary bacterial invaders. One suggestion is that the pneumonias and symptoms of cyanosis may have been due to an overly exuberant immune response involving the release of proinflammatory cells called cytokines. This phenomenon—known as a "cytokine storm"—was implicated in the deaths from Acute Respiratory Distress Syndrome (ARDS) that followed the H5N1 bird flu outbreaks in Southeast Asia in the early 2000s, and has also been observed with other epidemic viruses such as SARS.

Whether or not these pneumonias were primarily viral or bacterial, or a mixture of both, does not answer the question of why the Spanish flu proved so deadly to young adults in the prime of life, however. Here, present-day science has several hypotheses but no good answers. One suggestion is that older age groups enjoyed greater protection because they had previously been exposed to a similar virus. This fits with serological evidence suggesting that people born between 1830 and 1889 were also exposed to an H1. It was only after 1890 that this virus was replaced by a new pandemic virus, the Russian H3. In other words, those aged thirty-eight and over would have already possessed some antibodies to the H1N1 Spanish flu, and in the case of the very elderly—those born in 1834 who had been infants when they first encountered an H1—this protection would have been considerable.

Another suggestion is that the virus that was to become the Spanish flu (in a scenario where it acquired avian genes around 1915) may have begun life as an H1 that emerged shortly after 1900.[69] This could have been critical for those born in the first years of the twentieth century who would have been eighteen or younger at the time the pandemic struck, as it is thought that early life infection with influenza results in an immunological "blind spot." Usually referred to as "original antigenic sin," the idea is that antibodies to the first-encountered flu strain are more readily "recalled" and produced at the expense of new antibodies specific to newer flu strains.[70] It is even possible that through a process known as antibody-dependent enhancement, the older immune response might aid the virus to evade the body's defences and infect cells more readily. However, while the advantage of such hypotheses is that they help explain why, no matter where the flu struck, the mortality fell most heavily on twenty-to-forty-year-olds, most experts feel that without knowing the precise genetic identity of the 1890 virus and the viruses that came before and after, and the precise immunological profiles of the affected age groups, these hypotheses are somewhat speculative. As David Morens, a medical epidemiologist who works closely with Taubenberger, points out, it is equally possible that the W-shaped mortality pattern could be due to some as yet unidentifiable environmental exposure peculiar to young adults at the time.[71] We just do not know. Indeed, for all that new molecular techniques and a better understanding of the ecology and immunology of flu have brought new insights into the patterns of pandemics, Taubenberger and Morens argue that "we have moved ever further from certainty about the determinants of, and possibilities for pandemic emergence."[72] It is this uncertainty that makes flu—and the 1918 pandemic in particular—such an enigmatic and enduring object of scientific interest and source of anxiety.

But perhaps for the last word on the pandemic we should leave North America and turn to someone who viewed the spreading global morbidity and mortality from the periphery. In 1919, at the age of twenty, Frank Macfarlane Burnet was studying medicine at the University of Melbourne when he suffered an attack of influenza. Thankfully, the illness proved mild. Nevertheless, it left an indelible impression, igniting a lifelong fascination with flu and with what Burnet called "the natural history of infectious disease."[73] In 1931, Burnet arrived at the National Institute for Medical Research in London on a two-year fellowship to study the burgeoning new field of virus diseases. His arrival coincided with the discovery that ferrets could be infected with influenza, and on his return to Melbourne in 1934 he pioneered the technique for growing the virus in chick egg embryos. This would be the first in a series of contributions to influenza research by Burnet—research that would see him investigate variations in virulence between newly isolated and chick-cultivated viruses and lay the ground for future genetic insights into the emergence of pandemics.[74] Intrigued by Nicolle and Lebailly's findings in Tunis in 1918, in 1941 Burnet also conducted a series of trials in macaques, challenging the monkeys with several strains of egg-propagated virus. Although none of the monkeys developed a fever or other signs of illness when infected intranasally, several became ill when Burnet injected the virus directly into their trachea, and at autopsy one showed signs of extensive bronchopneumonia.[75] However, it was the epidemiology of influenza that fascinated Burnet most, and the more he studied the patterns of morbidity and mortality in 1918, the more convinced he became that it was the concentration of recruits from rural and urban districts in overcrowded barracks that held the key to the pandemic's unusual characteristics. Like Welch and the members of the pneumonia commission, Burnet was persuaded that the emergence of Spanish flu was, as he put it, "intimately linked to war conditions," and that it was the immunological profiles of American recruits, followed by their transfer to northern France, where they were able to mix freely with men from other nations, that accounted for the extreme virulence of the virus and the unusual age profile of its victims. "If the early American epidemics supplied the initial spark for the pandemic we can be certain that it was fanned into a flame in Europe," Burnet concluded.[76] But what struck Burnet as possibly even more significant from an immunological point of view was how many people had been *unaffected* by the pandemic. Two-thirds of the population had escaped infection altogether, and the overall mortality, as a measure of the total population, had been just 2 per cent. While that was twenty-five times higher than in a normal flu season, it was far lower than the mortality rate seen during outbreaks of cholera and pneumonic plague in the nineteenth century, and went some way to explaining why, except for the height of the killing wave in October, when hospitals had been flooded with pneumonia cases and the dead had become impossible to ignore, the pandemic had not provoked greater fear and panic. Yes, influenza had briefly presented as "some new kind of plague." But by November 1918 and the declaration of the armistice it was already once more on its way to becoming a familiar seasonal ailment. Unfortunately, that would not be true of other twentieth- and twenty-first-century epidemics caused by similar ecological imbalances and environmental disturbances.

2

PLAGUE IN THE CITY OF ANGELS

On 3 October 1924, Dr Giles Porter, a Los Angeles city health officer, was called to the home of a railroad worker in the heart of the Mexican quarter. A few days earlier, Jesus Lajun and his 15-year-old daughter, Francisca Concha Lajun, had fallen ill at their apartment at 700 Clara Street, and both were now running high temperatures. Francisca also had a spasmodic, rattling cough, while Jesus had a nasty swelling on his groin. Porter attributed Jesus's swelling to "venereal adenitis" due to syphilis, while Francisca's symptoms of fever and coughing, he thought, were most likely due to influenza. "This child was not considered to be in a serious condition," he recorded in his report. But Porter was wrong and two days later Luciana Samarano, the owner of a nearby boarding house who had been nursing Francisca, became so concerned about the girl's condition that she called an ambulance. Francisca died en route to Los Angeles General Hospital, a pathologist later listing the cause of death as "double pneumonia."[1] For an otherwise healthy teenager to suffer a severe attack of pneumonia was a highly unusual occurrence, but Clara Street was surrounded by brickyards and gas and electrical works, and even in fine weather the air was choked with pollutants. Taking into account the unpleasant odours emanating from the nearby meatpacking plants, it came as little surprise that Mexicans were the only people prepared to live in the environs of Clara Street or that a young life had been taken prematurely.

Built in 1895 on a vacant plot near the Los Angeles River, Clara Street had originally been an affordable white middle-class neighbourhood, but as the city expanded and a land and building boom brought a demand for brick makers and cheap agricultural labour, the Italian residents had moved out and the area had been colonized by Hispanics and migrant workers from south of the border. By 1924 some 2,500 Mexicans were packed into the 307 houses in and around Clara Street, an eight-block area bounded on the east by the Southern Pacific Railroad, on the west by Alameda Street, and on the south by Macy Street. Overcrowding was rife.[2] Many houses, such as Samarano's home at 742 Clara Street, had been subdivided into "apartments" or transformed into boarding houses in which up to thirty people resided at a time. Other guests bedded down in shacks appended to the rear of the simple clapboard dwellings. People were not the only lodgers. The crawl spaces beneath the floorboards also provided sanctuary for rats and, on occasion, ground squirrels. In short, it was a world away from the Los Angeles described by developers as the city "of eternal youth—a city without slums."[3]

In the 1920s, Los Angeles had a population of one million and was one of the fastest growing urban centres in the United States. Billed as the "climatic capital of the world," the city was in the midst of a real estate boom as Americans tired of the harsh midwestern winters and the overcrowded conditions in cities in the East flocked to Southern California, attracted by the promise of a new life in a land blessed by oil, palm trees, abundant farmland, and sunshine. Most of these settlers made for the new bedroom communities with names like "Petroleum Gardens" that were springing up on reclaimed desert just beyond the city limits. By contrast, Hispanics tended to congregate in Macy District—as the Mexican quarter was officially known—or the adjacent Mariana and Belvedere Gardens districts.

By 1924, Los Angeles's Hispanic population totalled around 22,000, and the signs of their labour were everywhere: it was Mexican hands, toiling in the clay pits adjacent to the Los Angeles River, that had fashioned the bricks for the high rises transforming L.A.'s skyline, and it was Mexicans who kept the grocery stores stocked with fresh fruit and vegetables and who scrubbed the floors of the posh downtown hotels. Yet for the city's majority Anglo-Saxon population, these brown-skinned inhabitants of the City of Angels were all but invisible. Sure, there may have been concerns from time to time about the diseases they were presumed to carry, or the demographic implications of the burgeoning Hispanic birth rate, but as Harry Chandler, the owner of the antiunion *Los Angeles Times*, and a prominent Californian landowner and power broker, reassured Congress: Mexicans "do not intermarry like the negro with white people. They don't mingle. They keep to themselves. That is the safety of it."[4]

Seven days after Francisca Lajun's death, her father Jesus also succumbed to the mysterious infection. Then, five days later, Luciana Samarano was admitted to County General, dying on 19 October of "myocarditis" or heart disease (six months pregnant at the time, Luciana's unborn child died with her). The next casualties were Samarano's husband, Guadalupe, followed by several mourners who had attended Luciana's wake, which, as per Catholic tradition, saw relatives filing past the open casket and kissing the corpse to pay their respects. As with Francisca Lajun, Guadalupe's death was listed as "double pneumonia."[5] By now, several other people who had attended Luciana's wake had also fallen ill with similar symptoms. However, it was only on 29 October that the hospital dispatched its chief resident, Dr Emil Bogen, to investigate. Bogen's first stop was a house at 343 Carmelita Street in Belvedere Gardens. "In the middle of the room," Bogen recalled, "an old Mexican woman was lying on a large double bed, crying between paroxysms of coughing, while along the wall was a couch on which was seen a Mexican man of about 30 years of age, restless and feverish, but not coughing." Several other people were also present, and one agreed to act as Bogen's interpreter. Bogen was told that the man had fallen sick the day before, that he had a pain along his spine, and that he was running a temperature of 104 degrees. He also had red spots on his chest. The old woman, meanwhile, "had been coughing for the past two days, expectorating a profuse bloody sputum, and had loud, coarse rhonchi."[6]

Bogen arranged for the couple to be transferred to an ambulance, then went with the interpreter to the adjacent house where another man and his wife and daughter were ill with similar symptoms. The wife informed Bogen that she felt better than previously while the daughter "insisted that she was not sick, only a little tired." Within three days, however, both the woman and the girl were in a critical condition at County General, and the woman's husband was dead. Only later did it emerge that he was Guadalupe Samarano's brother, Victor, and that both he and his wife had recently attended the wake at 742 Clara Street. There, Bogen found four desperately sick boys between the ages of four and twelve, the recently orphaned sons of Luciana and Guadalupe. "The four boys were brought to the hospital that same night, and during the following day six more cases were admitted from that neighbourhood," he recorded. "Soon after admission they developed signs of a severe pneumonia, with bloody expectoration and marked cyanosis."[7]

Samarano's home would subsequently be labelled the "death house." In all, thirty-three people who had attended Luciana's wake, who were related to the Samaranos or who had lodged at 742 Clara Street would contract plague, and thirty-one would die. The sequence of illnesses was laid out in an official report in which the casualties were listed according to their initials and their relationship to "L.S." or "G.S."[8] After the Samaranos, the next casualty was "J. F.," or Jessie Flores, a family friend and next-door neighbour who had nursed Luciana. Then came two of the couple's sons by different marriages, and both Luciana and Guadalupe's mothers. Even the family priest, Father Medardo Brualla, contracted the disease. Brualla had gone to 742 Clara Street on 26 October to administer the last rites to Guadalupe and Jessie, but a few days later he was also expectorating bloody sputum, and by 2 November he was dead.[9]

After Guadalupe's death, unsuspecting health officials had released his body so that his family could pay their respects. Once again, they held the service at 742 Clara Street, and once again, mourners who attended the wake fell ill soon after. By 30 October, some twelve people were in critical condition at County General. It was one of these, Horace Gutiérrez, a cousin of Luciana Samarano, who would provide the crucial evidence that would alert health officials to the identity of the pathogen and plunge the Los Angeles Chamber of Commerce and city hall into panic. In his summary, Bogen records that Gutiérrez had arrived at the hospital at around the same time as the four Samarano boys and, shortly after, had developed the same symptoms of pneumonia accompanied by bloody expectorations and cyanosis. As cyanosis had been a signature symptom of the Spanish influenza and the epidemic was still fresh in physicians' memories, the immediate suspicion was flu. In the end, however, the cases were attributed to "epidemic meningitis." Only the hospital's pathologist, Dr George Maner, thought differently, suggesting that perhaps they were dealing with plague.[10] Later, Maner decided to check his intuition by taking a sputum sample from Gutiérrez and examining it under a microscope. What he saw filled him with dread. Gutiérrez's sputum was packed with tiny rod-shaped bacteria that looked distinctly like the images Maner had seen in textbooks of *Pasteurella pestis*, the bacterium of plague.[11] Unsure of the bacteria's morphology and wanting to get a second opinion, Maner approached his predecessor as chief of pathology at Los Angeles General, a Scotsman by the name of Roy Hammack. Hammack had previously served in the Philippines, where he had treated several cases of plague, so he had the advantage of having seen the bacillus before. "Beautiful!" he supposedly exclaimed when he espied the familiar rod-shaped bacteria through his microscope. "Beautiful but damned."[12]

* * *

Pasteurella pestis, or *Yersinia pestis* to give the bacillus its proper name, is one of the deadliest pathogens known to man. Named for the Swiss bacteriologist

Alexandre Yersin, who isolated the microbe during the third plague pandemic in Hong Kong in 1894, *Y. pestis* is conservatively thought to have been responsible for 100 million deaths throughout history, perhaps as many as 200 million. Yet for all the horror evoked by the word *plague*, human infections are only incidental events in the life cycle of the parasite. The bacillus's natural reservoir is wild rodents, such as marmots, ground squirrels, and rats. Transmitted by the bites from infected fleas that live in the rodents' burrows, *Y. pestis* circulates for the most part harmlessly in these rodent populations. It is only when the relative immunity of rodent populations wanes, and there are sudden die-offs, leaving fleas temporarily homeless, or diseased rodents are brought closer to human habitations, that the existence of the zoonosis becomes visible and there is a risk of transfer of the infection to humans or some other animal host. From the point of view of the parasite and its survival, however, this is not a great strategy, as this "accidental" transfer usually results in the death of its new host, preventing further onward transmission of the bacillus.

The human disease takes three forms: bubonic, septicaemic, and pneumonic. The bubonic form occurs when a flea jumps from a rat or some other rodent and bites a human, injecting the plague bacilli under the skin (afterwards, human fleas or body lice may transmit bubonic plague to other individuals). As the victim scratches the site of the wound, the bacilli multiply and spread to the lymph glands in the groin (in the case of a flea bite to the leg) or the armpits (in the case of a bite to the arm). As the immune system struggles to contain the infection, the lymph glands become swollen and inflamed, giving rise to the painful egg-shaped "buboes" from which the disease takes its name. On average, plague takes three to five days to incubate, and another three to five days before the victim dies (untreated, bubonic plague is fatal in around 60 per cent of cases), the final stages being marked by extensive haemorrhaging and organ failure. In the most toxic form of bubonic plague, known as septicaemic plague, the skin becomes mottled with dark blue patches and the extremities may turn black, hence one possible derivation of the disease's name, "Black Death." In the last stages of the infection, victims often fall into a delirium and are unable to bear the slightest touch to their sores. The only mercy is that this form of plague usually kills quickly and is only transmissible by bites from fleas.

By contrast, the pneumonic form can be spread directly from person to person and can arise either from inhalation of *Y. pestis* or septicaemic spread of bacteria from the bubonic form of the disease. Typically, an originating case of pneumonic plague occurs when some of the bacilli escape the lymph system and migrate to the victim's lungs, causing oedema and secondary infection (this is particularly common when a bubo forms in the neck region). During this time, the victim is non-infectious but may exhibit a fever and rapid pulse. Within one to four days, however, the victim's condition suddenly deteriorates as the oedema spreads, triggering necrotizing pneumonia throughout the lungs and violent paroxysms. At this stage, the victim typically coughs or "spits" blood, causing the bed sheets to become spotted and stained crimson. Unless treated within twelve hours of the onset of fever, pneumonic plague is invariably fatal. Suspended in cough droplets or sputum, the bacilli can also be expelled as far as twelve inches, making it easy for someone lying on a nearby sofa or an adjacent bed to catch the disease. In cold weather and cool, humid conditions the bacilli can also become attached to water droplets and linger in the air for minutes or hours at a time. The bacteria can also survive for up to three days on hard surfaces, such as glass and steel, and for much longer in the soil and other organic material.[13]

It is difficult to be certain what proportion of deaths that occurred during historical outbreaks were due to the bubonic as opposed to the pneumonic form of the disease, because prior to modern bacteriological tests diagnosis was uncertain and rested on the interpretation of clinical symptoms and signs. The first plague pandemic, which began during the reign of the Byzantine emperor Justinian I, and which is estimated to have killed some 25 million people throughout the Mediterranean basin between 541 and 750, is thought to have been largely bubonic. However, the second pandemic appears to have been a mixed outbreak. Colloquially known as the Black Death, the pandemic began in 1334 in China before spreading along the great trade routes to Constantinople, Florence, and other European capitals in the middle decades of the fourteenth century, reducing Europe's population by approximately one-quarter to one-half between 1347 and 1353 and killing at least 20 million people, possibly as many as 50 million.[14] To judge by contemporary accounts, buboes and swellings, called *gavocciolo* by Italian chroniclers, were ubiquitous. However, in 1348, the first year of the Black Death in Europe, so were pneumonic symptoms. "Breath," wrote one Sicilian chronicler, "spread the infection among those speaking together ... and it seemed as if the victim[s] were struck all at once by the affliction and [were] shattered by it. ... Victims coughed up blood, and after three days of incessant vomiting for which there was no remedy, they died, and with them died not only everyone who talked with them, but also anyone who had acquired or touched or laid hands on their belongings."[15]

The news that a deadly pathogen from the Middle Ages had arrived in the City of Angels was not something anyone in Los Angeles wanted to hear in

1924, least of all business leaders. As William Deverell, a historian of California and the West, puts it, at a time when Los Angeles was selling itself as a hygienic retirement destination, "plague was not the sort of thing expected in the proud city of tomorrow."[16] Plague's presence in Los Angeles was also a considerable blow to the prestige of the US Public Health Service (PHS) and the Californian State Board of Health. Just ten years earlier, health officials had confidently declared that all "discoverable" plague had been eradicated from California.[17] This announcement was based on the new knowledge of plague's ecology that had been acquired following the outbreaks of bubonic plague in San Francisco in the early years of the century.

Introduced to the city in around 1900, most likely from black rats that had hitched a ride to San Francisco on a steamship from Honolulu, the plague was at first confined to Chinatown, where it killed 113 people. However, following the earthquake and fire that struck San Francisco in 1906, rats were displaced from their downtown runs and dispersed throughout the city, sparking new outbreaks in 1907–08 over a much wider urban area. In response, US Assistant Surgeon General Rupert Blue launched a massive rat extermination campaign. Whereas in 1903 Blue had concentrated on demolishing houses in Chinatown and baiting rat holes with arsenic, now he ordered his men to hunt down and kill rats wherever they found them. By January 1908, when the last two cases of bubonic plague were seen in the city, some two million rats had been exterminated and many thousands had been autopsied, giving Blue, and his chief laboratorian, George McCoy, new insights into the transmission of plague and its persistence in rodent reservoirs in interepidemic periods. Unlike in India and Asia, where the principal vector of plague was the black rat, *Rattus rattus*, Blue and McCoy discovered that in San Francisco the main vector had been the brown sewer rat, *Rattus norvegicus*. A prolific breeder, the brown rat's preferred habitat is sewers and cellars where it likes to lay out its run in the shape of a Y, with its food store hidden at one branch and its nest at the other—evidence, according to Blue, of the rodent's "sagacity" at evading predators.[18] This strategy had served the brown rat well, enabling it to spread from the waterfront in northeast San Francisco as far as the County Hospital in the southwest.

Although in 1908 no one had definitively demonstrated that fleas living on rats were vectors of plague, their incriminating role was widely presumed, and Blue routinely ordered his men to comb rats for fleas and count the number of ectoparasites.[19] He found that in winter his men could comb twenty rats and recover only one flea among them, but in warm weather the flea numbers multiplied, such that a healthy rat could harbour twenty-five fleas, while a sick one might host eighty-five. As long as these fleas fed on rats, he hypothesized, they posed little threat to human populations. It was only when rats were evicted from their runs and came into contact with people, or when plague-infected fleas killed their rodent hosts and began looking for a new blood meal, that humans risked being infected. However, there was much more to the ecology of plague than just rats and fleas.

In China, it had long been suspected that marmots acted as reservoirs of plague in interepidemic periods.[20] However, until Blue, McCoy, and William Wherry, a bacteriologist with the San Francisco Board of Health, began studying sporadic outbreaks of plague in counties on the east side of San Francisco Bay in 1908, no one had suspected that Californian ground squirrels and other wild rodents indigenous to the western United States might be similarly susceptible to infection with *Y. pestis* or might play a similar role in maintaining transmission of the parasite in interepidemic periods. Blue's suspicions had first been aroused five years earlier when a blacksmith from Contra Costa County died of bubonic plague at a hospital in San Francisco. On questioning his friends and family, Blue learned that the blacksmith had not visited the city in over a month, but that three to four days before the onset of his illness he had shot and killed a ground squirrel in the hills near his home. By July 1908 Blue was certain that there were no more infected rats in San Francisco. However, that same month he learned that the son of a rancher from Concord in Contra Costa County had contracted plague and died, prompting Blue to dispatch his top rat catcher, William Colby Rucker, to investigate. The scene that greeted Colby at the ranch had all the hallmarks of a classic epizootic, with bodies of dead rats littering the ground. In a barn on the ranch near where the boy had died, Colby also recovered a dead squirrel. Blue immediately ordered Colby and his men to collect squirrels from other ranches in the region and discovered that several were infected with *Y. pestis*.[21] As Blue later wrote to Washington, DC, this was "perhaps the first demonstration of the occurrence in nature of bubonic plague in the ground squirrel (*Citellus beecheyi*) of California."[22] McCoy speculated that the squirrels had caught the plague from rats that had migrated from San Francisco to Oakland and which had mingled with wild rodents in the hills behind Berkeley, exchanging ectoparasites in the process. Evidence for this hypothesis was supported by his discovery that the California ground squirrels were heavily infested with two species of flea, *Hoplopsyllus anomalus and Nosopsyllus fasciatus*. The latter was commonly found on rats and, together with *Xenopsylla cheopis*, the oriental rat flea, was thought to have been the principal vector of bubonic plague during the 1906 San Francisco outbreak.[23] However, McCoy observed that the squirrel fleas also readily attacked humans, writing that at one point his "squirrel stock room became so heavily infested that upon going into the room one was certain to be bitten by many of the parasites." McCoy also found that in the laboratory it was easy to transmit plague by means of the *H. anomalus* flea from squirrels to guinea pigs and rats, and vice versa, leading him to conclude that "it is not improbable that the conveyance in nature is in the same way."[24]

The discovery that squirrels might act as reservoirs of plague between rat epizootics and that their fleas might also be capable of transmitting the infection to humans caused Blue "considerable apprehension." However, it was thought that as long as the risk was confined to Contra Costa and Alameda Counties, there was little to worry about. Then in August, a report reached McCoy of the death of a ten-year-old boy in Elysian Park, in northeast Los Angeles, some four hundred miles to the south. On arriving at the boy's home, McCoy discovered that seven days before the onset of illness, the boy had come across a ground squirrel in his backyard and it had bitten him on the hand. Both the boy and a dead squirrel recovered from the property subsequently tested positive for plague. The boy's home, McCoy noted,* was just two miles from city hall and backed onto the yards of the San Francisco–Los Angeles line of the Southern Pacific Railroad.[25]

This was alarming news and prompted the PHS to cast its net wider. After writing to Washington for more rifles and ammunition, Blue sent hunting parties into nearby woodlands and hillsides to collect squirrels and bring them to McCoy's laboratory. By 1910, McCoy had examined 150,000 ground squirrels across ten California counties and discovered that 402, or 0.3 per cent of them, were infected with plague. These diseased squirrels had been recovered from as far south as San Luis Obispo and the San Joaquin Valley, many miles from the sea and the presumed original ports of entry to the United States. In response, Blue focused his efforts on the areas where infected squirrels had been found, poisoning their burrows with carbon bisulfide and sending hunting parties into the woods to shoot stray rodents. Blue's war on rodents made him a household name, and in 1912 he was elevated to surgeon general, the top medical position in the country. In his absence, oth-

---

* Though McCoy states that the squirrel had bitten the boy on the hand, he goes on to say that it is uncertain whether the boy contracted plague this way, speculating that he may have contracted it from infected fleas, which is the more usual transmission route of plague from squirrels to humans.

ers carried on the eradication work he had begun, and by 1914 ground squirrels had been recovered from twenty-one infected ranches and their burrows so thoroughly poisoned that officials were only able to find one infected squirrel when they repeated the survey, prompting Colby to claim that "danger of its further spread has been removed."[26] But Colby and his colleagues were wrong. The ecology of plague was far more complex than they could have anticipated—as one expert put it, writing in 1949, plague was "like following the different voices in a Bach fugue," the difference being that while the structure of a Bach fugue is known, with plague "the basic design is unknown."[27] The fact is, plague never entirely disappears from wild rodent populations. Rather, the pathogen circulates continually between fleas, squirrels, and other wild mammals, including chipmunks, marmots and prairie dogs.* Many of these rodents have genetic or acquired immunity so are resistant to illness. However, every few years, this resistance wanes and the host population crashes, leaving fleas without a source of food. It is at this stage that the fleas seek a new host, seizing upon whatever animal happens to stray into the vacant rodents' burrows. This could be another species of ground squirrel or it could be a wild rat or a field mouse, or even a rabbit. Regardless, the transfer usually results in a violent epizootic as these new and highly susceptible hosts fall victim to the disease for the first time—hence the rats that Colby found littering the grounds of the ranch in Concord.

Nonetheless, there was good reason why, by 1924, California health officials should have been on their guard, not only against renewed outbreaks of the bubonic form of the disease, but of pneumonic plague, too. Indeed, bacteriologists only needed to recall the outbreak of pneumonic plague that had occurred in Oakland five years earlier, killing thirteen people. The outbreak began in August 1919 when an Italian man named Di Bortoli went hunting in the foothills of Alameda County, returning with several squirrels for the table of his rooming house in Oakland. Within days, Di Bortoli was complaining of fever and pain in his right side and had reported to a doctor. Unfortunately, the physician attributed Bortoli's symptoms to influenza and even after Di Bortoli developed a painful bubo on his neck, the doctor did not think of plague. Most likely, it was septicaemic spread of plague from this bubo that sparked a tonsillar infection and secondary pneumonia. The result was that by

---

* Rabbits, pigs, coyotes, bobcats, badgers, bears, grey foxes and skunks can also be infected with plague, though they rarely exhibit symptoms. By contrast, domestic cats are highly susceptible.

the time Di Bortoli died at the end of the month, five other people, including his landlady and a nurse, had been infected and by 11 September, thirteen more people had contracted plague. In all, only one survived. Fortunately, thanks to the rapid hospitalization and isolation of the patients, the outbreak was self-limiting. Nevertheless, the fact that thirteen people had died and that the outbreak had begun following contact with a squirrel was extremely alarming, suggesting that, as with Siberian marmots, Californian squirrels might harbour fleas infected with highly virulent and potentially pneumotropic strains of the bacillus. As William Kellogg, the director of the State Board of Health Bureau's communicable disease division, observed, "Until plague-infected ground squirrels are entirely eradicated from California we shall always have a sword of Damocles hanging over our heads."[28]

Kellogg's concerns were born of bitter experience. In 1900 when plague had announced itself in San Francisco, it had been he who had taken samples from the lymph gland of the first presumed plague patient to Joseph Kinyoun at the United States' Marine Hospital laboratory on Angel Island for testing. After Kinyoun demonstrated that the tissues contained the plague bacillus, and that that organism caused guinea pigs to sicken and die, Kellogg then found himself thrust into the uncomfortable position of having to defend Kinyoun against a vitriolic campaign orchestrated by California's governor, Henry Gage, and local business interests. Angered by the imposition of the quarantine around Chinatown, Gage and his allies called into question Kinyoun's methods and findings, and alleged that the quarantine measures were a "scare." They also proposed that "it be made a felony to broadcast the presence of plague."[29] Kinyoun's findings were subsequently upheld by a commission of prominent bacteriologists appointed by the US Treasury, but Kellogg, whose competence came in for similar scrutiny and who faced similar vilification, felt that "for unexampled bitterness, unfair and dishonest methods" the campaign "probably never had been and never again will be equaled."[30]

Thankfully, the 1900 outbreak had been brought under control with just 121 cases and 113 deaths, and when plague revisited San Francisco in 1907 politicians and health officials no longer tried to pretend it was a fiction, moving swiftly to contain the disease by launching an extensive rat extermination campaign. Like other bacteriologists and officials who had been "blooded" by America's first experience of plague, Kellogg remained a keen student of the disease, and when in the winter of 1910 reports reached California of an outbreak of pneumonic plague in Manchuria, he followed news of the spreading outbreak keenly. Most likely sparked by tarbagans, a species of Mongolian and Siberian marmot valued for their fur, the epidemic appears to have begun at Manchouli, near the Chinese–Siberian border, in October 1910 before spreading via the trans-Manchurian railway to Harbin and other towns along the way. The principal culprits were inexperienced Chinese hunters who had been attracted to Manchuria by the high prices for pelts and did not take as much care as Manchurian trappers when handling sick tarbagans. As the Manchurian winter closed in and the hunters headed back to China, they mingled with returning agricultural workers and "coolies," crowding into packed railway carriages and inns. Soon, hospitals were overrun with patients, and by February 1911 some 50,000 people had died. Many of the bodies were cremated or dynamited in plague pits.[31] According to Wu Lien-Teh, a Cambridge-educated Chinese plague expert who made a detailed study of the epidemic, reports of buboes were entirely absent, but pneumonic symptoms were ubiquitous. Working with the American physician and tropical medicine specialist Richard Strong, Wu performed twenty-five autopsies and used bacteriological techniques to confirm the presence of *Y. pestis*, subsequently presenting the evidence at the International Plague Conference called by the Chinese in Mukden in 1911.[32]

At this time, most experts subscribed to the idea that plague was a rat-borne disease, most likely communicated by fleas, so the idea that the bacillus could be spread in droplet form to humans directly from tarbagans and marmots was controversial. But when the Chinese and Japanese authorities made a close examination of rats—some 50,000 were rounded up—they could not find any evidence of infection, and support for the theory grew. Some experts suspected the Manchurian strains were more virulent than those associated with previous bubonic outbreaks in India and elsewhere; others that the tarbagan-derived bacilli were pneumotropic, meaning they had an affinity for the lungs. This theory received a boost when Strong, who headed the Biological Laboratory in Manila (part of the Philippine Bureau of Science) and led the American delegation to the conference, demonstrated that plague bacilli could be cultured from agar plates on which patients had been allowed to breathe, and that tarbagans could also be infected with pneumonic plague if exposed to the organism in droplet form.

Another compelling theory concerned the weather. In Manchuria the average temperature during the three months of the epidemic had been −30°C, whereas in India, where plague had raged on and off since 1896 and had been largely bubonic, the average temperature had been 30°C. Hypothesizing that the failure of pneumonic plague to spread in India had been due to the higher average temperatures there, Oscar Teague and M. A. Barber, two bacteriologists attached to the Philippine Bureau of

Science, decided to perform a series of evaporation experiments with *Y. pestis* and other infectious bacteria. These showed that sprayed plague droplets disappeared very quickly from the atmosphere in conditions of low humidity, whereas the converse was the case in conditions of high humidity. "Such an atmosphere is, under ordinary circumstances, of common occurrence in very cold climates, whereas it is extremely rare in warm ones," they wrote. "Hence, since the droplets of sputum persist longer, the plague bacilli remain alive longer in the air, and there is a greater tendency for the disease to spread in cold climates than in warm ones."[33]

Not everyone was persuaded by this argument, however, or convinced that climate had been the decisive factor. Though impressed by the cold weather in Harbin in 1910, Wu did not think it had played a major part in the Manchurian outbreak, pointing out that there was "ample evidence" to show that pneumonic outbreaks also occurred in regions with hot climates, such as Egypt and West Africa. Instead, Wu believed that the decisive factor had been the overcrowding and the proximity to infectious patients, pointing out that "most infections occurred indoors, specially at night-time, when the coolies returned to their warm but crowded shelters." Nor did he accept another theory according to which the cold weather had resulted in the wide dispersion of *frozen* particles of plague-infected sputum. "If infection occurred in the open, it certainly was a direct one from patient to patient, and did not result from inhalation of frozen particles of sputum," he stated.[34]

Weighing the circumstances of the Oakland outbreak, Kellogg concluded that the health department had been fortunate that the outbreak had occurred in August, as the warm weather and low humidity meant that "conditions were not favorable for the transfer of infected droplets." The result was that "the drying and consequent death of the bacillus was so rapid that the ordinary measures of prophylaxis ... sufficed to check the progress of the infection." Had the weather been cooler or the atmospheric water deficit lower, then things might have been different, he acknowledged, but that had not been and was unlikely to be the case in California. While San Francisco and Los Angeles needed to be on their guard against further cases of bubonic plague sparked by stray squirrels, he concluded, it was cities in the East that should be most concerned about the pneumonic form of the disease. All it would take, he observed, was for someone to be infected by a squirrel and, while incubating the disease, journey to "some eastern state in winter time and [develop] an infection such as that of Di Bortoli." He concluded that while the persistence of sylvatic reservoirs of plague in California ground squirrels constituted a permanent risk of the bubonic form of the disease, the pneumonic form was "probably not a serious menace on the Pacific coast, owing to climatic conditions."[35]

* * *

The identification of *Y. pestis* in Horace Gutiérrez's sputum and the symptoms of severe pneumonia with bloody expectorations and cyanosis should have been a wake-up call that the improbable had happened and that pneumonic plague was at large in the Mexican quarter, even as Los Angeles broiled in a late autumn heat wave. But that is not what happened. Instead, fearing the political and economic repercussions, not to mention the panic that might attend an official announcement that the Black Death had arrived in the city of the future, health officials prevaricated. On being shown the slide packed with rod-shaped bacteria, the city's health commissioner, Dr Luther Powers, denied the evidence before his eyes, telling Maner the slide had been poorly prepared and that he needed to rerun the tests. Nevertheless, he took the precaution of sending quarantine officers to the Macy Street District, telling them there had been a "return of [Spanish] flu" in a virulent form in the Mexican quarter. By now, Maria Samarano, Guadalupe's 80-year-old grand-mother—the woman whom Bogen had examined at Carmelita Street—had been admitted to County General, and on 1 November she died, becoming the fourth victim of the outbreak. But still no one dared utter the "p" word in public. However, the evening before, the hospital's superintendent had sent a telegram to state and federal officials asking where he might obtain plague serum and vaccine. One of the telegrams was intercepted by Benjamin Brown, the PHS's senior surgeon in Los Angeles. Not sure that he could trust what he was reading, Brown called the hospital to inquire if there were plague patients on its wards, then wired the Surgeon General, Hugh S. Cumming, to alert him to the gravity of the situation. Encoding his telegram for secrecy, he dictated: "Eighteen cases ekkil [pneumonic plague]. Three suspects. Ten begos [deaths]. Ethos [situation bad]. Recommend federal aid." In response, Cumming ordered James Perry, a senior surgeon stationed in San Francisco, to proceed to Los Angeles and make discreet inquiries, but by now quarantine officers were roping off the eight city blocks that encompassed the death house at Clara Street and newspapermen had begun asking questions.[36]

Infectious diseases have long been objects of rumour and panic. When the identity of the pathogen is unknown or uncertain, and information about the outbreak is veiled in secrecy, these rumours—and the fears that attend them—can quickly spiral out of control. The first into print was the *Los*

Angeles Times, posting a report on 1 November that nine mourners who had attended the wake at 742 Clara Street had died of a "strange malady" resembling pneumonia. Listing the victims by name, perhaps so its readers would have no doubt that, for the moment, this was a Hispanic rather than an Anglo-Saxon problem, the paper went on to report that eight more people were confined to the hospital's isolation ward and that some of these were also "expected to die." The paper also revealed that the health authorities had "isolated a germ" but, like the *Herald Examiner* and other Los Angeles papers, the *Times* avoided mentioning the dreaded word "plague." Instead, the paper stated that there would be no official announcement until bacteriological studies had been concluded, and that for the moment patients had been given "the technical diagnosis of Spanish influenza."[37] Incredibly, it was this or a similar coded report in another California paper that seems to have alerted Kellogg's colleague, Dr William Dickie, the secretary of the State Board of Health, that something was amiss in the Mexican quarter. Dickie immediately sent a telegram to Dr Elmer Pascoe, Los Angeles's acting health officer, asking him to "Kindly wire immediately cause of death of Lucena Samarano [*sic*]." Pascoe, who had only just taken up the city's top health post following the sudden death of the previous occupant from a heart attack, kept his answer brief and to the point, "Death L.S. caused by *Bacillus pestis*."[38]

By now the quarantine had been extended to Belvedere Gardens, confining some 4,000 people within the plague zone, and the police and fire department had strict instructions not to let anyone in or out of the roped-off area. In addition, guards had been posted at the front and back of homes that were known to contain or that had formerly contained plague victims. Public gatherings were also prohibited, and parents were instructed to keep their children out of school and away from movie houses. Even Pacific Electric trolley cars, which continued to run along Macy Street, were banned from letting riders board or alight at stops near the quarantined area.

This was Los Angeles's shark-in-the-water moment. The sight of armed guards barring entry to the Mexican quarter was the equivalent of posting signs on the beach that it was no longer safe to enter the water. But rather than admitting the truth, city and health authorities, with the backing of local newspaper editors, sought to maintain the fiction that, as the *Los Angeles Times* put it, the outbreak was merely a "malignant form of pneumonia."[39] This infuriated *El Heraldo de Mexico*, the Spanish-language newspaper, which railed against "the hermetic silence in which authorities have locked themselves."[40] But it was a lone voice and no other paper in Los Angeles dared mention plague. Outside Los Angeles, however, it was a different story. "21 Victims of

'Black Death' in California," declared the Associated Press on 1 November. "Pneumonic Plague is Feared after 13 die in Los Angeles," announced the *Washington Post* on 2 November. "Pneumonic Plague takes seven more victims," reported the *New York Times* on 3 November.

The contrasting treatment of the outbreak in America's metropolitan dailies perhaps says more about the rivalries between East and West Coast business elites, and commercial concerns about the plague's economic impacts, than it does about the competence of Los Angeles health officials. Faced with the publicity nightmare of a disease from the Dark Ages appearing in twentieth-century Los Angeles, it is little wonder that the first instinct of the city's civic leaders and their press allies was to obfuscate. As George Young, the managing editor of the *Herald Examiner*, informed the Board of Directors of the Los Angeles Chamber of Commerce, Hearst newspapers "would print nothing we didn't think was in the interests of the city."[41] At stake was not only the viability of Los Angeles's tourism industry and future real estate sales, but the ambition to make the Port of Los Angeles at San Pedro the largest commercial harbour in the United States. Should federal health officials in Washington suspect plague was anywhere near the port, the surgeon general would have no choice but to close the harbour and impose a strict maritime quarantine. Once a quarantine had been instituted it would continue for at least ten days and could only be lifted when the authorities were sure the city was free of plague and there was no danger of the disease being reintroduced to wharfside areas by rats and other rodents. But by that point, of course, the damage to the city's reputation would have been done.

By contrast, for the New York newspapers there was nothing like plague to boost circulation, especially when the outbreak lay a safe 3,000 miles to the west. Besides, for years Los Angeles had boasted of its superior climate and quality of life, bombarding easterners with postcards adorned with sun-kissed orange groves and preternaturally happy couples. Never mind if reporting the truth fostered panic: it was worth it just to puncture the booster hubris and wipe the smirk off those sunny Californian faces.

* * *

In 1924 there was no treatment or cure for pneumonic plague. The best that physicians could offer were stimulants such as caffeine and digitalis, or depressants such as morphine. In theory, vaccines containing killed bacteria or convalescent serums containing antibodies from patients who had survived infection with plague might have made a difference, but only if convalescents with immunity to the disease could be found in time and the serums administered early enough in the infection to make a difference to the course of the disease. In the absence of such measures, 90 per cent of infections were fatal.

For those who had attended Luciana Samarano's wake, had boarded in her rooming house, or had helped care for one of her sick or dying relatives, it was almost certainly too late. But for those who had not yet been exposed to infectious sputum or blood from the Samaranos' extended family, there was one measure that was certain to break the chain of infections: quarantine and the rapid isolation of the sick. These measures had eventually halted the outbreak in Harbin in 1911, and they had also stemmed the outbreak in Oakland in 1919. Even without an official diagnosis of plague, physicians at County General were sufficiently wary of the infection and the alarming symptoms of cyanosis to place patients in an isolation ward and wear masks and rubber gloves when approaching their beds. However, the decision to quarantine Macy Street and Belvedere Gardens appears to have had little to do with infection control and everything to do with racism and prejudice.

Reconstructing the precise sequence of events is difficult given the incomplete documentation and the lack of transparency by the Los Angeles newspapers and Mayor George Cryer. But what is certain is that only Walter Dickie, the secretary of the State Board of Health, had the legal authority to order a quarantine of the Mexican quarter and he did not learn about the outbreak until 1 November, by which time, of course, the area had already been roped off. Instead, it seems that the decision was made by the county health chief, J. L. Pomeroy, acting on his own initiative. Though Pomeroy was a qualified doctor, his decision appears to have had less to do with his knowledge of plague than his experience of previous quarantines and his low regard for Mexicans. By the 1920s ethnic quarantines, spurred by fears of smallpox and typhus being introduced by migrants from across the border, had become a routine measure in Los Angeles and other southern Californian towns. According to Pomeroy, special guard details were "the only effective way of quarantining Mexicans," and he ordered his men to institute the quarantine by stealth so as not to spread alarm. To this end, Pomeroy conscripted seventy-five police officers and positioned his men discreetly at the boundaries of Macy Street and Carmelita Street in Belvedere Gardens. To avoid "a general stampede," he instructed the guards to wait until after midnight when they were certain all residents had returned home. It was only then that ropes were strung around the zone and the "quarantine was [made] absolute." The measures, which were in force for two weeks, would eventually extend to five urban districts in which Hispanics were known to reside. However, only two of these, Macy Street and Belvedere, had verifiable cases of plague. As Deverell puts it, "the others had only verified cases of ethnicity. In other words, Mexicans lived there."[42]

Though judged by today's standards Pomeroy's methods were discriminatory, they appear to have been extremely effective. With the exception of an ambulance driver who ferried one of the patients to the hospital, all the casualties, bar one, came from within the quarantine zone and could be traced to the Samarano clan or to mourners who had been present at one of the wakes. Indeed, Pomeroy's decision to impose a quarantine seems to have been prompted in part by the questioning of boarders who shared the house at 343 Carmelita Street with Guadalupe's elderly mother, Maria Samarano. This was the address that Bogen had visited two days earlier and where he had discovered Maria and Guadalupe's brother, Victor, lying deathly ill. By the time Pomeroy arrived at Carmelita Street, Victor was dead of suspected "meningitis." However, on quizzing the other boarders and learning that Victor had recently attended his father's funeral, Pomeroy immediately posted armed guards at the front and back of the house. Next, he discovered that one of Luciana Samarano's cousins had died at another house in Belvedere Gardens and that his wife was also ill with what was presumed to be the same disease. This was the flag that appears to have convinced Pomeroy to draw a wider line around Macy District and extend the quarantine to Belvedere Gardens, even though it lay across the city line in Los Angeles County.

Waking the following morning to find that they were effectively prisoners—"inmates" was the official term used by the health authorities—must have been a terrifying experience for the Mexican residents and anyone else caught up in the dragnet. Indeed, no sooner was the quarantine in place than the authorities began house-to-house inspections. Those who were sick or were suspected of having been in contact with sick persons were removed to the isolation ward at County General, while those left behind were told to prepare a mixture of hot water, salt, and lime juice, and gargle with it several times a day. The chamber of commerce refused to requisition additional funds to provide provisions for the trapped residents of the plague zone. Instead, it was left to local charities to deliver packages of food and milk to stricken families.

Confined to their homes, waiting to see who would be next to succumb to the *Muerto Negro*, as Spanish speakers referred to the disease, one can only imagine the images that flashed through people's minds and the thoughts that they clung to for comfort. As Camus reminds us, in such situations "we tell ourselves that pestilence is a mere bogy of the mind, a bad dream that will pass away."[43] But the plague was not a bogy, it was real and it could strike, without warning, at any time. The only mercy was that the worst suffering took place far from the quarantine zone, inside the isolation ward at County General. There, in a desperate effort to halt the course of the disease, doctors placed patients on an intravenous drip of Mercurochrome solution, a mercury-based antiseptic used to treat minor cuts and bruises that was almost certainly useless against plague.* The first to receive the treatment was ten-year-old Roberto Samarano, the eldest of Guadalupe's three sons. He was hooked up to a Mercurochrome drip on 28 October and given three successive injections, only to die two days later, his body "practically riddled with plague infection." Roberto's death was followed by that of his younger brother, Gilberto, and Alfredo Burnett, Luciana Samarano's son from an earlier marriage (Alfredo died on 11 November after a heroic thirteen-day struggle with the disease that saw him slipping in and out of a "restless delirium").[44] By now two boarders at 742 Clara Street had also died. Incredibly, the only member of the Samarano clan to survive the death house was the Samaranos' second son, Raul. The eight-year-old was evacuated from Clara Street at the same time as his siblings, but, unlike his brothers, was given plague serum.[45] He lived, growing up to enjoy a career in the navy and the Los Angeles Army Corp of Engineers. Another notable survivor was Mary Costello, a nurse who had attended Guadalupe Samarano at Clara Street. Costello was admitted to County General on 29 October. By Halloween both her lungs were showing signs of consolidation and she was bringing up "bloody expectorations," but after being given Mercurochrome solution Costello showed a slight improvement, and a few days later she also received plague serum. It was this that may have made the difference.

Incredible as it might seem today, Angelinos in other parts of the city appear to have been largely ignorant of the outbreak and the significance of the quarantine. One man recalled the plague as "a big hush-up," while his father, who lived within walking distance of Macy Street and was a regular reader of the *Los Angeles Times*, admitted he had known little about the outbreak.[46] This is not surprising when you consider that the *Los Angeles Times* and other municipal papers did not refer to the disease by its proper name until 6 November, by which time the epidemic had more or less run its course. Even then, they sought to justify their evasion by adding that pneumonic

---

* Mercurochrome is the brand name for dibromohydroxymercurifluorescein, sometimes called merbromin. Its use was discontinued by the FDA in 1998 because of fears of potential mercury poisoning.

plague was merely the "technical term" for malignant pneumonia. Plague was "not a new phenomenon in California," Dickie pointed out truthfully, if a little disingenuously. "While an outbreak of plague is always a potential menace ... there is no reason for public alarm."[47]

Outside of Los Angeles, however, it was a different story, as newspapers competed to keep their readers abreast of the latest developments. The call for plague serum and the news of its dramatic journey received particular attention, not least of all because the manufacturer, Mulford Laboratories of Philadelphia, used Los Angeles's plight as a marketing opportunity to issue regular press updates on the progress of the serum from the West to the East Coast. Pascoe's appeal for serum had reached Mulford on 3 November, prompting the company to dispatch several vials by automobile to Mineola airfield in Long Island. The following day the serum was transferred to a mail plane and flown 3,000 miles to San Francisco and thence to Los Angeles, reaching the city health department on 5 November. "Serum for plague speeds by plane to Los Angeles," reported the New York *Evening World News* on 5 November; "5000 more doses of serum go west," added the *Public Ledger* of Philadelphia a few days later.[48] Mulford did its best to play up the "thrilling" story of the vaccine's bicoastal journey, describing how within thirty-six hours of receiving the appeal, "the vials of serum were brought to the front lines where the battle is on against the Terror." Speed laws were "forgotten" as the precious vials were rushed to Mineola and, though the mail plane was briefly delayed by a storm at Salt Lake City, it was not long before "the messenger of mercy had right of way" again. Reading Mulford's sensational, self-serving prose must have been an uncomfortable experience for Los Angeles's own boosters. "It was pneumonic plague or Black Plague—the scourge of the fourteenth century," declared an announcement in the Mulford company journal, "the dread disease which numbered its victims by the millions."[49] But Los Angeles business leaders were nothing if not adept at inoculating negative publicity, and soon they were putting their own spin on the episode, reassuring easterners that, as William Lacy, the president of the Los Angeles Chamber of Commerce, put it in an article in the *Los Angeles Realtor*, the city had suffered "a slight epidemic of pneumonic plague" and there was no reason for anyone to cancel their vacation plans.[50]

If the outbreak challenged Los Angeles's carefully cultivated image as an idyllic holiday destination, it was no less of a headache for the State Board of Health and the PHS. In Washington the sensational newspaper reports were read with mounting alarm, leading to demands for reassurance from Congress that federal health officials were doing their utmost to ensure that plague did not spread to other harbour cities. The problem was that, technically, the outbreak in the Mexican quarter was the responsibility of the Los Angeles City Health department and the State Board of Health. Unless and until the outbreak reached the Port of Los Angeles, the PHS had no authority to intervene and could only serve in an advisory capacity. In theory, cooperation was in the interests of bureaucrats at the local, state, and federal level, but the city health commissioner was a political appointee who reported directly to the mayor George Cryer, who in turn answered to the board of the chamber of commerce. This placed Pascoe in an impossible position, since Cryer was acutely sensitive to any statement that adversely impacted the city's image and its commercial prospects. Indeed, when Pascoe overstepped his authority by confirming to the eastern papers that the outbreak was due to pneumonic plague, Cryer passed him over for promotion and appointed a more pliant official to head the department.[51] However, Dickie valued Pascoe's expertise and when, on 3 November, at a meeting in Cryer's office, Dickie was put in charge of the plague clean-up operation, he insisted that Pascoe join his team. It would seem that Cryer had little choice but to accede to this demand; nor could he prevent Dickie offering a place on the advisory committee to James Perry, the PHS surgeon who had been dispatched from San Francisco to monitor the situation, despite the board's paranoia about word reaching Washington that plague might be encroaching on the environs of the port at San Pedro. Perry found himself in a similarly awkward position vis-à-vis his superiors in Washington, as he had to balance the surgeon general's concerns that local officials were not up to the job against interventions that might be seen as interfering with the state's jurisdiction and undermining Dickie's authority. Indeed, it would seem that Perry may have gone too far in accommodating local officials, because on 7 November, after being reprimanded for not transmitting information to Washington quickly enough, he explained that Dickie was "keenly desirous" of taking full control himself and that, in any case, there had been some doubt as to whether the outbreak was due to pneumonic plague. Interestingly, it would appear that Perry's scepticism was also the opinion of other experts, including Kellogg, who had accompanied him to Los Angeles and who had insisted on preparing fresh bacteriological slides before accepting Maner's diagnosis. Once it became clear that the outbreak was plague and deserved to be treated as such, however, Perry found himself increasingly at odds with Dickie. At the heart of their differences was the question whether the outbreak in the Mexican quarter was due to squirrels or rats, or some combination of both, and the implication that this might have for other parts of the city, including the port. Dickie and his colleagues in the county health department believed the epidemic would eventually be traced to infected squirrels, as had been the case with the Oakland outbreak, meaning that it should end when the last infectious patient had been isolated in the hospital. Indeed, when, at the suggestion of Karl Meyer, a bacteriologist who directed the Hooper Foundation for Medical Research in San Francisco and who had visited McCoy's plague laboratory to familiarize himself with his techniques, they combed rats in the Mexican quarter for fleas, they discovered a fair number harboured *H. anomalus* plus another species, *Diamanus montanus*, more commonly found on ground squirrels. Recalling the case of the boy in Elysian Park who had died of plague after exposure to a squirrel in 1908, Meyer suggested that this meant the outbreak had probably originated in the "hinterland," not the port.[52] Perry thought otherwise and, responding to increasingly stern telegrams from Washington, insisted that the outbreak had been due to rats and that only a well-financed rodent eradication campaign targeting both the Mexican quarter and the port would be certain to rid Los Angeles of the disease. This was not a verdict the chamber of commerce wished to hear, for obvious reasons. Nevertheless, in mid-November the chamber granted $250,000 to finance rodent extermination measures, with the promise of more money should it be needed. The pivotal decision came at a meeting of the chamber and the city council on 13 November when, standing in front of a map of greater Los Angeles studded with black pins representing pneumonic plague cases, Dickie warned: "I realize that the dream of Los Angeles and the dream of officials and the chamber of commerce is the harbor. Your dream will never come true as long as plague exists in Los Angeles and as long as there is any question of doubt in reference to the harbor." Unless San Pedro received a clean bill of health "half of the commerce of your harbor will quickly vanish," Dickie predicted, before concluding that "no disease known has such an effect upon the business world as the plague."[53]

Los Angeles business leaders must have hoped that by granting substantial monies for anti-plague measures, they would convince officials in Washington they were serious about addressing the rat problem and avoid the need for San Pedro to be quarantined. If so, their hopes were dashed. This had little to do with the enthusiasm with which Dickie and the City Health Department prosecuted rodent extermination, and everything to do with the PHS's concern for its reputation and its suspicion of California politicians and local business leaders. During the rat clean-up campaign in San Francisco, federal health officials had watched aghast as local newspapers, encouraged by Gage, had questioned Kinyoun's scientific competence. In the end, the reappearance of plague in San Francisco in 1907 had forced Gage to bow to the authority of the federal plague commission and cooperate with the PHS, but the experience had left Blue and Hugh Cumming, his successor as surgeon general who had been a protégé of Kinyoun's, suspicious of local city health departments and state-appointed health officials. In an attempt to foster closer cooperation between state and federal officials and improve the flow of information to Washington, in 1923 Cumming divided the country into seven public health districts and appointed experienced officers to each. One of the key postings was at the quarantine station at Angel Island, a position which went to Cumming's close friend and confidant, Assistant Surgeon General Richard H. Creel. From San Francisco, Creel would oversee quarantines for all ports along the United States' western seaboard, including Los Angeles, and keep a close eye on the progress of Dickie's campaign, feeding the information back to Cumming in Washington.[54]

Determined to show that the State Board of Health was up to the task, Dickie moved into the new Pacific Finance Building off Wilshire Boulevard, where he fashioned himself "commander-in-chief." There, surrounded by colour-coded maps studded with pins recording the locations of trapped rodents (red for rats, yellow for squirrels), he presided over 127 rodent exterminators.[55] Under Dickie's direction, the campaign took on the trappings of a military exercise. One team of rat catchers was assigned exclusively to the harbour, with orders to inspect every arriving vessel and tag any rodent found in the vicinity of the port. The rats would then be removed to the city laboratory on Eighth Street for testing. At the same time, other squads fanned out across the Mexican quarter, performing "plague abatements." Modelled on the campaign in San Francisco's Chinatown in 1900, these involved removing the sidings from houses in and around Clara Street and raising the dwellings eighteen inches off the ground, so that dogs and cats could freely enter the buildings and flush diseased rodents from their lairs. At the same time, premises were ruthlessly stripped of furniture, clothing, and bedding, and funeral pyres made of tenants' belongings. These slash-and-burn tactics culminated with fumigation with petroleum, sulphur or cyanide gas, measures that guaranteed that no creature foolish enough to return to the properties would survive long in the poisoned rooms. Running alongside these plague abatement measures was an equally ferocious rodent trapping and extermination campaign. Squares of bread baited with phosphorus or arsenic were scattered in suspect neighbourhoods both inside and outside the quarantine zone. The city health department also offered a bounty of $1 for every dead rat or squirrel brought for counting and testing to its laboratory at Eighth Street. When this did not yield a sufficient bounty of rodents, the health department offered men a fixed salary of $130 a day. For First World War veterans this was considerably more than they could hope to earn in civilian employment, and soon the hunting parties were swelled by former infantrymen eager to demonstrate their sharpshooting skills. It was not long before Macy District echoed to the continuous pop of rifles, and when the hunting parties ran out of rodents within the city limits they fanned out to Belvedere Gardens and other areas in the county. "These surveys may take us a hundred miles or more from Los Angeles before we find the guilty rodent," Dickie warned.[56]

Ironically, this campaign turned up far fewer rats in the Mexican quarter than had been expected, and virtually none in the harbour area. Indeed, by 22 November, not one of the 1,000 rats trapped in the harbour had tested positive for plague.[57] By contrast, to the embarrassment of the chamber of commerce, rats were readily trapped in the downtown blocks that housed the city's premier hotels and department stores. Meyer, who accompanied health officials on several of their inspections, recalled how at one downtown rice-cake factory run by a Japanese gentleman he had only to drop a crumb on the floor to "see a rat come up and pick it up." To Meyer, the scene was like something out of "Zanzibar" with the smart facades concealing a "jungle." The only way to ensure that such premises were rat-proof, he observed, was to pour concrete over the dirt floors, but that was expensive (and not always effective).[58]

By the end of the year, Dickie could boast that his men had trapped more than 25,000 rats and 768 squirrels. In addition, flooring and planking had been removed from countless buildings in and around Clara and Macy Streets, and poison laid at 1,000 premises. However, for all the intensity of the plague abatement measures, Perry was unimpressed by Dickie's efforts, informing Cumming that the Board's campaign had been "casual and periodic" and that its laboratory work could not be trusted. "It is apparent that Dr Dickie does not appreciate the gravity of the situation, or the importance of enlarging the scope of the campaign, or of increasing the efficiency of the operations," Perry informed Cumming in mid-December. "This is evidenced by his non-acceptance of the proffered, concrete Service aid." Instead, he urged Cumming to dissociate the PHS from the state's programme, warning that unless the PHS took charge of the campaign there was a "grave" danger the disease could spread to other countries.[59] This was the one thing that Cumming could not allow, as under the provisions of the 1922 International Sanitary Convention the United States had a duty to ensure that "adequate measures" were being taken to prevent the spread of plague to other jurisdictions, failure to do so running the risk that foreign governments would impose quarantines against American shipping. Adding to Cumming's concern was the discovery of plague-infected rats in both New Orleans and Oakland. In the case of New Orleans, it was suspected the culprit had been the *Atlanticos*, a coal-steamer that had reached the Crescent City at the end of October after sailing from Oran, a notorious Algerian plague port that would be immortalized in Camus's 1947 novel. On board was a stowaway with a swelling on his groin. The stowaway was hospitalized and the ship fumigated, but soon after, eight plague rats were found on the waterfront, prompting the Louisiana State Board of Health to request the PHS begin a rodent survey. In the case of Oakland, there was no evidence of foreign introduction of plague. Instead, the alarm was raised by the discovery on 13 December of a plague rat on a garbage dump close to the waterfront.

In Los Angeles, by contrast, no plague-carrying rats had been found in the immediate vicinity of the harbour. However, by the end of December thirty-five had been retrieved from ranches within a mile of the port, and nearly twice as many again from other areas within a forty-mile circumference of San Pedro. In addition, survey squads had established that 64 per cent of rats in the Los Angeles area were colonized by squirrel fleas and, although hunting parties had failed to turn up any infected squirrels in or around the city, eight squirrels retrieved from a ranch in San Luis Obispo that had been the focus of previous plague epizootics also tested positive for *Y. pestis*. At the same time, ranchers reported having observed epizootics of squirrel plague in San Benito and Monterey Counties the previous summer, suggesting that, as Meyer put it, 1924 had "truly [been] a sylvatic plague year in California."[60] However, it was the reports from Europe of a new outbreak of rat plague at several Mediterranean ports that persuaded Cumming the PHS was facing a world-wide recrudescence of the disease and prompted him to finally institute quarantines at San Pedro and other "plague-infected" American ports.[61]

Cumming's decision prompted a subtle but significant shift in the medical language. It was no longer the threat of domestic American squirrels transmitting the pneumonic form of the disease that was to be feared, so much as foreign introductions by "bubonic rats."[62] That hysterical conjunction was sufficient to panic Congress into voting an emergency appropriation of $275,000 to support the PHS's renewed campaign against its old enemy. At first, Los Angeles's chamber of commerce protested the decision, accusing Cumming of "discriminatory" action since no plague rats had been found at San Pedro. In any case, it argued, while the harbour was the Fed's fiefdom, the port was the jurisdiction of the state and the city health department.[63] For a while Cryer tried to argue the case for his new appointee, city health officer George Parrish. However, when Cryer got his wish and the city council authorized Parrish to take over the eradication campaign from Dickie, it also slashed his budget, forcing Cryer to swallow his pride and go cap in hand to President Calvin Coolidge to request that the PHS be allowed to assume responsibility for the plague clean-up work. As far as Cumming was concerned, there was only one man for the job, his predecessor Rupert Blue, who was promptly recommissioned into the Service and dispatched to Los Angeles. For Blue it was an opportunity to finish the work he had begun in 1908, and by July he was once again in his element, probing Los Angeles's downtown rat runs, overseeing the concreting over of basements and taking other abatement measures. "Nine suspicious rats and five ground squirrels have been found since June thirteen in widely separated sections, extending from Hollywood north to West Washington Street south," he wired Cumming on 26 June. "Should these prove positive for plague we may expect several human cases to occur at any time. Seasonal conditions highly favorable for a return of the epidemic."[64]

It is hard to say who deserves most credit for the eventual eradication of plague in Los Angeles, Blue or Dickie. The last reported case of pneumonic plague occurred on 12 January 1925, and, despite Blue's ominous telegram, the last plague-infected rat was recovered from eastern Los Angeles on 21 May, in other words two months before Blue took charge. And while Dickie may have been guilty of colluding in the press cover-up, he never doubted that the outbreak was serious. Moreover, his prompt action in quarantining Macy District and directing the plague clean-up efforts, however harsh and unfair the measures must have seemed to the area's Mexican residents, ensured that pneumonic plague did not spread to other parts of the city. Indeed, it could be argued that the Board's response might have been even more effective had the city health department alerted Dickie to the outbreak sooner, rather than waiting for him to learn about it from a newspaper. As Dickie observed in his official report on the outbreak,[65] physicians and bacteriologists at County General were also culpable in failing to recognize the symptoms of plague in Jesus Lajun.* Though official figures probably did not reflect the full extent of the outbreak, in total there had been just forty-one cases of pneumonic plague and thirty-seven fatalities. In addition,

---

* The swelling in Jesus's groin was almost certainly an inguinal bubo that had been allowed to drain for three weeks before anyone thought to examine it for plague bacilli. A culture subsequently revealed "bipolar organisms," and when a laboratory animal was inoculated with the culture it died within twelve hours.

there had been seven cases and five deaths from bubonic plague and a single fatal case of septicaemic plague. Most important of all, perhaps, it was the last recorded outbreak of pneumonic plague anywhere in North America.

* * *

The Los Angeles outbreak upset the assumptions of Kellogg and other plague experts, challenging the wisdom that California's mild, year-round Mediterranean climate was a protection. Instead, it demonstrated that conditions of low humidity and warm weather made little difference to the transmission of the pneumonic form of the disease and that in Southern California the pathogen could assume as deadly a form as plagues during earlier historical periods.[66] Indeed, the crucial factor was not the weather but the close proximity of the sick to the healthy. In the overcrowded conditions of the Mexican quarter the bacillus had found the ideal conditions for spread via respiratory droplets. Plague's explosive potential had been further amplified by burial rituals—in particular, the Catholic custom of holding open wakes—which brought mourners into close contact with infectious cadavers and those who might be incubating the infection. The Los Angeles outbreak had another legacy too: it shattered the belief that plague was largely a rat-borne disease of urban areas and that to eradicate it all you needed to do was clean up the places where rats bred. Though it was never proven that squirrels were the source of the 1924 outbreak, the discovery of squirrel fleas on rats recovered from the greater Los Angeles area, together with the fact that no plague-infected rat was found between the port and the Mexican quarter, suggested that Meyer had been right and that the disease had most likely found its way to the Mexican quarter from the hinterland. Looking back, the signs had been there in 1908 when the boy in Elysian Park, thirty miles from the port, had died of plague after handling an infected squirrel in his backyard. It was around this time that squirrel die-offs had been reported in San Luis Obispo, a phenomenon that was repeated in 1924 when similar epizootics were observed in several counties in Southern and Northern California. Perhaps squirrels had originally caught the bug from rats rummaging in garbage dumps in Oakland, or that had hitched a ride south on the Southern Pacific Railroad. Or perhaps ground squirrels and other wild rodents had been harbouring the plague bacillus for decades without anyone noticing. Whatever had been the case, the Los Angeles outbreak prompted Meyer and others to take a closer look at the role of squirrels in the persistence of plague between epidemics and the role of their fleas in the transmission of the disease to rats and other wild rodents.[67] With Dickie's help Meyer examined the records of previous outbreaks, trying to see if there was a relationship between epizootics observed in squirrels and human outbreaks. In 1927, when the state resumed responsibility for plague control work, Meyer and Dickie joined forces to survey ranches and woodlands suspected of harbouring plague-infected squirrels. By the mid-1930s, state survey crews had trapped tens of thousands of squirrels and combed their fur for fleas, returning the rodents and their ectoparasites to Meyer's laboratory at the Hooper Foundation. Although many of these squirrels appeared perfectly healthy, Meyer discovered that some harboured latent infections and that their ground-up organs could be used to communicate plague to guinea pigs. Many were also infested with plague fleas. In addition, crews recovered diseased fleas from burrows that were known to have harboured infected squirrels twenty years previously but which were now occupied by other rodents, suggesting that in certain parts of the state ground squirrels constituted a hidden "reservoir" of disease. It was the beginning of a new ecological approach, one that by the mid-1930s would see Meyer adopt the term *sylvatic plague* to describe the preservation of the disease by forest-dwelling rodents.

By 1935, the PHS had joined the survey effort and established that sylvatic plague was endemic to eleven Pacific coast and Rocky Mountain states and that its reservoirs included eighteen species of ground squirrel, plus chipmunks, prairie dogs, marmots, wild rats, white-footed mice, kangaroo rats and cottontails.[68] By 1938 more than 100,000 squirrels had been trapped and shipped to the Hooper Foundation for examination. However, when Meyer came to autopsy the rodents he found that only a small percentage were infected with *Y. pestis*. He also observed that no sooner had the squirrels been eliminated than field mice took up residence in the empty burrows where they promptly became infested with the same plague fleas and "peddled" the infection to other rodents. Eradication was doomed to failure because sylvatic plague was "independent of the usual lines of communication," he concluded.[69] The challenge was to keep sylvatic plague at a low level by periodically culling the squirrel populations that harboured *Y. pestis*. Of course, every now and again, someone might be bitten by a squirrel flea and contract the disease, but such events were rare, and as long as squirrels were prevented from infecting urban rat populations, sylvatic plague posed little threat to people living in built-up areas.

This is pretty much the approach employed by the CDC today. From its wildlife station in Fort Collins, Colorado, the CDC monitors the incidence of plague in prairie dogs, thought to be a key reservoir of plague in the western

United States, and the spillover of the disease into squirrels and other wild rodents.[70] In the Pacific Coast and Rocky Mountain states the principal vector is a species of flea called *Oropsylla montana*. Unlike in the rat flea *X. cheopis*, the midgut of *O. montana* gets blocked only rarely when it takes a blood meal, but it is known[71] to unleash rapidly moving epizoonotics among Californian ground squirrels and rock squirrels through an "early-phase" transmission system.* When plague levels are considered dangerously high, warnings are posted in state parks and campgrounds showing a squirrel in a red circle with a diagonal slash through it. At such times hikers are warned not to feed squirrels and pet owners are advised to keep an eye on cats and other domestic animals lest they cross paths with a squirrel and accidentally become infested with their fleas. In spite of these precautions, every year about three people in the United States are infected with plague and in some years, as in 2006, there have been as many as seventeen infections.[72] Prompt treatment with a powerful antibiotic, such as doxycycline of ciprofloxacin, is usually sufficient to clear the plague bacillus from the system.** Nonetheless, newspapers continue to run panicked headlines about the deaths of Americans from "bubonic plague" and the threats posed by squirrels and other wild rodents, as occurred in 2015 when an elderly Utah man died from the disease.[73]

No one is sure what causes these periodic flare-ups, but climate and topography are thought to be important factors. Plague persists in relatively small geographical pockets, such as the high plateaus and grasslands of New Mexico, Utah, and Colorado, and the coastal fog belts of Northern California, where the weather tends to be cool and damp year-round. Indeed, in California, only the dry, central desert region is completely free of sylvatic plague. By contrast, in Yosemite National Park and other wilderness and coastal areas, plague is nearly always present. In such locales, it finds the ideal ecological balance between climate, flea vectors and rodent hosts. It is only when unusual rainfall levels boost plant growth or some other factor increases the rodent and flea populations that the balance between parasite and host is disturbed and plague risks spilling over into other animals.[74]

---

* Plague bacilli multiply rapidly in *X. cheopis*, sometimes causing blockages that prevent ingested blood from reaching the flea's midgut. These blockages cause the flea to feed more voraciously, thereby increasing the chances it will retransmit the infection.

** In patients treated with antibiotics the average fatality rate is 16 per cent. In the untreated, it ranges from 66 per cent to 93 per cent.

Indeed, with the ongoing encroachment of residential developments into these wild habitats, the animal that most threatens to disturb this balance today is humans, which is why in the future we should expect further small outbreaks of plague, in its bubonic form at least. However, it is highly unlikely that Los Angeles or any other American city will ever again be confronted with an epidemic of pneumonic plague, much less a pandemic on the scale of the Black Death.

THE GREAT PARROT FEVER PANDEMIC

On 6 January 1930, Dr Willis P. Martin paid an urgent house call to a family in Annapolis, Maryland. Lillian, her daughter Edith, and Edith's husband Lee Kalmey, the owner of a local auto repair shop, had begun to feel feverish shortly after Christmas, and all three were now deathly ill. At first, they attributed their symptoms to influenza and the depressive effects of the recent stock market crash, which had hit Kalmey's business as hard as any, but in the first week of the new year their condition had taken a decided turn for the worse. To the chills and generalized aches and pains typical of influenza was now added an irritable dry cough, accompanied by constipation and exhaustion that alternated with headaches and insomnia. For large parts of the day, Lillian, Edith, and Lee lay somnolent as logs, the silence broken only by their intermittent mutterings. By contrast, when awake they would be restless and prone to fits of violent excitement. The most worrying symptom of all, however, was the rattling sound coming from deep within their lungs.

Dr Martin suspected pneumonia, possibly mixed with typhoid fever. However, Lillian's husband, who had eaten the same meals as the rest of the family, was perfectly well, which tended to rule out a food-borne illness. The only other member of the household who had been sick was a parrot that Lillian's husband had purchased from a pet store in Baltimore and which Edith and Lee had kept at their home in the run-up to the Yuletide festivities so as to present the bird to Lillian as a surprise on Christmas Day. Unfortunately, by Christmas Eve the parrot's plumage had grown ruffled and dirty and the creature was showing signs of listlessness. Come Christmas Day the parrot was dead.[1]

Dr Martin was baffled by the family's symptoms and shared his bewilderment with his wife. At first, Mrs Martin was similarly puzzled. Then Dr Martin mentioned the dead parrot. It might be a coincidence, she said, but the previous Sunday she had been reading about an outbreak of "parrot fever" in a theatrical troupe in Buenos Aires. According to the newspaper report, the disease was being blamed for the death of two members of the company, who, in common with other members of the cast, had been required to interact with a live parrot on stage. That bird was now dead and pet owners throughout Argentina were being warned to report sickly psittacines—birds in the parrot family—to the authorities.[2]

It sounded unlikely, ridiculous even, but Martin was not the type to take a chance. Instead, he sent a telegram to the PHS in Washington, DC:

> Request information regarding diagnosis parrot fever ... What information available regarding prevention spread of parrot fever. ... Can you place supply parrot fever serum our disposal immediately. Wire reply.[3]

Martin was not the only doctor puzzled by the sudden appearance of mysterious pneumonias accompanied by typhoid-like symptoms in the United States that winter. By now similar telegrams were arriving at the PHS from Baltimore and New York, and health officials in Ohio and California were fielding similar requests for information. Like Martin's telegram, these communications ended up on the desk of Surgeon General Hugh S. Cumming, who passed them on to his subordinate, Dr George W. McCoy, the director of PHS's Hygienic Laboratory. A veteran of the bubonic plague investigations in San Francisco, McCoy was renowned for discovering tularaemia—dubbed the "first American disease" because the bacterium was first identified in McCoy's lab in California—and was then the most celebrated bacteriologist in America.[*] If anyone could solve the outbreak, Cumming figured, it was McCoy. But when McCoy read Martin's telegram he could not help smiling. *Parrot fever?* It sounded like the sort of diagnosis you might encounter in the medical columns of the yellow press or a joke in the funny pages. Certainly,

---

[*] McCoy first isolated the bacterium of tularaemia in 1911 while examining squirrels for plague lesions in Tulare County, California. Transmitted by ticks, mites and lice, tularaemia is endemic to every state in the US, the principal reservoirs being wild rabbits and deer. In humans, the tick or deer fly bites can result in ulceration and swelling of the lymph glands; hence its confusion with plague.

McCoy had never heard of parrot fever. But then McCoy was a busy man—America was in the grip of an influenza epidemic, a recrudescence, it was feared, of the Spanish flu, and he and his deputy, Charlie Armstrong, were working day and night on a serum for post-vaccinal encephalitis, a "sleeping sickness" that affected some individuals who'd received the smallpox vaccine. Nevertheless, McCoy thought it best to check with his colleague.

"Armstrong, what do *you* know about parrot fever?" McCoy demanded. "What do I know about it? I don't know a *thing* about it," Armstrong admitted.[4]

Within days, however, McCoy and Armstrong would come to rue their ignorance as one by one laboratory workers tasked with investigating whether parrots were implicated in the outbreaks seen in Annapolis and elsewhere fell ill. Indeed, by February Armstrong and several other personnel at the "Hygienic," as the ramshackle red-brick laboratory overlooking the Potomac was known, had been removed to the nearby US Naval Hospital. By the time the outbreak concluded in March, Armstrong's long-time assistant, Henry "Shorty" Anderson, was dead. In the end, it fell to McCoy to conduct the critical passage experiments on parrots in the basement of the Hygienic in an attempt to isolate the "virus" of psittacosis and develop a serum. But the tests were inconclusive and in the end McCoy had been forced to chloroform the birds and fumigate the Hygienic from top to bottom to prevent the putative virus from escaping the building. As the science writer Paul de Kruif put it in his book *Men Against Death*, McCoy "never smiled nor even muttered" as he performed this grim task, "but just killed and killed and at the end of it swashed out every last cage with creosol, and gave all the dead bodies of those assorted unhappy experimental creatures a decent and thorough burning in the laboratory incinerator."[5]

* * *

Today few people recall the hysteria surrounding the great parrot fever pandemic of 1929–30, but in an era when parrots were all the rage and itinerant peddlers went door-to-door with "lovebirds" for widows and bored housewives, the idea that one's pet parrot or parakeet might be harbouring a deadly pathogen from the Amazon was the stuff of domestic nightmares and a story few newspaper editors could resist. Indeed, were it not for the yellow press, and the Hearst newspaper group in particular, it is unlikely that the connection between parrots and psittacosis would have come to light so fast, or that the PHS would have reacted so quickly. The story about the Argentine theatrical troupe had appeared in the 5 January edition of the *American Weekly*, a lavish supplement distributed with the Sunday editions of the *New York American* and other papers in the Hearst group, under the headline "Killed By A Pet Parrot." Mrs Martin probably read the story in the *Baltimore American* sandwiched between an article about a well-to-do twice-divorced couple and the "astonishing confessions" of a slave trader. Morrill Goddard, the editor of the *American Weekly*, had spotted the tale about the troupe in an obscure Argentine scientific journal the previous November and had wired the paper's Buenos Aires correspondent, asking for further details.[6] The correspondent found the theatre where the troupe had been performing shuttered, but managed to trace the surviving cast members. The most prominent victim had been Carmen Mas, the show's star and a well-known Argentinian comedian. Her leading man, Florencia Paravincini, had also been felled by the disease, but, according to the Hearst correspondent, after "17 days of agony" had recovered. Nevertheless the "bacillus passed from the parrot" had exacted a considerable toll. Prior to the attack Paravincini had been a "big, heavy-set man with hair as black as leather." Now, he weighed less than one hundred pounds and his hair was "as white as snow." It was a doctor at the hospital who had put two and two together. After speaking to the company's prop man, he learned that the actors had been required to pet the parrot on stage and that said bird had since died. As a result, an alert was issued by the *Asistencia Publica*, the Argentine National Health Board, and soon reports of similar outbreaks connected to sickly parrots but wrongly diagnosed as typhoid or influenza were coming to light. In Cordoba, fifty cases were traced to a parrot dealer who had set up shop in a local boarding house. His birds were promptly slaughtered but too late to prevent the distribution of other suspect psittacines. According to the correspondent, the outbreaks in Argentina were entirely avoidable and would not have occurred had dealers observed some simple precautions familiar to indigenous forest peoples accustomed to living alongside wild birds in their natural habitat.

> In semitropical parts of Argentina where the parrots are caught, the parrot disease is well known among the natives, who never have the creatures for pets, and keep away from them unless they make a business of catching and shipping them to the cities. The professional parrot catcher takes care not to get hold of a sick bird. If by mistake he does catch a "quiet one" he knows it is deadly and lets it go as well as any healthy captives with which it may have come in contact.[7]

The outbreak in Cordoba was subsequently traced to a consignment of 5,000 parrots imported from Brazil that had been kept in unsanitary conditions in overcrowded crates. By the time Goddard came to learn of the outbreaks, the connection between psittacosis and Brazilian parrots was well known in Argentina and the authorities had outlawed the trade. However, passengers on cruise ships calling at Buenos Aires were largely ignorant of the ban, creating an opening for unscrupulous dealers to offload their sickly birds on unsuspecting tourists. It was this practice that most likely led to the introduction of psittacosis to the United States.

As the term "pandemic" implies, the United States was not the only country affected. In the summer of 1929, four cases of suspected psittacosis were reported in Birmingham, England, and by March of the following year one hundred cases had been recorded across England and Wales. One notable early victim was a ship's carpenter who had purchased two parrots in Buenos Aires, only to see them perish on the voyage to London (when he presented at the London Hospital in December 1929, the carpenter's symptoms were mistaken for typhoid, just as with the Martins in Annapolis). Although most cases seemed to involve sustained exposure to live birds, British researchers observed that this was not always the case, one example being a man who had merely stopped for a beer in a public house in which a sick parrot had been present. By January 1930, similar outbreaks were also being reported in Germany, Italy, Switzerland, France, Denmark, Algeria, Holland and Egypt. There were even reports of an outbreak in Honolulu.[8]

During the first week of illness, most patients appeared comparatively well in spite of running high temperatures. After five or six days, however, headache, insomnia and an irritable cough would set in, and they would complain of profound exhaustion, their symptoms often being accompanied by lung consolidation. Soon after, many patients slipped into delirium and became semi-comatose. This was the critical period, with death often following soon after. However, in other cases, just as it looked as if the illness was about to take a fatal turn, the patient's temperature would fall and his condition would suddenly improve. Full recovery might take a further week or two, and sometimes as long as eight. During this protracted convalescence period, physicians had to constantly monitor their patients' temperatures, as relapses were frequent.

It was not until much later, of course, that doctors would become familiar with the typical course of the illness and recognize it as psittacosis. Instead, it was the story in the *American Weekly* and Dr Martin's telegram that appears to have alerted Cumming to the outbreak and prompted him to put McCoy and Armstrong onto the case. By then, psittacosis was widely seeded in cities on the eastern seaboard of the United States and had already been communicated via dealers to other caged birds popular with American consumers, such as shell parakeets (Australian budgerigars). The result was that as parrot fever spread from Annapolis to Baltimore, New York and Los Angeles, the outbreak became a headline writer's dream. "Parrot Fever Hits Trio at Annapolis," declared the *Washington Post* on its front page on 8 January 1930. "Parrot Disease Fatal to Seven," reported the *Los Angeles Times* three days later. "Woman's Case Brings Parrot Victims to 19," announced the *Baltimore Sun* on 16 January.

For widows and bored housewives, caged birds were the FM radios of their day. The chirping of canaries provided a soothing background music, punctuating the drudgery of household tasks, and, in the case of parakeets—parrots' smaller, sprightlier cousin—their facility for words and humorous phrases provided a facsimile of human conversation. Estimating that New York City alone was home to some 30,000 parrots, the *National Geographic* dubbed Amazons and African grays "the ballyhoo barkers of birddom, the noisy, clever, side-show performers of the tropical forest."[9] Their pint-sized cousin, the parakeet or lovebird (genus *Agapornis*), had a reputation for similarly buffoonish behaviour, and with their talent for hanging upside down or dancing on their owners' shoulders were a source of endless amusement for children and an entertainment for house guests. Little wonder then that in 1929 nearly 50,000 parrots, parakeets and lovebirds, and some 500,000 canaries, were imported to the United States.[10] These birds arrived not only from Brazil and Argentina, but from Colombia, Cuba, Trinidad, Salvador, Mexico and Japan. The majority entered the United States via New York, the centre of the East Coast bird trade. However, in the case of Australian budgerigars, the main ports of entry were San Francisco and Los Angeles. Indeed, following the Wall Street crash in 1929, a huge bird breeding industry had grown up in Southern California, with hundreds of independent breeders raising lovebirds in their backyards to supplement their incomes. To the naked eye these birds appeared perfectly healthy. However, when they were packed into crowded aviaries or containers and shipped across state lines, many began to shed the virus and transmit the infection. It would prove an invisible and combustible combination.

* * *

Despite its name, parrot fever or psittacosis is not confined only to parrotlike birds but has been isolated from some 450 other bird species, including canaries, finches, pigeons, doves, and kestrels.* Moreover, although human infections are typically acquired by exposure to parakeets, bird-to-human

---

* In nonpsittacine birds, the infection is known as ornithosis.

transmission has also been documented from poultry and free-ranging birds. The culprit is a tiny intracellular parasite, *Chlamydophila psittaci*, a member of the same family of bacteria that transmits chlamydia, a common infection of the eye and genital tract. In the wild, psittacosis lives in equilibrium with its host. Hatchlings are usually infected in the nest through contact with mature birds who harbour the bacillus in their guts. Under natural conditions this contact results in a mild infection that confers lifelong immunity. However, under conditions of stress, such as when food becomes scarce or birds are packed into small crates or confined to cages for long periods, immunity can wane and the infection can be reignited. Typically, a bird's feathers become rough and dirty, and instead of squawking and clawing at the bars of the cage it becomes listless and inert. Sometimes, bloody fluid may leak from its beak and nose, but the most common symptom is diarrhoea. It is the faeces that pose the principal threat to humans, especially when they become dry and powdery, as occurs in cool conditions. Then, all it takes is a flap of the birds' wings or a sudden breeze from an open window for the particles to be wafted into the atmosphere. The final stage comes when a person enters the same space and inhales the aerosolized particles, allowing the psittacosis bacillus to lodge in the respiratory tract from where it is free to colonize the lungs. Sickness usually occurs six to ten days later, the first sign being a fever accompanied by headache, an irritable dry cough and, on occasion, discharges of bloody mucus from the nose.

It is likely that aboriginal peoples from South America suffered psittacosis from time to time, particularly given the fondness of the Awa and other Brazilian tribes for headdresses featuring brightly coloured feathers from macaws, parrots, and toucans. However, it is unlikely that they would have noticed sudden die-offs due to epizootics, since birds falling from the trees in the jungle would have been camouflaged by vegetable debris on the forest floor or rapidly consumed by insects and other scavengers. By contrast, sudden die-offs of birds in captivity are highly visible and difficult to ignore.

No doubt European aristocrats who started the vogue for importing exotic birds from Africa and elsewhere noted such occurrences as early as the eighteenth century, but it was not until 1872 that Jakob Ritter, a Swiss physician living in Uster, near Zurich, gave the first detailed description of the disease when an outbreak occurred at his brother's house, infecting seven people and killing three. Ritter named the disease "pneumotyphus" and blamed it on a consignment of parrots and finches caged in his brother's study that had recently been imported from Hamburg. This was followed, in 1882, by a second outbreak in Switzerland, this time in Bern, in which two people died.

On that occasion, suspicion fell on some sick parrots imported from London. However, the outbreak that attracted widest comment occurred in Paris in 1892 and centred on the homes of two bird fanciers who had recently shipped some five hundred parrots to the French capital from Buenos Aires. During the sea crossing, 300 birds had died, and people coming into contact with the survivors had rapidly developed symptoms of influenza. On this occasion the outbreak had a mortality rate of 33 per cent, prompting the interest of Edmond Nocard, a young assistant of Pasteur. Nocard was unable to get hold of any live birds implicated in the outbreak. Instead, he examined a packet of dried wings taken from parrots that had died during the voyage. From their bone marrow, he was able to cultivate a small Gram-negative bacterium. He then injected or fed the organism to a wide variety of test animals—parrots, pigeons, mice, rabbits and guinea pigs—and demonstrated that in all cases it caused a fatal illness similar to the human disease. Nocard named the microbe *Bacillus psittacosis*, psittacosis being the Greek word for parrot. However, other researchers found it difficult to cultivate Nocard's bacillus from the blood, lungs, urine, or faeces of presumed human cases, and as agglutination tests proved similarly negative or inconsistent, doubts gradually grew as to the bacillus's aetiological role.[11]

Scientists were right to question Nocard's claim: in fact, the organism he had isolated was a type of salmonella and had nothing to do with psittacosis. Unfortunately, this would not become known until after the 1929–30 outbreak. In the meantime, just as with Pfeiffer's erroneous claim about the bacterial aetiology of influenza, Nocard's error spread confusion, making medics and public health officials reluctant to accept that parrots had anything to do with the human cases of typhoid-like illness.* This only compounded the uncertainty and fears about the source of the epidemic.

Scientists were not the only ones to fail the public. Reflecting on the parrot fever pandemic in 1933 in his best-selling book, *Men Against Death*, Paul de Kruif would describe the outbreak and the panic that accompanied it as "one of our American hysterias."[12] If so it was a hysteria that he and other journalists helped engender. This was a pity, as de Kruif ought to have known better. Before turning to science writing de Kruif had worked as a bacteriologist at

---

* The ease with which people contracted psittacosis in the presence of parrots was seen as further evidence that the infective agent must be an intestinal parasite, even though in many cases patients had not touched sick birds or handled their faecal matter but had merely been in the same room as them.

the University of Michigan and during the First World War had served as a captain in the US Sanitary Corps, where he helped develop an antitoxin for gas gangrene. Afterwards, he joined the Rockefeller Institute, but just as it looked as if he were set for an illustrious career as a medical researcher, de Kruif wrote an ill-advised book, *Our Medicine Men* (1922), containing thinly disguised portraits of his Rockefeller colleagues. The book cost him his position at the Rockefeller Institute but launched his career as a science journalist. In 1925, he teamed up with Sinclair Lewis to write *Arrowsmith*, a runaway best seller about a country doctor turned research scientist that fired the imaginations of a generation of American medical researchers. This was followed in 1926 by *Microbe Hunters*, a nonfiction book profiling the pioneers of microbiology, such as Koch, Pasteur, and the Nobel Prize-winning physiologist Paul Ehrlich, who had reversed centuries of medical superstition by applying laboratory techniques to the study of infectious disease.[13] But successful as these books were, de Kruif's bread and butter was "scare" stories about obscure microorganisms that posed a theoretical threat to American housewives. "In American milk today there lurks a terrible, wasting fever, that may keep you in bed for a couple of weeks, that may fasten itself on you for one, or for two, or even for seven years—that might culminate by killing you," he informed the readers of *Ladies Home Journal* in 1929.[14] De Kruif was referring to undulant fever, or brucellosis, a disease of cattle that, while it might cause cows to abort prematurely, in truth posed little threat to people. However, in an era before pasteurization when many housewives still drank "raw" milk drawn from local dairy herds, undulant fever was a perfect candidate for a germ panic, fitting the template of what medical historian Nancy Tomes calls the "killer germ genre of journalism."[15] Drawing on the latest microbiological discoveries and Progressive Era messages about the importance of sanitation and personal hygiene, this genre played on the dangers that lurked in everyday objects, such as coins, library books, or drinking cups. Dust and insects were targets of similar scaremongering, hence the advertisements urging housewives to mop regularly with disinfectants and spray their homes with insecticides. By the 1920s, as Americans adopted new germ-conscious regimes, even handshaking and kissing babies came to be frowned upon.

These fears were not only used to sell bleaches, detergents, and bug sprays, but they were also a way of selling newspapers; hence Goddard's decision to hype the story about the Argentine theatrical troupe. In a germophobic era, even the normally level-headed *New York Times* was not immune to the parrot panic. "Many have long had the feeling that there is something diabolical about the parrot tribe," opined a columnist at the height of the scare. "More than one family pet, known by its owners to possess the amiable and gentle disposition of a kitten, is regarded with fear and trembling by visitors. Until more has been learned about the nature of the malady the safest course seems absolute ostracism for recent immigrants of the parrot family."[16]

Within days of that editorial, however, the *New York Times* was quoting the opinion of a Viennese expert who thought the scare "baseless" and that Americans were victims of "mass suggestion."[17] Two days later, psittacosis—or parrots, at least—had become a laughing matter as the paper regaled its readers with the story of Secretary of State Henry Stimson's pet parrot, "The Old Soak." Stimson's bird had been caught misbehaving while his master was overseas, cursing at tourists and their guides as they entered the Pan-American Building. The bird, apparently, was "quite a linguist," and was said to have learned the profanities "during his days in the Philippines." As a punishment, The Old Soak was confined to the basement of the Pan-American building where he could curse without giving offence.[18] However, no joking could hide the fact that America's microbe hunters had missed something that had been known to their medical colleagues in Argentina since the previous summer, and that had most likely been incubating under their noses since the autumn of 1929. How had this been possible, and who would be the person to restore the reputation of the US Public Health Service?

* * *

Charlie Armstrong is a type that has almost disappeared from American medicine today: a scientist equally at home in the laboratory and the field, who combined serious medical research with a career devoted to fighting infectious disease and improving public health. A graduate of Johns Hopkins Medical School, Armstrong's interest in public health was fired by his early experiences as medical officer in the US Marine Hospital Service on Ellis Island in 1916, where it was his job to examine immigrants suspected of introducing diseases like trachoma and typhus to the United States. Two years later, as an assistant surgeon on the *Seneca*, a US coast guard cutter on escort duty in the Atlantic, he had witnessed the first wave of Spanish flu when an outbreak occurred on his boat off the coast of Gibraltar, prompting him to hoist the yellow quarantine ensign. Later, while serving at the Fore River Shipyard, near Boston, Armstrong had also treated sailors affected by the deadly second wave. It was an experience he would never forget. Asked years later what the flu was like, he told a reporter: "with influenza you think you are going to die and afraid that you won't [sic]."[19] After the war, Armstrong was posted to the Ohio Department of Health, where he continued his investigations into influenza and honed his epidemiological skills. Then, in 1921, he was posted to the Hygienic. He would remain there until his retirement in 1950, a period in which he would also contract malaria, dengue fever, encephalitis, Q fever and tularaemia. Despite the risks that his laboratory work exposed him to, however, Armstrong was a tireless investigator. His most notable contribution to scientific research came in 1934 when he isolated a new neurotrophic virus—a virus with affinity for nerve tissue—which he named *lymphocytic choriomeningitis*, from the spinal fluid of monkeys artificially infected with material from the 1933 St. Louis encephalitis epidemic. This was followed, in 1940, by the first transmission of a polio virus from monkeys to rats and mice, an experimental innovation that laid the ground for subsequent investigations into the immunology of the disease and the development of human polio vaccines. Awarded the Sedgwick Memorial Medal of the American Public Health Association the following year, Armstrong was hailed as someone who had made "a distinct contribution to the knowledge of every disease with which he has worked."[20] In short, he was the epitome of the microbe hunter. As de Kruif put it, Armstrong was "thick set, with reddish hair and round china-blue eyes set wide apart in a face that couldn't keep from smiling," and definitely not the sort of man who would "own a parrot let alone kiss it."[21] In spite of his scepticism about parrot fever, however, when McCoy summoned him to his office, Armstrong immediately agreed to drop his vaccine experiments and travel to Annapolis to see if there was any truth in the rumour.

According to de Kruif, by now requests for information about the mysterious new disease were pouring into Washington, and Cumming's desk was piled with "stacks of yellow and blue slips."[22] For once, de Kruif was not exaggerating. In her history of the PHS, Bess Furman reports that by early January thirty-six cases of suspected psittacosis had been reported to the surgeon general, and his desk was "deluged" with urgent telegrams.[23] Like all good disease detectives, Armstrong headed to the scene of the crime: Lillian's bedside. Her pet parrot had long been buried but she still had the cage and, miraculously, it still contained some of the bird's droppings. Following protocol, Armstrong shared some of the cleanings from the cage with William Royal Stokes, the head of bacteriology at the Baltimore Department of Health, so that he could conduct independent tests. Before returning to Washington, Armstrong warned Stokes to be careful when culturing organisms from the material, reminding him that many people suspected that psittacosis "might be a virus," not a bacterium.[24] Stokes promised to heed Armstrong's warning, but within a matter of weeks he would be dead.

By 8 January 1930, Lillian and her daughter and son-in-law were not the only ones thought to have parrot fever. Four employees of the pet store at North Eutaw Street were also ill, as was a woman who had bought a parrot at another store in southeast Baltimore. Then, on 10 January, came the fatalities. The first victim was a Baltimore woman, Mrs Louise Schaeffer, whose death had originally been attributed to pneumonia; it was only when Baltimore health officials questioned her family that it emerged she had been in contact with a parrot several days earlier. However, it was the second death that really alarmed health officials because it occurred in Toledo, Ohio, nearly five hundred miles to the northwest of Baltimore. The victim was Mrs Percy Q. Williams. She had died at Toledo's Mercy Hospital three weeks after her husband had returned from Cuba with a gift of three parrots (one of the parrots had died shortly after his return). It was the first indication of the true extent of the epidemic and the challenge facing state and federal health officials. Cumming had previously avoided making a public statement. Now he had no choice. He "did not fear an epidemic," he said, as it was generally believed that psittacosis was transmitted "only from bird to human being, and not from person to person." Nevertheless, he advised Americans to avoid handling recently imported parrots until the completion of Armstrong's investigation. "There is at present no indication of widespread prevalence of the disease, but I would urge that people avoid contact with possible conveyors, the birds."[25]

Cumming's statement was all that newspapers needed to run with the story. Even the *New York Times* displayed the reports prominently. "Parrot Fever Kills 2 In This Country," it declared on 11 January, placing the story at the top of page 3. "Woman in Baltimore and Another in Toledo are Victims of Rare Disease. Eleven others are ill," continued the subhead. The following day, with reports of further suspect cases in Ohio involving several clerks in the poultry department of a Toledo store, the paper promoted the story to page one. "Hunts For Source of 'Parrot Fever," it declared, above a report describing the efforts of Baltimore state health officials and the Bureau of Animal Industry and Biological Survey to confirm the source of the parrots sold in Baltimore pet shops. "We do not consider it practical to place an embargo on importation before making sure where the sick parrots are coming from," stated Cumming in a game attempt to reassure an increasingly nervous public.[26]

By the middle of January, Baltimore officials working with colleagues from the state health department had visited seven pet stores in the city and the homes of thirty-eight people who had recently purchased parrots. Of these, thirty-six were ill with the same symptoms as Mrs Martin. This so alarmed

Daniel S. Hatfield, the director of the Bureau of Communicable Diseases, that he ordered an immediate moratorium on the sale of parrots and the isolation of all birds seized in Baltimore pet stores. However, Hatfield was not so cautious when it came to protecting his own health, and on 19 January, while assisting Stokes, he contracted psittacosis and was rushed to Baltimore's Mercy Hospital. Hatfield was lucky. Unlike Stokes, who by now was autopsying parrots daily and, presumably, exposing himself to massive amounts of the virus, he had a mild case of the disease and survived.

If there was any doubt before about the role of foreign birds, the Baltimore investigations dispelled it: out of the seven pet shops investigated, four were shown to be the source of diseased parrots. Nearly all were traced to shipments from Central or South America that had come via dealers in New York. If that was the case, it was highly likely that those same dealers had sold diseased birds to pet stores in other cities. Sure enough, when Armstrong wired public health officials across the country he was inundated with information, and birds, both dead and alive, began arriving from Baltimore, Maine, Chicago, New Haven and Los Angeles. And as more and more cases came to light, so the death toll crept up. Women, many of them widows, constituted the majority of victims, most likely because they were the principal recipients of lovebirds. Peddlers usually sold the birds singly to facilitate their bonding with their owners. Women were also most likely to kiss the birds affectionately, or care for them when they fell sick. By the final week in January, more than fifty cases had been reported nationwide, including fourteen in New York, where, under pressure from the city's health commissioner, bird dealers were forced to accept a voluntary embargo. Soon, orphaned birds began turning up all over the city, including in the vestibule of a house in East Elmhurst, Queens. Taking pity on the young foundling, which had a chipped beak, the householder turned it over to the Society for the Prevention of Cruelty to Animals. "Fear of psittacosis," reported the *New York Times*, "is thought to be the reason for the abandonment of the bird."[27]

At this point, the only persons interested in collecting parrots were Armstrong and his assistant, "Shorty" Anderson (so called because he stood just five feet six inches tall). By 16 January, Armstrong and Anderson had everything they needed to conduct bacteriological tests: parrots both dead and alive, the scrapings from Lillian's birdcage, and blood from human patients. Well aware that the birds were highly contagious and that they were probably dealing with a "filter-passing" virus, Armstrong decided to confine the experiments to two small dark rooms in the basement of the Hygienic. According to de Kruif, these rooms were "dank, frowsty little holes hardly bigger than coal bins, [and] an insult to offer to any self-respecting microbe hunter for a laboratory." Worse, the healthy birds were "clawing green devils," who were constantly scrabbling to escape their cages or scattering food and faecal droppings onto the floor.[28] To try to contain them, Armstrong and Anderson placed the most violent birds in cages they'd rigged from metal garbage cans enclosed with wire mesh covers. In addition, they kept the birds behind moist curtains soaked in disinfectant and put troughs containing creosol in the doorways. They also periodically scrubbed the walls with disinfectant and wore heavy rubber gloves and aprons when extracting birds from their cages. Nevertheless, de Kruif considered the Hygienic one of the most "odiferously untidy" buildings he had ever visited.[29] The Rockefeller virologist, Thomas Rivers, a leading authority on filterable viruses, concurred, remarking that the only thing hygienic about the building was its name.[30]

Despite this unpromising working environment, however, within days Armstrong had succeeded in communicating the disease from sick to healthy birds using either the droppings from infected birds or ground-up tissue from a dead parrot (according to de Kruif, the deceased bird came from Stokes in Baltimore). Armstrong also observed that while some of the sick birds died, many survived inoculation with infective material, after which they became asymptomatic carriers.* According to de Kruif, Anderson was particularly adept at grabbing the parrots without getting "gaffed" by them. Just days before, both men had considered themselves "parrot ignoramuses." Now, "by a little jab of next to nothing through a needle," the birds were sitting hunched in their cages "with their heads bent forward," and Armstrong and Anderson had the feeling they were "getting control of this weird disease."[31] Try as they might, however, they could not isolate the bacillus described by Nocard, or culture any other organism from the ground-up material. It seemed increasingly likely that psittacosis was a filter-passer that could only be transmitted from bird to bird or from bird to human by close contact. But how precisely the virus was conveyed from parrots and whether people were also capable of transmitting it independently of birds, was anyone's guess. Perhaps patients communicated the virus via the respiratory route when they coughed infectious material? If that was the case, it might become as transmissible as flu.

---

* This was an important clue to the natural history of the disease, one that helped explain why wild birds were not continually dropping dead of psittacosis and epizootics were rare. However, the significance of the finding would only become apparent to researchers in the mid-1930s. See discussion below.

Clearly, it was imperative to make a serum before the unthinkable happened and psittacosis became a true pandemic.

Armstrong would need that serum sooner than he anticipated. Based on the initial results of his investigation, on 24 January President Herbert Hoover issued an Executive Order prohibiting "the immediate importation of parrots into the United States, its possessions and dependencies from any foreign port" until such time as the causative organism and its means of transmission could be ascertained.[32] Unfortunately, when Armstrong strode into the "old red brick building on the hill" to resume the investigation the following morning he found Shorty slumped over his desk, complaining of a high fever and a "rotten headache." Normally, when work was going well Shorty was "all smiles and cheerful profanity." A born "lab-swipe," Shorty was never happier than when he was microbe-hunting, claimed de Kruif. "Now he looked awful." It was not difficult to diagnose the cause of his malaise. Armstrong arranged for him to be admitted to the US Naval Hospital, where X-rays showed a sinister cloud at the base of his left lung. It was at this point that McCoy stepped in and, over the objections of his employees and family, joined Armstrong in the basement. As McCoy tried to mimic Shorty's technique of gaffing the birds, Armstrong rushed back and forth between the laboratory and the hospital to check on his assistant's condition. There was little sign of improvement, and in desperation Armstrong drew blood from Shorty's veins and collected expectorations from his bedsheets in order to inoculate the fluids into parrots and other test animals. At the same time, to see how parrots became infected, he and McCoy also placed parts of dead parrots in cages along with healthy birds. Armstrong may have thought that by co-opting Shorty into the experiments, he would buy his assistant some more time. But though he was able to confirm that psittacosis was a filter passer, he could not forestall the inevitable and on 8 February Shorty died. Scrupulous about paying his bills, his last request was that Armstrong settle his outstanding debts.

Unfortunately, it was a request Armstrong was unable to honour as that very day he was also admitted to the hospital. As Shorty was laid to rest in Arlington National Cemetery with full military honours (he was an ex-navy man), Armstrong's temperature spiked from 102° to 104°F. The following day, an X-ray showed a white shadow enveloping his left lung, confirmation that he had pneumonia and was almost certainly infected with the same bug. When McCoy saw the X-ray he decided to take a gamble by using a method of unknown and questionable value: namely, the administration of convalescent blood serum. It had been known since the 1890s that survivors of diphtheria and other bacterial diseases were immune to reinfection, and that their immunity was associated with antibodies circulating in their blood. Moreover, if their blood was purified and the antibodies separated from the red corpuscles, the resulting serum could also be used to protect immune-naïve individuals from the same diseases. By the 1920s, this principle was also being applied to viral diseases, such as influenza and polio, but although the transfer of passive serum from survivors of flu and polio sometimes appeared to confer protection, it was far from clear if this protection was due to the serum or some other factor. Moreover, since there was no way of screening blood for impurities in the 1920s, physicians had no way of knowing whether or not passive serums contained active viral material or some other undiscovered virus, such as hepatitis. Ironically, one of the biggest serum sceptics of all was McCoy. Hardly a month went by without a claim from some fly-by-night pharmaceutical firm that it had developed a serum for pneumonia or meningitis. As the head of the Hygienic, it was McCoy's job to examine these requests and deny licences to those he considered questionable. Now, he threw caution to the wind and instructed Roscoe Spencer of the Rocky Mountain Laboratory to head the search for potential serum donors. Spencer had recently developed a vaccine against spotted fever, a tick-borne disease endemic to Montana and some midwestern states—an endeavour for which he would be awarded the gold medal of the American Medical Association—and was quite happy to turn errand boy to help a fellow microbiologist stricken in the line of duty. According to de Kruif, the serum came from an elderly Maryland lady who graciously refused payment for her blood. Others report Spencer procured the precious serum from a physician at Johns Hopkins Hospital in Baltimore. What is not in dispute is that within hours of the serum entering his veins, Armstrong rallied and his condition improved.

Over the next two weeks, as Armstrong grew stronger, McCoy continued his investigation, mashing up the livers and spleens of dead parakeets before passing them through filters and inoculating the filtrate into healthy birds. Fearing further infections, McCoy forbade his staff from entering the make-shift laboratory in the basement of the north building of the Hygienic Laboratory, and from 7 February insisted on conducting the autopsies of parrots and disposing of their carcasses in person. At this point, it was still not known whether psittacosis could be communicated from person to person or whether the microbe was also conveyed as an aerosol in dust particles. To minimize the risk of accidental contamination, the only person McCoy allowed to approach the basement laboratory was the general foreman whose job it was to bring sandwiches for McCoy and feed for the birds. He usually handed these items to McCoy at the threshold and did not enter the rooms himself. To reduce the chances of the sick birds accidentally spreading the infection to healthy parrots, McCoy also strung a muslin curtain across the archway between the laboratory rooms and wetted the floor each morning with creosol. Nevertheless, on occasion, McCoy would find diseased parrots, who had somehow freed themselves from the cages, wandering in a room reserved for healthy birds.

Despite these precautions, within eight days of Armstrong's illness several other staff at the Hygienic had also fallen ill. The first casualty was the north building's night watchman, Robert Lanham, who came on duty at midnight and left every morning at 8am, a period when laboratory work was suspended and no autopsies were being carried out. Lanham's only risk was that he had briefly been in the same room as Anderson on 27 January, the day Shorty fell ill. However, Lanham had fallen sick eighteen days later, which was well outside the presumed incubation period.

The next person to contract psittacosis was a laboratory assistant, whose symptoms became apparent on 28 February. Unlike Lanham, she had never breathed the same air as someone incubating psittacosis. However, her office was next door to the basement room where McCoy kept the healthy birds, and she had also handled material for culturing the organism, though since her principal role was to look for salmonella and streptococci McCoy thought it unlikely that she could have been exposed to psittacosis this way. However, the next group of casualties left McCoy in no doubt that his precautions had failed and that the north building was thoroughly contaminated. The first to fall ill was a medical officer whose office was on the side of the corridor opposite the autopsy room. The next day, 11 March, the general foreman was also taken ill, followed in quick succession by two cleaners and two bacteriologists engaged in research on other diseases. Except for McCoy, no one escaped the disease. Even Ludvig Hektoen, a distinguished pathologist and chairman of the National Research Council, who was doing private research at the Hygienic and had merely spent his afternoons in one of the rooms, was admitted to the hospital.

All told, between 25 January and 15 March, eleven people at the Hygienic were hospitalized with psittacosis. Despite drawing a floor plan of the infections, McCoy could discern no pattern in the cases, leading him to speculate that psittacosis may have been transferred to the upper floors by mice or cockroaches.[33] The other possibility, of course, was that the organism had been aerosolized and the building was full of infectious fomites. Either way, drastic action was needed. So it was that on 15 March McCoy ordered everyone to evacuate the building and shut the laboratory. Experimental animals not involved in psittacosis research were removed to temporary lodgings. Then McCoy entered the basement for the last time and exterminated all those that remained—a menagerie of parrots, guinea pigs, mice, rats, pigeons, and monkeys. Next, he burned their bodies in the incinerator and scrubbed their cages with creosol, and methodically worked his way through the building to seal the windows on each floor. Finally, when he was sure there was no living thing left inside the Hygienic, he ordered a fumigation squad to blitz the building with cyanide. The legend goes that so much gas was used that sparrows flying fifty feet above the Hygienic stopped in mid-flight and plummeted to Earth. The next day, the headline in the Sunday edition of the *Washington Post* read, "Parrot Fever Panic Seizes Laboratory."[34]

McCoy was not the only one panicking. By now, Roscoe Spencer was rushing up and down the East Coast in search of serum. The flasks of blood he brought back to Washington were used to treat the Hygienic personnel, and by April all the building's staff had recovered, Armstrong included. Others were not so fortunate, however. Stokes got two transfusions of Roscoe's serum but died on 9 February, the day after Anderson.[35] For those stricken with psittacosis there was good reason to be afraid. The infection often proved fatal, with thirty-three deaths recorded in the United States between November 1929 and May 1930. Of the 167 cases where the sex of the victim was known, 105, or two-thirds, had been women.[36] Another badly affected country was Germany, with 215 cases and 45 deaths. Indeed, at one point Berlin Zoo had been forced to bar its gates to frightened parrot owners desperately looking for a temporary refuge for their birds. In all, some fifteen countries were affected. By the time the pandemic ended in May 1930, eight hundred cases had been recorded worldwide, with an average mortality rate of 15 per cent.[37]

Armstrong and McCoy were not the only researchers puzzled by the sudden appearance of psittacosis and the failure to find Nocard's bacillus. Soon, researchers in other countries were also convinced the pathogen must be a filter passer and that Nocard had mistaken it for salmonella, the bacterium that causes typhoid. The first to succeed was a team led by Samuel Bedson, a senior researcher at the London Hospital.[38] Taking parrots associated with human cases, Bedson and his colleagues emulsified the dead birds' liver and spleen, passed the material through a Chamberland filter, and then inoculated budgerigars with the filtrate. The budgerigars died within five days. Next, Bedson's group showed that by passaging filtered material from diseased budgerigars every few days, the organism gradually lost its virulence. Bedson's conclusion was unequivocal: "the aetiological agent of psittacosis in parrots is a virus which cannot be cultivated on ordinary bacteriological media, and which is capable of passing through some of the more porous filters."[39]

Soon after, Charles Krumwiede, a researcher at the New York Board of Health, demonstrated that the virus could be readily transferred from parakeets to white mice. This greatly facilitated laboratory study of psittacosis as white mice were far less infectious than birds. Nevertheless, Krumwiede was forced to suspend his studies when he fell ill, resulting in his research being taken up by Thomas Rivers. Aware that psittacosis was highly infectious, the Rockefeller researcher left nothing to chance, insisting that his team wear full body suits, with glass goggles in the helmets and rubber gloves attached to the sleeves—precautions that foreshadowed measures that would become standard in Biosafety Level Four laboratories used to study Ebola and other hazardous pathogens sixty years later. Rivers also demonstrated that psittacosis could be transferred to rabbits, guinea pigs, and monkeys. However, in monkeys the infectious material only produced typical pneumonia if introduced via the trachea. To Rivers, this suggested that the principal transmission route in humans was via the respiratory tract, not through scratches or parrot bites—a view soon adopted by other researchers.[40]

Although psittacosis was beyond the magnification range of optical microscopes at that time, by now Ralph Lillie at the Hygienic Laboratory, A. C. Coles of the Lister Institute in London, and Walter Levinthal of the Robert Koch Institute in Dahlem, Germany, were reporting distinctive clusters of inclusion bodies in the cytoplasm of patients who had died of psittacosis. Dubbed "Levinthal-Coles-Lillie" or "LCL" bodies, these could be observed through an ordinary optical microscope, where they appeared as microcolonies on the surface of the cell, making the diagnosis of psittacosis and the development of agglutination tests far easier.[41] The only point that remained uncertain was the exact mode of transmission. Handling an ill or dead bird was certainly a risk, but there were also plenty of cases in which patients had merely been in the same room or house as a sick parrot. There were even cases in which people had contracted psittacosis after visiting a pet shop or, in the case of baggage handlers, sharing a railway carriage with a sick bird. This was not a message that pet shop owners or bird breeders wished to hear. On the contrary, many refused to accept that the reports of pneumonia and typhoid-like illness were due to parrots or parakeets at all, much less that psittacosis could be spread via the atmosphere from bird to man. Otherwise, they claimed, breeders and people who worked in pet shops would be ill all the time, but according to dealers the opposite was the case. "So far as it is aware," declared the newly formed Bird Dealers Association of America at a meeting held in New York's Commodore Hotel at the height of the pandemic, "no bird dealers whose hourly contact with feathered pets presumably would render them likely to contract psittacosis if it is communicable to humans, have been affected." Nor could reports of pet owners catching psittacosis directly from imported birds be believed as "any one putting his face near enough a newly imported parrot to catch a disease would be sure to be bitten by the untrained bird." In short, the parrot fever "scare" was down to "the active imagination of a Baltimore newspaper man."[42]

One can hardly blame bird dealers for wanting to fight back. America's six leading pet dealers, all of which were based in either New York of Philadelphia, stood to lose $5 million annually from Hoover's import ban. And, in many ways, they were right, for as the panic over imported parrots subsided, foreign birds no longer constituted the principal threat. Instead, it was home-reared birds—parrots and parakeets raised in backyard aviaries—that posed the biggest risk to pet owners, particularly in Southern California where conditions were perfect for breeding birds outdoors year-round. This time it would not be a newspaperman who would spot the danger, however, but a Swiss-trained veterinary pathologist whose laboratory sat near the summit of a chilly, fog-shrouded hill overlooking the Golden Gate Bridge.

* * *

In the summer of 1930, while researchers on the East Coast were developing tools for visualizing psittacosis and refining agglutination tests, Karl Friedrich Meyer was focused on a mysterious "sleeping sickness" affecting horses in California and other western states. Educated in Basel and Zurich, Meyer's interest in animal diseases bridged by multiple insect and arthropod vectors was born in 1909 in South Africa, when, as an assistant to Arnold Theiler (the father of the Nobel Prize winner Max Theiler), he became the first person to elucidate the life cycle of the plasmodium of East Coast Fever, a tick-borne disease of cattle. Soon after, Meyer contracted malaria and was forced to return to Europe, but he did not stay long. By 1911 he had secured a teaching position at the University of Pennsylvania's veterinary school. There, Meyer became acquainted with the leading lights in American pathology and bacteriology, including Theobald Smith, whose ground-breaking study of Texas Cattle Fever was to provoke a rethinking of germ theory and the role of parasitical infections generally, and Frederick Novy, the director of the University of Michigan's Hygiene Laboratory, who had headed the official inquiry into the 1901 bubonic plague outbreak in San Francisco. Through Smith, Meyer was also introduced to Simon Flexner, the director of the Rockefeller Institute. But rather than take a job in New York, Meyer decided to head west, lured by the offer of an assistant professorship at Berkeley and the prospect of a research position at the newly formed George Williams Hooper Foundation for Medical Research in San Francisco.[43]

Housed in a three-story brick building in the former veterinary school on Mount Sutro in Parnassus Heights, the Hooper Foundation had been established by Hooper's widow in 1913 with a generous $1 million bequest and was the first private medical research institution to be attached to any American university. Although Flexner warned Meyer that in joining the Hooper, he risked "disappear[ing] in the Pacific Ocean, because the intelligentsia of the United States lives within a hundred miles from New York," the Hooper offered Meyer a degree of intellectual freedom that would have been impossible in the East.[44] Besides, as Meyer acknowledged, he was a "typical Basel squarehead" with a stubborn streak as wide as the Rhine. In his interactions with colleagues and other scientists, this stubbornness could come across as arrogance—an impression not helped by Meyer's Teutonic bearing, thick German-accented English, and intolerance of errors, particularly ones that occurred in his laboratory. However, when it came to tracking and identifying the source of new diseases there was, apparently, no more indefatigable opponent of microbes. Indeed, in a special tribute published in *Reader's Digest* in 1950, de Kruif hailed Meyer, then in his 60s, as "the most versatile microbe hunter since Pasteur." In a career spanning three decades, Meyer had helped eradicate brucellosis from Californian dairy herds; had demonstrated that botulism, a deadly food-borne pathogen, was a highly resistant spore found in soils across America; and had shown how sylvatic plague was endemic to ground squirrels and other wild rodent populations across the western United States. In short, declared de Kruif, Meyer was "an outdoor scientist living in a state of permanent outdoor emergency ... [and a] master among the world's microbe hunters."[45]

History does not record whether Meyer was pleased or embarrassed by de Kruif's gushing tribute—interviewed in the 1960s, Meyer said that his former wife suspected de Kruif of trying to "belittle" and "besmear" him.[46] However, although de Kruif was an alcoholic and had a turbulent personality, he and Meyer maintained a friendship for more than three decades, and twice a year de Kruif would make a point of visiting Meyer in San Francisco, where the pair enjoyed solitary moments hiking together on Mount Tamalpais, discussing the latest medical breakthroughs and exchanging gossip about their bacteriological colleagues.[47]

A member of the Sierra Club, Meyer traced his fascination with infectious disease to his boyhood excursions in the Swiss Alps, where he fell into conversation with British climbers recently returned from the plague spots of India; De Kruif was right to link his passion for microbe hunting with his enthusiasm for adventure and outdoor living. So it is little wonder that when reports reached the Hooper of a massive horse epizootic in the San Joaquin Valley, Meyer raced from his laboratory to investigate.[48] There, he found horses wandering aimlessly in circles or listing from side to side. Meyer's veterinary colleagues thought the horses' staggering symptoms were the result of "forage poisoning" due to botulism. However, the San Joaquin epizootic had broken out in June—the wrong time of year for botulism—and vets who visited affected ranches noted that the majority of the victims of "staggers," as the disease was known, were free-ranging horses, not those that had been fed on silage or stacked hay. At autopsy Meyer noted that the horses' brains were inflamed and scarred by microscopic haemorrhages, leading him to suspect that the neurological impairment was caused by a virus. Unfortunately, by the time he came to examine the horses, the virus had disappeared. What Meyer needed was to autopsy the brain of a recently infected horse. His opportunity came later that summer when one of his colleagues located a sick horse on a ranch in Merced. The rancher wanted nothing to do with Meyer's experiment, so Meyer bribed his wife with $20 and, when she signalled that her husband was asleep, snuck into the stable and decapitated the horse, hot-tailing it back to San Francisco in the middle of the night with its severed head sticking out of the trunk of his car. That very same morning, Meyer extracted the horse's brain, mashed it up, and injected the material into guinea pigs. Soon the guinea pigs' bodies were racked with tremors. Next, they curled up into balls or hunched up like cats, dying four to six days later. After repeating the experiment in rabbits, monkeys, and horses with the same results, Meyer and his colleagues announced that they had isolated a new filter-passing virus. It would be several years before researchers would confirm that, as Meyer had suspected, the virus was a type of encephalitis communicated to horses by mosquitoes breeding in nearby irrigation ditches, and would be able to divine its arboreal life cycle.[49]

Though preoccupied by equine encephalitis, Meyer had followed the parrot fever outbreaks and Armstrong and McCoy's efforts to passage the virus. However, it was not until the following year that he had reason to initiate his own studies and became interested in the involvement of bird breeders. The impetus came when three elderly women, who had attended a coffee club in Grass Valley in the Sierra Nevadas shortly before Thanksgiving in 1931, died.

Local physicians were baffled as to the cause, attributing the women's deaths to, variously, typhoid fever, dysentery, and "toxic pneumonia." However, on reviewing the medical reports and learning that the husband of the woman who had convened the gathering was also ill, Meyer realized that the common denominator was the room where they had gathered. He instructed the local health officer to see if there was a sick or dead parrot there. Meyer's intuition was partially correct: there was no parrot, but on going to the woman's home in Grass Valley the health officer discovered a healthy shell parakeet still in its cage, and another one which had recently died. Meyer immediately ordered the official to disinter the parakeet and send its carcass to the Hooper, together with its live mate. That same evening, at around 10pm, Meyer was astonished to see a driver in a face mask pull up outside his laboratory. It was the official, and on the back seat was the surviving parakeet chirping in its cage. "He was scared out of his wits that he might pick it up," Meyer recalled, "because it was generally known that because it was air-borne this was a highly contagious disease."[50]

To verify his hunch that the bird was infected, Meyer began with a simple exposure test, taking a healthy Japanese ricebird (finch), which he had read was highly susceptible to psittacosis, and placing it in a bell jar with the parakeet. Within two to three weeks the ricebird was dead. The parakeet, meanwhile, appeared "perfectly normal" and continued to shed sufficient virus such that if it was transferred again to a clean bell jar with another ricebird, that bird also became ill and died.[51] When Meyer finally sacrificed the parakeet on 16 January 1932, and inoculated the bird's mashed-up spleen into mice in his laboratory, the mice died within three to four days, suggesting that the "agent was exceedingly virile."[52] To be sure, Meyer repeated the experiment, removing the parakeet from the glass jar every time a finch died and transferring it to a new jar with another finch. After six months, Meyer had his proof: it was the desiccated droppings from the parakeet that were spreading the infection.

In the meantime, in January, the woman's husband had also died. Concerned that there might be a state-wide problem, Meyer had pressed the health department to issue a press release. The resulting publicity brought further reports of suspicious deaths involving parakeets from as far south as Tehachapi. Questioning itinerant peddlers who made a living selling parakeets door-to-door, Meyer and his assistant Bernice Eddie discovered that most of the birds had come from backyard aviaries in the Los Angeles area. Many of these breeding establishments belonged to war veterans and had been funded by the bonuses they had received under Depression relief. It was a low-tech and highly profitable business as the birds bred astonishingly fast. All an amateur breeder needed was lumber, wire netting and a breeding box. Within weeks the pens were full of young hatchlings or "crawlers." These young birds were very popular with pet owners; they could be trained to sit on their fingers and pick seeds. Rather than allow the nestlings to mature, amateur breeders had quickly sold them on to the trade. Indeed, over the Thanksgiving period and in the run-up to Christmas, Meyer discovered peddlers had crisscrossed the state offering lovebirds as gifts for housewives and widows.

Meyer put out a call to pet shops throughout California requesting that they send him other birds that were visibly sick or were associated with a householder who had recently been hospitalized with psittacosis. Soon, birds were arriving at the Hooper Foundation from as far north as Santa Rosa and as far south as San Luis Obispo. At first glance, the parakeets appeared perfectly healthy, but when Meyer examined their spleens he discovered their organs were swollen and scarred with lesions characteristic of psittacosis. The final proof came when he inoculated mice with the mashed-up bird spleens and the rodents fell ill. The more Meyer and Eddie quizzed peddlers and pet shop owners, the greater became their fear that birds all over California might be harbouring these asymptomatic, latent infections. From Pasadena, they obtained twenty-two birds, only to find that nine had enlarged livers and spleens. In some of the breeding pens, Meyer reported, the birds were visibly diseased and "so weak that they were actually crawling on the floor."[53]

Concerned that as many as 40 per cent of birds raised in backyard aviaries and professional breeding pens might be carriers of psittacosis, Meyer warned that California could be harbouring a huge reservoir of infection. He urged health officials to take action. In particular, he worried that when Californian parakeets were packed into crowded containers and shipped across state lines, the stress caused them to shed the virus, running the risk that they would reignite the epidemic. In other words, Argentine parrots were no longer the main danger: it was Californian birds that now posed the principal threat.

The State Department of Health had previously been blissfully unaware of the extent of California's bird breeding industry and the implications for public health. Now, it declared it was imposing a quarantine and placed an embargo on the transportation of lovebirds across state lines. The measure sparked uproar among California's breeders, particularly as Hoover's embargo on imported parrots the previous year had led to pent-up demand for parakeets, and pet stores in the East were increasingly looking to California to supply the market. Estimates as to the value of this market varied: breeders put it at $5 million; Meyer thought it was worth one-tenth of that. What was not in doubt was that Southern California's temperate year-round Mediterranean climate provided the ideal conditions for bird breeding and that upwards of 3,000 individuals now depended on the trade. What was needed was a system of inspecting pens and checking the condition of birds. However, it was a completely unregulated industry, and no one seemed willing to assume responsibility. Meyer scented an opportunity. When the botulism scare had hit the sales of Californian sardines and other canned foods in the 1920s, the canners had hired Meyer to advise on heat sterilization, establishing safety procedures that soon became standard across America. Now, he proposed a similar technological solution for Californian bird breeders.

His opening came in March 1932 when 125 leading breeders were summoned to a meeting at the Associated Realty Building in Los Angeles. Opening the proceedings, Dr Giles Porter, the director of the State Department of Public Health with whom Meyer had previously collaborated during the pneumonic plague outbreak in Los Angeles, introduced Meyer as a world authority on psittacosis and someone who could "prove to you, that this is not just a 'scare' but ... a really serious matter." Meyer began with a review of medical knowledge of psittacosis prior to 1930, then presented the evidence obtained during the pandemic that psittacosis was a filterable virus. "Probably there is a lot of 'hokus-pokus' talk about psittacosis that is not true," he told breeders, but there was no doubt that it was a "highly contagious infection" that could be spread aerially from bird to man via droppings or mucal discharges. This had been proven by the "sad experience" at the Hygienic Laboratory, where nine people had contracted psittacosis merely after passing along a corridor close to cages containing desiccated material. "Probably the wind blew the dust from these cages through a crack in the door and in this way the contact was made," he said. Next, he briefly detailed his own investigations in San Francisco. Then, pointing to a chart, he directly addressed the problem of infections in bird breeding establishments.

Let us say, for the sake of argument, we have one hundred birds. In this group of one hundred birds, the disease, parrot fever, breaks out. Probably—let us say—ten of the birds will die. Now these ten birds should have been examined. Unfortunately, nothing of this sort is usually done, but so far, we examine these birds and find ten have the parrot fever. There are ninety birds left. You would probably assume that these ninety birds ... are practically safe. My answer is NO! NO!

The difficulty was that every pen contained a certain percentage of "carriers"; that is, birds whose spleens showed evidence of prior infection but who did not appear sick or visibly diseased. These healthy-looking birds might harbour the virus for six months or longer without infecting other birds in the same pen. However, if such birds were exposed to cold or sudden climatic changes, then these infections could "become activated," and the birds might "secrete the virus," infecting other birds with whom they were confined. In particular, Meyer speculated, there was a good chance they would pass the virus to young birds or "runts." Nor was that the end of the danger. "Convalescent birds," that is birds recovering from infection, might also secrete the virus for four to six weeks. In all probability, the only birds that were safe were those with inherited immunity, or older birds that had acquired immunity during previous outbreaks or through exposure to the virus in the nest.

The only way to know for sure whether a flock was infected or not was for breeders to turn over 10 to 20 per cent of their stock so that Meyer could examine them for latent infections. In this way, Meyer would be able to give those aviaries that were free of disease a clean bill of health, and there would be no need for further embargos or quarantines. However, Meyer warned, autopsying the birds was dangerous and expensive work, and, in return, he would expect breeders to pay him for his services. He suggested that $10,000 would be sufficient.

> This is a disease which has caused in every laboratory they work with cases of psittacosis; and we have to almost put our foot in the grave, so to speak, in order to solve the problem. I took this responsibility to work with you. I therefore solicit from you your earnest cooperation—or, I give it up. It is not my business to die for a disease like psittacosis.[54]

Not surprisingly, the breeders balked at Meyer's offer, feeling his price was too steep. Instead, they tried to convince health officials that such tests were unnecessary and that once birds reached the age of four months they no longer presented a health risk. Next, they proposed that officials introduce a permit system. Porter refused to budge, but the breeders lobbied the governor, who relented and lifted the embargo. As the trade resumed in the summer of 1931 and parakeets were sent from California to markets in the East, Meyer feared a revival of the pandemic. Once the parakeets reached dealers in New York, there was no telling how many flocks might be infected or in which state or country a psittacosis carrier might turn up next. By the end of the year, Californian lovebirds had been scattered to every state in the union. They proved particularly popular at country fairs in Wisconsin and Minnesota, where they were raffled as prizes. Then, on 22 September 1932, came the news that Mrs William E. Borah, the wife of the senator from Idaho, was seriously ill at her home in Boise, Idaho. On investigation, her physician discovered she was a collector of parakeets and had recently acquired a set of lovebirds from California. Suspecting parrot fever, her husband, the senator, wired Washington to send serum immediately. Thus began another extraordinary chapter in the history of the Hygienic.

* * *

Two months after McCoy's fumigation of the north building, Congress had passed an act changing the laboratory's name to the National Institute of Health (NIH) and establishing fellowships for research into basic biological and medical problems. The Randsell Act, named after Senator E. Randsell, a Democrat from Louisiana, was seen as a reward for the PHS's investigations of psittacosis and the heroism of its research staff, and marked a sea change in American attitudes to the public funding of medical research.* Unfortunately, when Senator Borah's request arrived on McCoy's desk, the NIH's stores of serum had been exhausted. It was at this point that Armstrong volunteered his services. Having made a full recovery, it was likely his blood still contained antibodies. Why not make use of it? Armstrong's personal physician performed the phlebotomy, then stayed up all night separating out the serum. Because of the urgency, there was no time to check that it was sterile. Instead, the serum was dispatched directly to a waiting plane. The story of the mercy flight was a media sensation, with the Associated Press and national and local newspapers publishing hourly logs of the serum's progress from Washington to Boise, Idaho. By now Mrs Borah was close to death and her doctors were doubtful the serum would make a difference. But they decided it was worth a try and administered all twelve ounces (350 ml) in a single transfusion. Five days later she was on the road to recovery and by the following February she was fit enough to travel to Washington. Her first stop was the NIH. "I came to thank you for saving my life," she told Armstrong. "I have some of your blood flowing through my veins."[55]

If Mrs Borah's recovery was good news for the NIH, it was bad news for Californian bird breeders, as no sooner had his wife recovered than Senator

---

* It also appears to have been motivated by the 1928–29 influenza epidemic, the worst flu outbreak since the 1918 pandemic, and chemists' desire to apply their knowledge to medical problems. In 1948, the institute's name was pluralized to National Institutes of Health.

Borah urged President Hoover to reinstate the embargo, but this time on Californian rather than Argentine birds. Hoover forwarded the request to the PHS, prompting Cumming to issue an order banning the interstate transport of Californian parakeets. However, he indicated that if California could find a procedure for demonstrating that its birds were free of psittacosis then he might make an exception. The previous March, breeders had done everything they could to avoid submitting their birds to testing. Now, as the embargo bit, denying them access to lucrative markets in the East, they came around to Meyer's proposition.

By 1933 Meyer and Eddie had inspected sixty-six aviaries containing nearly 2,000 lovebirds. In these aviaries, they found that anywhere from 10 to 90 per cent of birds classed as healthy by their owners might be carrying latent psittacosis. However, they observed that while many of these infections were of an "eminently chronic character," they did not spread to parakeets in adjacent pens. Contrary to breeders' claims that they never fell ill, Meyer and Eddie discovered many had antibodies to psittacosis, suggesting they had been previously exposed and had suffered mild infections which had been misdiagnosed. The principal risk came from handling dead birds or direct contact with their nasal discharges and excreta, or from bite wounds. However, on occasion, psittacosis could be contracted simply by inhaling desiccated droppings. Indeed, Meyer found that such droppings were highly efficient aerosols and could be scattered over a wide area simply by the flapping of a bird's wings when it became agitated. In such circumstances, the environment is "charged with virus and becomes a menace to human beings who inhale it."[56] For this reason, they warned, psittacosis presented a particular threat to bird breeders and pet store owners, or those with close attachments to lovebirds.

They also found that the LCL bodies of psittacosis could be readily observed on a microscopic slide simply by taking a smear from the spleens of diseased birds and adding an appropriate stain. In other cases, the size of the spleen provided a rough-and-ready approximation of the degree of a latent infection in a pen. In particular, medium-sized spleens measuring three to five millimetres were more likely to produce "a typical, acutely fatal, or latent" illness in inoculated mice than spleens measuring seven to ten millimetres. Meyer and Eddie also found proportionately more enlarged spleens (six millimetres or greater) in young, immature birds than in the older capped birds, suggesting that parakeets typically contracted psittacosis early in their development and that enlarged but noninfective spleens in the older caged birds were evidence of an old sterilizing infection. Their conclusion was unequivocal: "In general, 'noncapped' immature birds are more frequently carriers of the virus than the 'capped' old birds."[57] The implications were clear: birds needed to be observed until they were at least four months old to be sure that they had cleared the infection and no longer presented a danger of transmitting the mycobacterium.

By 1934 Meyer and Eddie had tested nearly 30,000 parakeets and certified 185 Californian aviaries as psittacosis-free. The program was a valuable source of income for the Hooper Foundation, and soon Meyer was using the funds to investigate other scientific questions. Meyer was not only a bacteriologist and veterinary pathologist, he also considered himself a biologist and nascent ecologist. Though trained in the German tradition, by the 1930s he was growing disenchanted with bacteriology's narrow focus on microbes. Instead, as he considered the phenomenon of latent infections, he found himself drawn to the language of "hosts" and "parasites" and wider evolutionary questions about the relationship between virulence and immunity to disease. In particular, he wished to discover whether wild parakeets showed the same susceptibility to psittacosis as birds bred in captivity. To find out, Meyer paid a barber on a Pacific liner to bring him two hundred wild shell parakeets from the Australian bush. As psittacosis had never been reported in Australian parakeets before, Meyer assumed that these birds would possess a high susceptibility to the virus and lend themselves to comparative exposure and immunity tests. Imagine his astonishment, then, when within four weeks of his quarantining the Australian parakeets, one of them died. On examination he found its spleen riddled with the same lesions as those in the Californian birds. Perhaps the most significant finding, however, came when Meyer allowed the Australian birds to mingle freely with Californian parakeets, half of which he knew to be latently infected: none of the Australian parakeets died of the disease, and when he sacrificed the birds and performed autopsies, Meyer was unable to recover virus from the birds' spleens.

In an example of Meyer's use of international scientific networks, he immediately shared his findings with the Australian virus researcher Frank Macfarlane Burnet, prompting Burnet to launch a parallel study in which he found that psittacosis was an endemic infection of wild Australian parakeets and had probably been "enzootic amongst Australian parrots for centuries."[58] Burnet hypothesized that it was most likely Australian parrots and parakeets from Japanese dealers, not Argentine parrots, that had been the source of the outbreaks of psittacosis in California in 1931. In a letter to Meyer, Burnet explained that in the wild, young birds were typically infected in the nest, but these natural, mild infections could also flare up under the stress of close confinement, resulting in the birds' losing their acquired resistance and shedding the virus. By questioning importers, Meyer established it was common practice for shippers to mix wild unbanded birds with clean birds, greatly facilitating the spread of the virus. He concluded that in the wild, these virus strains were highly adapted to their avian hosts, but conditions in shipping containers and Californian aviaries had greatly increased the virulence of psittacosis and, as he put it, "shifted the balance in favor of the virus"—hence the spillovers of enzootic psittacosis infections seen in Californian birds and people in the early 1930s.[59]

* * *

Today, psittacosis no longer presents a pressing health threat and parrot fever has once again disappeared from public view. The disease's retreat from popular consciousness is due in large part to Meyer. Following the discovery of Aureomycin in 1948, Meyer approached the Hartz Mountain Distribution Company, then the largest supplier of milled bird seed in the United States, to develop a line of medicated millet. By the middle 1950s another easy-to-administer antibiotic, oral tetracycline, had also become available and chlortetracycline-impregnated seed had become standard in the bird breeding industry. To be sure, there were still occasional outbreaks, but these tended to occur on turkey farms or in poultry processing plants, where exposure to psittacosis was, and still is, an occupational hazard. In most cases, all it took was a properly administered course of tetracycline to clear human infections and return a flock to health.[60]

Unfortunately, today, as in the 1930s, some breeders refuse to believe their aviaries are latently infected. Instead, they dilute the seed or fail to administer a full course of antibiotics, resulting in the persistence of subclinical infections of psittacosis in domestic bird flocks. Should these birds be shipped to a pet store and mingle with imported birds emerging from quarantine, there is a risk they will communicate the organism and spark fresh outbreaks of parrot fever. Indeed, the principal lesson of the 1930 pandemic is that imported birds were merely the fall guys. The main culprits were domestic lovebirds bred in Californian aviaries. Once this was realized, parrots and parakeets ceased to be a source of fear and hysteria, and the control of psittacosis became a largely veterinary problem. However, without the simultaneous worldwide outbreaks sparked by Argentinian parrots and the press coverage that accompanied them, it is unlikely that anyone would have noticed the unusual pattern of pneumonia deaths, and Nocard's misconception that psittacosis was due to a type of salmonella would have taken longer to dispel.

There was another lesson, too, one that would become increasingly apposite in the second half of the twentieth century as other little-known or neglected pathogens emerged to spark new epidemic scares. And that is that in nature parrots and parakeets pose little threat to human populations. Sure, there might be occasional mass die-offs deep in the Amazonian rain forest or the Australian bush, but, in Burnet's words, psittacosis was "not intrinsically a very infectious disease." On the contrary, he argued, the parasite's primary function was to return wild bird populations that had grown too large or too dense for their ecological niches to a state of equilibrium. The problem was that when man disrupted these biological and ecological processes by packing parakeets into overcrowded crates, he created the ideal conditions for the propagation of the virus and its transfer from bird to man. "It is reasonably certain that cocka-toos, left to a natural life in the wild, would never have shown any symptoms of their infection," Burnet observed, following an outbreak in Melbourne in 1935. "In captivity, crowded, filthy and without exercise or sunlight, a flare-up of any latent infection was only to be expected."[61]

Indeed, by the 1940s Burnet was worrying that these spillover events were becoming more common and that overpopulation, coupled with international trade and jet travel, was disrupting natural ecologies in new and unpredictable ways, leading to virulent outbreaks of vector-borne diseases such as yellow fever. While a world in which everyone and everything was more closely linked in a biological sense should favour a "virtual equilibrium" between humans and microbial parasites, Burnet warned that "man ... lives in an environment con-stantly being changed by his own activities, and few of his diseases have attained such equilibrium."

Meyer also worried about the way that rapid economic and industrial change was disrupting the balance between humans and microbes. However, in the case of psittacosis he placed the blame squarely on bird breeders and their stubborn insistence that psittacosis did not pose a threat, even as the disease claimed the lives of pet owners and medical researchers in Baltimore and Washington. Perhaps the most important factor of all, however, had been the popularity of lovebirds with American consumers and the lucrative interstate trade that saw itinerant peddlers going door-to-door offering parakeets to widows and housewives. In 1930, the idea that these cute American-bred birds might be the avian equivalent of Trojan horses was too disturbing to contem-plate. Far easier to blame feathered green immigrants from the southern hemisphere.

4

THE "PHILLY KILLER"

"The outbreak ... has presented a number of unusual and complex features. ... It has run counter to our expectations that contemporary science is infallible and can solve all the problems that we confront."

David J. Sencer, Director, Center for Disease Control, Atlanta,
24 November 1976

At the junction of Walnut Street and South Broad Street—or what Philadelphians now call the "Avenue of the Arts"—stands a well-appointed modern business hotel. With its spacious guestrooms boasting "pillow top" mattresses and its wood-panelled nineteenth-floor restaurant with sweeping views over Center City, the Hyatt at the Bellevue effortlessly combines contemporary luxury and old-world charm. That charm is evident the moment you step from Broad Street into the lobby area and glide across the polished floor to the reception desk, taking in the glittering chandelier overhead and the curved staircase with its elegant hand-worked marble-and-iron rails. However, if you care little for decor and have important business to attend to, the hotel also offers state-of-the-art conference rooms, plus an indoor jogging track, a full-length swimming pool, and a 93,000-square-foot sports club. For allergy sufferers or the hyper-health-conscious, the Hyatt at the Bellevue even has spotless "hypo-allergenic" rooms equipped with a high-tech air purification system designed to filter out allergens and other airborne irritants. "Enjoy a better night's sleep and make the most of your travels in a Hyatt PURE room," purrs the hotel's marketing blurb.[1]

What is not mentioned anywhere on the hotel's website is the thing the building is best known for, at least among members of Philadelphia's baby boom generation. For in 1976, the Bellevue-Stratford, as the hotel was then known, was the site of one of the most baffling infectious disease outbreaks

99

in history—an outbreak centred on the hotel's air conditioning and water cooling systems.

The "Legionnaires' disease" affair began on Wednesday, 21 July, when 2,300 delegates from the Pennsylvania section of the American Legion and their families (some 4,500 people in all) began arriving at the Bellevue-Stratford for their annual four-day jamboree. It was the summer of the American Bicentennial celebrations, and the Legionnaires—many of them veterans of World War II and Korea—were looking forward to partying in style. Those who could afford it—perhaps five hundred in all—had checked into the Bellevue, taking advantage of the discounts on rooms negotiated by the Legion's state adjutant, Edward Hoak, whose job it was to preside over the convention that year and glad-hand delegates.

Formed from the shell of the Stratford, which used to stand at the southwest corner of Stratford and Broad, and the Bellevue, which used to overlook the northwest corner, the Bellevue-Stratford had opened its doors to guests in 1904 after a two-year refit costing a staggering $8 million (about $20 million in today's money). Billed at the time as the most luxurious hotel in America, it was designed in the French Renaissance style, with the most magnificent ballroom in the United States, four restaurants, 1,000 guest rooms, and lighting fixtures by Thomas Edison. By the 1920s, "the Grande Old Dame of Broad Street" had become a fixture of Philadelphia society and a favourite haunt of celebrities, royalty and heads of state. Former guests included Mark Twain, Rudyard Kipling, Queen Marie of Romania and General John J. Pershing. Every US president from Theodore Roosevelt on had stayed there, including President John F. Kennedy, who had visited the hotel in October 1963, the month before his assassination in Dallas. However, by the 1970s the Bellevue had fallen out of fashion and was struggling to compete with the new luxury chains. Indeed, despite the discounts negotiated by Hoak, many delegates complained that the food and drinks were overpriced. They also thought the air conditioning in the hospitality suites was substandard and did not like the attitude of the "snooty" staff.[2]

Those who could not afford the Bellevue had opted for the nearby Ben Franklin hotel and other cheaper midtown options. However, nearly everyone had visited the Bellevue's lobby to register and as all the principal conference events, from the Keystone Go-Getter Club Breakfast on the opening day to the Commander's Bicentennial Ball on the final evening, were held at the hotel, conventioneers and their families soon became familiar with its bars and hospitality suites. The Legionnaires loved a drink at the best of times, and with temperatures in Philadelphia that week in the high nineties, the suites were soon packed with delegates seeking to quench their thirst and cool off. To keep costs down, Hoak had arranged for delegates to supply their own alcohol and snacks, but he could do little about the hotel's creaking air conditioning system or the ice supplies, which soon ran out.

The first intimation Hoak had that Legionnaires had been visited by something worse than a hangover came a week later when he arrived in Manor, Pennsylvania, a small town two hundred miles west of Harrisburg, for the swearing-in of new officers of Post 472 and was informed that six Legionnaires in the area were ill and that one had died. There was further grim news when Hoak returned to his home near Harrisburg and found a letter waiting for him from the wife of a close colleague informing him that her husband was ill with pneumonia and was not responding to treatment. A few hours later Hoak received word from his secretary that the man was dead. Next, Hoak called his assistant adjutant in Chambersburg concerning another matter only to learn that he was attending the viewing of Charles Chamberlain, commander-elect of St. Thomas Post 612 in south-central Pennsylvania, who had died suddenly following the convention. When Hoak called the former state commander of Williamsport to inform him of the three deaths, he learned that six other people from Williamsport who had also attended the convention were seriously ill in area hospitals. In theory this was not unusual. After all, the Legionnaires formed an elderly demographic and many were also heavy smokers and drinkers with underlying health problems. But three deaths and more than six hospitalizations in the space of a week struck Hoak as more than a little odd, and when he made further calls and learned that other delegates across the state were also ill, his alarm deepened.[3]

Hoak was not the only person becoming concerned that weekend. On Saturday, 31 July, Robert Sharrar, chief of Acute Communicable Disease Control for Philadelphia, had taken a call from a physician in Carlisle worried about a patient who had recently attended the Legion convention and who was complaining of a fever and a dry, hacking cough. A chest X-ray indicated the patient had bronchopneumonia of the lower right lobe. Sharrar told him it sounded like mycoplasmal pneumonia and advised him to draw blood and send it for testing to the state laboratory when it reopened on Monday. In the meantime, he recommended the doctor treat his patient with a fast-acting antibiotic. Sharrar was about to end the conversation when the doctor asked whether he knew of any other cases of pneumonia in Philadelphia in the past few days. Sharrar did not. That was when the doctor said that he had heard that a patient had recently died of pneumonia in Lewisburg, in northwest Pennsylvania. Sharrar immediately called Lewisburg Hospital and asked to be put through to the resident pathologist, who informed him that the victim was a Legionnaire and that the cause of death had been "acute viral ... hemorrhagic pneumonia."[4]

Two cases of pneumonia in a city the size of Philadelphia was not unusual—in an average summer week Sharrar could expect twenty to thirty deaths from the disease. Nevertheless, the cases gave Sharrar pause for thought. In February, a new strain of swine flu had been isolated at a US Army base at Fort Dix, New Jersey, thirty-five miles northeast of Philadelphia. The flu had claimed the life of a young private and gone on to sicken several soldiers on the base. Tests showed the strain was closely related to the H1N1 virus responsible for the deadly "Spanish flu" pandemic. Fearing that the Fort Dix outbreak was the harbinger of a new pandemic wave, David Sencer, the director of the CDC in Atlanta, had urged the Ford administration to immunize the entire US population. As a CDC-trained epidemiologist, Sharrar had fully supported Sencer's recommendation and was determined that Philadelphians would be among the first to get the flu shots. All he was waiting for was for Congress to approve the administration's $134 million funding request and for politicians in Washington to agree to insurance to cover vaccine manufacturers worried about their liability should the vaccine prove to have adverse effects.

* * *

In the late Victorian and Edwardian periods, pneumonia had been the most feared disease after tuberculosis and was nearly always fatal, particularly in the case of the elderly or those with compromised immune systems. Indeed, prior to antibiotics, lobar pneumonia had accounted for between one-quarter to a third of all deaths.

However, this changed with Dubos's discovery in 1927, in Avery's laboratory at the Rockefeller Institute in New York, of an enzyme that decomposed the polysaccharide capsule of the pneumococcus, making it vulnerable to phagocytosis. Together with the isolation of the first sulpha drugs in the 1930s, treatment and survival rates for pneumonia gradually improved. The wider availability of penicillin in the late 1940s, and the discovery of new antibiotics such as erythromycin and doxycycline in the 1950s, coupled with better respiratory technology in hospitals, saw further strides in treatment and convalescent care. By the early 1970s the rate of hospital fatalities had fallen to around 5 per cent, the level at which it remains today.[5] The result was that pneumonia ceased to be an interesting field of research for young medical scientists. Instead, believing that the "conquest of epidemic disease" was imminent, researchers focused on cancer and chronic diseases associated with genetic conditions and modern lifestyles.[6]

As the outbreak in Philadelphia would demonstrate, this was a mistake. While most bacterial pneumonias are due to the pneumococcus, pneumonia can also be caused by several other common bacteria, for example, *Yersinia pestis*, the bacterium of plague, and *Chlamydia psittaci*, the bacterium of psittacosis. Another common source of atypical pneumonias is *Haemophilus influenzae*, the bacillus that Pfeiffer blamed for the Russian and Spanish influenza pandemics, and *Mycoplasma pneumoniae*, a tiny organism midway between a bacterium and a virus. In addition, there had been several outbreaks of pneumonia for which a causal agent had never been identified. These unsolved outbreaks included an incident in 1965 at St. Elizabeth's Mental Hospital in Washington, DC in which fourteen people had died, and an outbreak at a health department building in Pontiac, Michigan. Dubbed "Pontiac Fever," the latter had caused an influenza-like illness in 144 workers and visitors to the building, including a team from the CDC. Although there had been no deaths and no recorded cases of pneumonia, guinea pigs exposed to aerosols of unfiltered water from the building's air condenser unit developed nodular pneumonia. That suggested the presence of a bacterium-sized infectious agent. Unfortunately, all attempts to culture the pathogen from the water or from the lung tissue of guinea pigs failed, much to the CDC's frustration. The result was that while the Pontiac and St. Elizabeth's outbreaks were known to epidemiologists, the cases had never been written up.[7] By contrast, everyone knew about the swine flu outbreak at Fort Dix because there was such a panic about it and the newspapers were full of the government's vaccination plans. Perhaps that was why, on 2 August, a physician from the Veterans Administration Clinic in Philadelphia telephoned CDC headquarters and asked to speak with someone from the National Influenza Immunization Program. He was put through to Robert Craven, a young Epidemic Intelligence Service (EIS) officer who, together with his colleague, Phil Graitcer, was manning the desk in Auditorium A, the "war room" set up by the CDC in expectation of a nationwide epidemic of swine flu. The physician had grim news: four Legionnaires admitted to his clinic had died of pneumonia over the weekend. All of them had attended the state convention in Philadelphia. In addition, some twenty-six other people who had been at the convention were also showing signs of "febrile respiratory disease."[8]

At first Craven and Graitcer dismissed the reports: four deaths from pneumonia was to be expected among such a large gathering of elderly people. However, within the hour the CDC officers had fielded several more calls from doctors and health officials in Pennsylvania telling a similar story, and by mid-morning the death count from pneumonia had reached eleven. This was certainly unusual. As it happened, one of their colleagues, another young EIS officer named Jim Beecham, had recently been posted to the headquarters of the Pennsylvania State Health Department in Harrisburg. When Craven got through to him he learned that earlier that morning Hoak had issued a statement saying that at least eight of his members were dead and some thirty other Legionnaires who had attended the convention were ill with "mysterious symptoms." Reporters wondered whether the cases were connected to swine flu.

Influenza typically has an incubation period of one to four days, and most healthy adults are able to infect others up to five to seven days after becoming sick. If the Legionnaires had caught swine flu at the convention in Philadelphia, then the first illnesses would have shown themselves around 28 July. It also meant that officials could expect a second wave in the first week of August. Was that what was now happening? Had the long-feared swine flu outbreak begun? No one was sure, but with rumours mounting and pharmaceutical companies months away from being able to supply sufficient doses of vaccine, it was imperative that the CDC answer the question quickly. If nothing else, David Sencer's reputation depended on it.

The person to whom it fell to investigate the outbreak was David Fraser, a 32-year-old graduate of Harvard Medical School who bore a striking resemblance to Bobby Kennedy. Tapped as a future director of the CDC, Fraser had recently been appointed head of the CDC's Special Pathogens Branch and occupied a small windowless office five floors above the swine flu war room. There he presided over a crack team of epidemiologists, including the latest cohort of EIS graduates. Established in 1951 as an early warning corps against biological warfare, EIS is the CDC's elite disease detection squad. As befits a group that takes pride in its ability to investigate outbreaks in any part of the world, its symbol is a globe with a worn-out shoe sole. Every year, between 250 to 300 applicants compete for the privilege of seventy-five places in the EIS's intensive, two-year training program. Candidates are recruited from every area of medicine and include doctors, veterinarians, virologists, nurses and dentists. The emphasis is on applied epidemiological procedures, biostatistics, and the management of an outbreak investigation. Particular emphasis is placed on the study of old case files and the compilation of "line lists," or charts, detailing each case and the distribution of infections in time and space. In addition, trainees are expected to learn how to gather pathology and serology specimens.

In keeping with the vision of EIS's founder, Alexander D. Langmuir, the emphasis was on learning on the job. As Langmuir once told an interviewer, he liked nothing better than throwing EIS candidates "overboard" to see if they could swim; and if they couldn't, he was happy to "throw them a life ring, pull them out, and throw them in again."[9] In short, EIS graduates would stop at nothing to get to the bottom of an outbreak. A few years earlier, for instance, Fraser had helped solve the mystery of a Lassa Fever outbreak in Sierra Leone that had very nearly killed one of his colleagues who tramped through villages trapping rodents in search of the presumed reservoir of the virus (he eventually traced it to a local species of brown rat). Another reason Sencer had picked Fraser was his reputation for diplomacy, something that Sencer knew would be needed when Fraser arrived in Harrisburg, the Pennsylvania state capital, and local health officials learned of the CDC's interest in the case.

The first thing epidemiologists are taught in the event of an outbreak is to draw up a working case definition in order to verify the diagnosis. The second is to look at the frequency of exposure among people with illness and those of comparable groups who are not ill (so-called controls). Only then is it possible to say whether the identified cases constitute an epidemic. As Fraser left for Harrisburg on 3 August, he knew there were one hundred suspected cases and that there had been nineteen deaths. He also knew that all the cases involved Legionnaires who had attended the state convention in Philadelphia. However, that could merely be an artefact of the reporting: the American Legion was a close-knit group with efficient communication networks, so it was only natural that cases occurring among Legionnaires would come to attention first. Moreover, the press was already showing a keen interest in the outbreak, something that was likely to further skew the reporting. To know if there really was an epidemic underway in Pennsylvania, Fraser would need to establish whether any other groups or individuals had also fallen ill with pneumonia in the relevant time period and whether they had also been in Philadelphia or somewhere else. He would also need to establish how many Legionnaires and their families had attended the convention so as to obtain an accurate denominator with which to gauge the attack rate. Ideally, he would also need line lists detailing the name, age, and address of each patient, and, in the case of Legionnaires, the dates they had attended the convention and the hotels they had stayed at. These charts would also need to include key medical and pathological information, such as the date of onset of illness and, in the case of the deceased, the cause of death. Clearly it was a big job, and before it had ended thirty EIS officers had fanned out across the state, inter-

viewing the families of victims or, in the case of those who had been hospital-
ized, the institutions where they had received treatment. In anticipation of
this effort, on 2 August the CDC had dispatched Craven and Graitcer to
Pittsburgh and Philadelphia respectively, and a recently qualified EIS officer,
Theodore Tsai, to Harrisburg. In addition, Fraser would be joined in
Harrisburg by two other newly qualified EIS officers, David Heymann, a
future director of Emerging and Communicable Diseases at the World Health
Organization, and Stephen Thacker, who would go on to become an assistant
surgeon general in the US Public Health Service.

The other priority was to establish whether or not the outbreak was due to
swine flu. This task would largely fall to Graitcer, whose job it was to liaise with
state laboratories and forward throat washings and sera to the CDC's laboratory in Atlanta. There, a team of specialists was on hand to see if the sera
cross-reacted with the H1N1 swine flu, dubbed A/New Jersey/76, that had
been isolated at Fort Dix in February. At the same time, CDC technicians
would test for antigens to the most prevalent strain of flu then circulating in
the northern hemisphere, an H3N2 virus known as A/Victoria/75, as well as
other common infectious agents associated with pneumonia.

Within forty-eight hours of arriving in Harrisburg, Fraser had the answer
to the first question: it was not swine flu. And within seventy-two hours technicians confirmed it was not the A/New Jersey or A/Victoria strains either.
That left several other possibilities. At the top of the list was *Chlamydia psittaci*, the bacterium of psittacosis, and *Coxiella burnetii*, the bacterium of Q
Fever, a disease of cattle, sheep, and goats which was also known to cause
pneumonia in humans. Another more remote possibility was *Histoplasma*, a
fungal infection transmitted by birds and bats. Testing for these pathogens,
Fraser knew, would take weeks and possibly months, and would have to be
combined with the calm and careful collection of other evidence, such as dust
and water samples from the Bellevue, and the examination of pathology specimens from deceased Legionnaires. But arriving at the offices of Leonard
Bachmann, the secretary of health for Pennsylvania, and his chief epidemiologist, William Parkin, Fraser found the atmosphere anything but calm. Already,
the phones were ringing off the hook with panicked callers, while in the press
room next door newspapermen were demanding to know whether the outbreak might be something more sinister, a deliberate act of poisoning perhaps
by anti-war radicals intent on sabotaging the Bicentennial celebrations or
sending a message to Gerald Ford, who two years earlier had controversially
pardoned Richard Nixon for his alleged crimes in connection with the
Watergate break-in. The press could be forgiven for asking such questions; in

the run-up to the convention, Philadelphia's mayor Frank Rizzo, a tough-talking former policeman and close friend of Nixon's, had deliberately stoked fears of a terrorist attack by posting undercover officers in and around the downtown area. Following the outbreak, Rizzo's official spokesman, Albert Gaudiosi, had raised even more bizarre conspiracy theories, including the possibility of a covert operation by the CIA using chemical and biological weapons. Gaudiosi's statement struck many as a blatant attempt to divert attention from the mayor's failure to resolve a long-running garbage collection dispute—a dispute that had gone on for three weeks and had seen mounds of refuse collect on city streets.[10] Those garbage mounds were a magnet for rats and other vermin. Might those rats be infested with plague fleas, wondered journalists? Could plague be the source of the Legionnaires' peculiar pneumonic symptoms?

While CDC scientists were testing sputa and examining lung tissue and other pathology specimens, EIS officers were extending their investigations across Pennsylvania. Each officer drove an average of 450 miles, interviewing ten patients in over six hospitals. By now, a clear clinical picture was emerging. Typically, a case of Legionnaires' disease began with a feeling of malaise, muscle aches, and a slight headache. Within twenty-four hours, patients would exhibit a rapidly rising fever, chills, and a dry cough, as well as, on occasion, abdominal pains and gastrointestinal symptoms. Two or three days later, the patients would have a raging fever of 102–105°F, and a chest X-ray would show patchy pneumonia. Accordingly, a case was defined clinically as any person with a cough and a fever of 102°F or higher, or any fever and chest X-ray evidence of pneumonia. In addition, investigators included an epidemiological criterion (a case must have attended the American Legion convention or been inside the Bellevue-Stratford between 1 July and 18 August). At this point, the cases listed at the State Department of Health consisted entirely of people who had attended the convention or who had been at the Bellevue, so this clinico-epidemiological definition made sense. However, it was also possible that the line lists had been skewed by the publicity surrounding the outbreak at the Bellevue and that people had not thought to report other cases that might warrant inclusion, so the Department of Health also set up a hotline and invited members of the public to report possible epidemic cases regardless of association with the convention or the Bellevue.

By the first week of August it was clear that the epidemic had peaked and the disease was not contagious, there being no secondary cases. Tracing the epidemic curve back in time, it was evident there had been a rapid upswing in cases from 22 to 25 July, followed by a plateau through 28 July and a somewhat slow decline through 3 August. Moreover, there had been no cases prior to the convention, suggesting that, whatever the agent, the incubation period was two to ten days. In all, in a four-week period up to 10 August, there had been 182 cases and 29 deaths, giving a case fatality rate of 16 per cent. The infection had proved particularly dangerous to cigarette smokers and older age groups, with those aged sixty or more twice as likely to suffer fatal outcomes. Almost all were Legionnaires who had either resided at the Bellevue or had attended events in its lobby and hospitality suites. However, there were also a few clinically compatible cases among non-Legionnaires. These included a Bellevue air conditioner repair man, a bus driver, and several pedestrians who had merely passed by the hotel's imposing frontage on Broad Street. Were these Broad Street pneumonias part of the same epidemiological event? And why was it that, with the exception of the air conditioner repair man, hardly any of the Bellevue's employees appeared to have fallen ill?

Though epidemiology aspires to be an exact science, it also contains a large element of induction. As Wade Hampton Frost, a former professor of epidemiology at Johns Hopkins and one of the pioneers of the field, once put it: "Epidemiology at any given time is something more than the total of its established facts. It includes their orderly arrangement into chains of inference which extend beyond the bounds of direct observation."[11] In other words, the raw data can only be parsed so far. To get a feel for Legionnaires' disease, Fraser realized he needed to go to the focus of the outbreak. Obtaining rooms at the Bellevue was not a problem: by now, most guests had cancelled their bookings for fear of contracting the disease, and on 10 August Fraser and ten of his officers moved into the hotel and began exploring the lobby area and hospitality suites.[12] Was there a pattern, he wondered, some sort of clue in the way that the Legionnaires had used the hotel's facilities?

To verify how many of the 10,000 registered Pennsylvania Legion members had actually attended the convention and to reconstruct their movements, Fraser distributed questionnaires to Legionnaires across the state. As well as confirming their attendance in Philadelphia, Legionnaires were asked to provide details of which hotel they had stayed at, and how many hours they had spent inside the Bellevue or on the sidewalk outside. The two-page questionnaires also contained checklists about key convention activities and functions. Had they gone to the Keystone Go-Getter Club Breakfast on the morning of 23 July in the Rose Garden on the eighteenth floor of the Bellevue? Had they attended the ticket-only Commander's Bicentennial Ball in the Bellevue's lavish second floor ballroom that same evening? Fraser also quizzed them about their consumption of food, coffee and alcohol, and whether they had added ice and mixers to their drinks or bought anything from street vendors during the Legion parade through downtown. In addition, officers interviewed other guests and non-conventioneers who had stayed at or visited the Bellevue during the same period. Finally, EIS officers interviewed Bellevue staff to establish whether they had suffered any illnesses. To help with the surveys, Rizzo even provided Fraser and Sharrar with a team of homicide detectives. According to Sharrar, the detectives "did not miss a trick" and proved particularly adept at quizzing Legionnaires about their interactions with female sex workers, many of whom had passed themselves off as hotel guests in order to gain access to the hospitality suites.

It quickly became apparent that nearly everyone had spent time in the first floor lobby area, where the registration desk was set up, talking to other delegates running for election or chatting to family and friends. And nearly everyone had ridden in the elevators, either to visit the rooftop restaurant or to visit the bars and hospitality suites. Typical cases included Jimmy Dolan and John Bryant Ralph—"J.D." and "J.B." in the anonymous line lists. Members of the Williamstown Legion post, Dolan and Ralph were thirty-nine and forty-one respectively and had been buddies since childhood. To save money, the pair had stayed at the Holiday Inn in midtown with Jimmy's cousin, Richard Dolan, the 43-year-old commander of Pennsylvania Legion Post 239. Well built and with a reputation for partying, all three had attended the Commander's Bicentennial Ball, drinking until well past midnight. The trio had also spent many hours in the lobby area, but had avoided the hotel's bars and restaurants. Within days of returning to Williamstown, both Jimmy Dolan and Ralph were complaining of fever, head-aches and coughs, and on 29 July Jimmy Dolan was admitted to the hospital. He died three days later, the pathologist recording the cause as "bilateral consolida-tion lungs, bloody sputum terminal." The day after, 2 August, Ralph also suc-cumbed to the mysterious disease, the cause of death being listed as "gross mas-sive bilateral lobar pneumonia." By contrast, Richard Dolan had suffered no symptoms of illness.[13]

Three "statistically significant" factors emerged from the questionnaires. First, ill delegates had spent on average four or five more hours in the Bellevue than had healthy delegates, and considerably more time in the lobby than controls. The correlation between the amount of time spent in the lobby and illness applied particularly to those who had slept at the Bellevue, but also held for Legionnaires who had stayed at other hotels. However, this correla-tion did not hold for hotel staff who worked in the lobby area and had spent as much if not more time there than Legionnaires. Indeed, with the exception of an air conditioning repair man, who had developed flu-like symptoms on

21 July and had returned to work four days later, there was no evidence of illness or disease in any of the hotel's thirty full-time employees. Second, there appeared to be a small correlation between illness and visits to hospitality suites, with delegate cases visiting on average 2.6 hospitality rooms as compared to 1.8 visited by nondelegate cases. However, no one hospitality room had been visited by more than one-third of cases. Third, while cases were more likely to have drunk water at the Bellevue than non-cases, only two-thirds admitted to drinking water in any form, presumably because they preferred to quench their thirst with alcohol and/or carbonated drinks. In short, as Sharrar put it, the typical case "was most likely to be a friendly, thirsty, elderly, male delegate who hung around the hotel lobby."[14]

In any outbreak investigation, once the existence of the epidemic has been confirmed and the diagnosis established, the next questions are who, where, when, how, and what? Following the surveys, there could be little doubt that Legionnaires were the who, the convention was the when, and the Bellevue was the where. But that left the how and what wide open. Had Legionnaires' disease been triggered by exposure to a fomite, such as dust or ash particles, or was it due to some kind of gas? Alternatively, could the pathogen have been water- or food-borne? Moreover, if the common denominator was the Bellevue, how did one explain the apparent immunity of the hotel's staff? Was it possible that the conspiracy theories were right and the outbreak had been a deliberate act of espionage?

By now, speculation was rife, with several newspapers suggesting the Legionnaires had been poisoned with paraquat, a weed killer known to cause pulmonary edema and breathing problems. Another suggestion was phosgene gas, a pulmonary agent that had been deployed by the Germans, and later the Allies, in World War I, which causes choking and shortness of breath. Other suggestions were that the Legionnaires' symptoms could be due to poisoning with nickel carbonyl, a highly toxic liquid that can trigger chemical pneumonitis and cardiorespiratory failure, or else cadmium poisoning from the cadmium pitchers that the bar staff had used to mix the Legionnaires' drinks. Fraser asked CDC technicians to screen pathology specimens from the deceased Legionnaires for traces of these toxins and poisons and instructed EIS officers to examine the restaurants, bars, rooms, and hospitality suites for traces of the same chemicals. If the pathogen had been phosgene, Fraser reasoned, it could have been added to the Legionnaires' drinks or sucked in gaseous form via the elevator shaft, from where the constant motion of the elevators would have distributed it to the upper floors of the hotel. That could be why the survey had turned up no association between the illness and

Legionnaires' presence in a particular hospitality suite. However, everyone had ridden the elevators and had gotten in and out at the lobby. Phosgene is also rapidly excreted from the body, making it an ideal poisoning agent. However, it usually causes severe kidney damage, and none of the kidneys from Legionnaires exhibited signs of trauma. Nor did any of the specimens contain paraquat. By contrast, traces of nickel were found in the lungs, liver, and kidneys of six Legionnaires and two of the Broad Street pneumonias. However, these were well within normal levels and were not elevated compared to those of controls.

As the obvious candidates were excluded, Fraser began to consider more remote possibilities, including the air conditioning system. Most modern hotels boast rooftop chiller units, as cold air settles and it is impossible to drive cold air upwards. However, the Bellevue employed an old cold water system operated via two Carrier refrigeration machines located in the subbasement. Installed in 1954, these chillers had a capacity of 800 and 600 tons respectively and used Freon 11 refrigerant to cool the water. This chilled water was then pumped up to the roof of the hotel from where it was circulated downward to some sixty air-handling units (AHUs). Most of these used approximately 75 per cent recirculated air and 25 per cent outside air, but in the case of the AHU located directly above the lobby desk, all of the air was recirculated.

At the same time, a separate system, using "cooled" water from a cooling tower on the roof, was employed to condense the refrigerant. In the event of accidental leakage, the chilled water system was designed to be replenished automatically via a float valve in a nearby water expansion tank. Unfortunately, due to a fault in the valve, the water pipes at the top of the hotel had become filled with air, resulting in the failure of one of the AHUs serving the Rose Garden restaurant on the eighteenth floor. To rectify this, staff had hooked up a temporary connection using a garden hose that ran from the water tower to a pipe leading to the AHU. This makeshift system solved the problem of the faulty float in the expansion tank, but if the valves at either end of the hose were left open or leaked and various safety valves malfunctioned, it was conceivable that water from the water tower could have found its way into two steel tanks, also located in the roof, that supplied the hotel's drinking water. Since the water in the tower had been treated with chromate to preserve the pipes, this made it a potential contamination risk. The water tower was also uncovered and exposed to the elements, meaning it would be very easy for droppings from pigeons roosting on the balconies to get into the potable water.

Another potentially worse hazard was the 800-ton basement chiller unit. The unit had been leaking F-11 coolant continuously since May, prompting the Bellevue's management to put in repeated calls to the Carrier company to fix the problem. However, these repairs had been only partly successful, and with the summer conference season imminent, management had opted to postpone further servicing until later in the year. Unfortunately, air from the subbasement exhausted directly onto Chancellor Street on the southern side of the hotel. In theory the exhausted air could have contained F-11 coolant from the faulty chiller in a gaseous state. In addition, piped vents from the chillers also discharged air onto Chancellor Street just three feet away from the exhaust fan, meaning it was possible that some of this air could have been sucked back into the subbasement via an air shaft adjacent to the point of exhaust. Fraser was unable to determine the "ultimate fate of this air," but as the subbasement was also served by two large fans that exhausted air via another shaft that extended up to the roof, he could not discount the possibility that contaminated air had been circulated throughout the hotel.[15] Fuelling Fraser's suspicions about leaking chiller coolant was the fact that an air conditioner repair man had signed off sick on 20 July, the day before the convention opened. As the man reported having a cough and a temperature of 102°F, his name had been included in the line list. However, he did not develop pneumonia and on 24 July was well enough to return to work. Later, it was discovered that his wife and two daughters had been sick with a respiratory illness at the same time, prompting Sharrar to argue that he should never have been included in the line list and that his illness was probably due to flu, not Legionnaires' disease.[16]

By the end of August, EIS officers had combed the hotel from top to bottom. Samples removed to Atlanta for testing included Freon II and chilled water from the air conditioner system; dust from the AHUs, carpets, draperies, and hotel elevators; water from the hotel drinking fountains and ice dispensers; rodent control chemicals; bleaches and housekeeping supplies; and a variety of convention mementos including mugs, hats, badges, and packs of Merit cigarettes that had been included in the convention gift bags. Noticing that ventilation grilles from the subway discharged onto Broad Street, Fraser had also ordered inspections of the underground concourse. Finally, mindful that no epidemiological survey could be considered complete without a record of the weather, Fraser ordered up meteorological readings for the period from 21 to 25 July. These showed that the convention had opened to sweltering conditions and that on 22 July there had been a sharp temperature inversion. The result was that rather than temperatures decreasing with elevation above ground level, as is usual, air at the upper levels of the hotel, including the roof, had become superheated. This unusual effect had lasted for a day and a half, ending at around noon on 24 July, and, Fraser discovered, had been accompanied by slightly higher levels of carbon monoxide and other atmospheric pollutants.

From the beginning, one of the most popular theories was that the outbreak had been due to psittacosis. Although in 1976 the great parrot fever pandemic of 1930 was a distant memory, ornithologists and veterinary specialists had continued to study the epidemiology of the disease and its natural history. As tighter regulation reduced the incidence of outbreaks in bird breeding establishments and pet stores, the focus had shifted to occupational settings, such as turkey farms and poultry processing plants. At the same time, serological studies and a better understanding of the role of latent infections had brought a new appreciation of the disease's wide host range. Indeed, in 1967, Karl Meyer had tabulated 130 species of bird that carried the disease. These included homing pigeons raised in backyard lofts and the pigeons in New York's Central Park, half of whom were found to be harbouring the chlamydia bacterium.[17]

Fraser noted that the upper floors and roof of the Bellevue were popular pigeon roosts. In addition, a local Philadelphia character, known as the "pigeon lady," had been seen scattering bread crumbs on Broad Street. Then, there was the report from a guest that she had heard a parakeet chirping in one of the rooms. Fraser's task was not made any easier by the support given to the psittacosis theory by prominent medics. The most vocal was Dr Gary Lattimer, a specialist in infectious diseases at the Sacred Heart Hospital in Allentown. In early August, Lattimer had examined four Legionnaires and, believing they had psittacosis, treated them with tetracycline, a broad-spectrum antibiotic that was known to be effective against psittacosis and rickettsial diseases.* The Legionnaires' symptoms had immediately improved, prompting Lattimer to urge Fraser to issue a directive recommending tetracycline to other patients. Fraser refused, citing the absence of scientific proof and saying it would be irresponsible to recommend tetracycline over erythromycin and rifampicin.[18] However, Lattimer would not back down. Instead he began holding press conferences and writing to well-known chlamydia experts, including Julius Schachter, Meyer's formal pupil and a professor of epidemiology at UCSF.[19] In support of his theory, Lattimer cited the fact that psittacosis had a variable incubation period of three to eleven days, similar to the two to ten days' period for Legionnaires' disease. The mortality rate and

---

* *Rickettsia* is the name for a family of bacteria transmitted by the bites of chiggers, ticks, fleas and lice. The best known rickettsial diseases are typhus and Rocky Mountain spotted fever.

symptoms were also similar, and, as with psittacosis, there appeared to be no secondary transmission. Finally, Lattimer pointed out that histopathological examinations revealed extensive alveolitis or inflammation of the air sacs of victims' lungs. Together with the changes seen in the liver and spleen, these were "compatible in all aspects with those reported from previous human chlamydial epidemics."[20] Unfortunately for Lattimer, in September a panel of expert pathologists tasked with reviewing the autopsy evidence disagreed. Although the panel found that five of the core Legionnaires' cases and the three Broad Street pneumonias showed patterns of "acute diffuse alveolar damage," it ruled that such alveolar damage could also be the result of exposure to toxins. "No pathologic diagnosis could be made on the basis of these findings," they concluded.[21]

All hope of solving the mystery now rested on the microbiology studies. As the leading federal agency for disease control and a WHO reporting centre for influenza, the CDC's laboratories in Atlanta were considered second to none. Staffed by 625 scientists and technicians, the laboratories, which were located on the main Clifton Road site adjacent to Emory University, covered seventeen separate disciplines, including bacteriology, toxicology, mycology, parasitology, virology, vector-borne diseases and pathology. Here technicians could use electron microscopy to directly observe infected tissue, culture bacteria on appropriate media, and inoculate diseased material in cell cultures, eggs and small laboratory animals. In addition, they could screen sputa and sera for antibodies to a range of antigens.

By the end of August, CDC technicians had scanned hundreds of tissue samples and used fluorescent antibodies against over a dozen different microbes. With the exception of one patient, who tested positive for mycoplasmal pneumonia, none of the sera showed significant antibody responses. Nor did tests of nasal and throat washings reveal the presence of chlamydia, *Y. pestis*, or more exotic bacteria and viruses, such as Lassa and Marburg. At one point, technicians got excited when three guinea pigs died of a mixed bacterial infection after inoculation with a lung suspension from a patient. However, it later transpired that the bacteria were typical of those found in patients after treatment with antibiotics or in post-mortem overgrowth,[22] and when the lung suspension was passed through a bacterial filter in an effort to exclude everything except a virus, it was no longer pathogenic for guinea pigs.* As the tests came up blank,

---

* Many bacteria will continue to grow in tissue post-mortem, hence the importance of embalming and cold storage to prevent putrefaction. However, most bacteria that cause disease cannot survive more than a few hours in a dead body.

the scientists tried different methods. One was to put blood samples in test tubes with antibodies against various microbes and look for a positive reaction. Mindful of the toxic chemicals theory, the scientists also subjected lung, liver, and kidney samples from deceased Legionnaires to radioactive assays for poisoning with twenty-three heavy metals, including mercury, arsenic, nickel and cobalt.

After influenza and psittacosis, the next most likely suspect had been Q fever. Caused by *Coxiella burnetii*, an obligate intracellular parasite midway between a bacterium and a virus, Q fever used to be classed as a type of rickettsia.[23] However, unlike other rickettsial diseases, such as typhus and Rocky Mountain spotted fever, which are transmitted by the bites of arthropods, humans typically get Q fever when they breathe in dust infected by contaminated animals (the principal animal reservoirs are cattle, sheep, and goats). Common symptoms are fever, severe headache, and a cough. In about half of patients, pneumonia ensues, and hepatitis is frequent enough that the combination of pneumonia and hepatitis is usually considered diagnostic. Unlike with typhus, a rash is rare and, though Q fever is an acute illness, patients usually recover even in the absence of antibiotics.

The researchers to whom it fell to test for Q fever were Charles Shepard, the head of the CDC's Leprosy and Rickettsia Branch, and his assistant, Joe McDade. A bespectacled, blue-eyed scientist with a reputation for meticulous research, McDade had only just joined the CDC a year earlier. Thirty-six years old, he had previously been stationed with a Naval Medical Research Unit in North Africa, where he had worked on rickettsial diseases. In theory, this made McDade the perfect person for the job. However, at the time he had no experience of public health microbiology and looked to Shepard and other more experienced CDC hands for direction.[24] After his overseas posting, McDade found the work in Atlanta laborious and a little dull. Departing from standard tests and other procedural deviations was not encouraged, he recalled. Instead, he was expected to follow prescribed algorithms and testing procedures, entering the results in a matrix that would hopefully line up with the epidemiological evidence and bring about a resolution of the mystery. Working with lung tissue from deceased Legionnaires, McDade's first job was to grind up the autopsy material and inoculate it into guinea pigs. Q fever has an incubation period of a week to ten days, so the next stage was to wait. If a guinea pig developed fever, McDade euthanized the animal, removed some of its tissue, and injected it into an embryonic egg. In this way, he hoped to obtain sufficient numbers of bacteria that could be stained and examined.

Part of the reason for McDade's lack of enthusiasm was that at the time "everyone was looking for influenza or known causes of bacterial pneumonia," and there was no evidence that the Legionnaires had been exposed to live-stock, making Q fever highly unlikely. Sure enough, when he inoculated the material into guinea pigs they developed fever within two or three days, far earlier than if the organism had been *C. burnetii*. Modifying his procedure, McDade euthanized the guinea pigs prematurely and removed a section of their spleens. He then made impression smears on glass slides and stained them to see what organisms he could observe through the microscope. At the same time he used some of the tissue to prepare a suspension and streaked it on an agar plate to see if anything would grow on the media. Finally, he added anti-biotics to the mixture to inhibit the growth of any contaminants that might be lurking in the tissue and inoculated the material directly into embryonated eggs so as to grow rickettsia should they be present.

He found no evidence of rickettsia; all the eggs remained perfectly healthy for more than ten days. Nor was he able to recover any bacteria from the agar plates. However, as he peered at the smears through the microscope, McDade would occasionally spot a rod-shaped, Gram-negative bacterium, "one here and another there." Distrusting his observations, McDade shared the slides with more experienced colleagues, only to be told that guinea pigs were "notori-ously dirty animals" and what he had seen was most likely an "experimental contamination." "I was told there was an accumulating body of evidence that no bacteria were involved and what I had was an anomalous observation," he recalled. Instead, McDade was told to look for a virus.[25]

As McDade and Shepard's efforts faltered, other scientists, abetted by politi-cians in Washington, revived the toxic metal and chemical contaminant theories. The leading advocate of the toxic metals theory was Dr William F. Sunderman Jr., the head of laboratory medicine at the University of Connecticut School of Medicine. Early on in the outbreak, Sunderman and his father, William Sunderman Sr., professor of pathology at the Hahnemann Medical College, Philadelphia, had urged the public health authorities to collect urine and blood samples from suspected cases so they could be analyzed for toxic substances. The leading suspect in the Sundermans' view was nickel carbonyl. A colourless, odour-less metal, nickel carbonyl is widely used in industrial operations and is highly toxic. Symptoms can present themselves anywhere from one to ten days after exposure and typically include a severe headache, dizziness, and muscle pains. In the first hour after exposure, victims may also complain of shortness of breath and a dry cough. Without treatment, exposure can result in acute pneumonitis and bronchopneumonia with high fever.

In mid-September, the younger Sunderman had studied six lung tissue samples from patients with Legionnaires' disease and found that five contained unusually high levels of nickel. However, while this suggested the patients may have inhaled a toxic substance, nickel concentrations in other tissues and organs, such as the liver and kidney, were normal. To exclude the possibility that the elevated readings were due to accidental contamination, he would also need to test urine and blood from Legionnaires, but unfortunately, in the confusion of the early days of the outbreak, public health officials had failed to collect and preserve specimens for future testing. Despite these caveats, at a congressional hearing in November chaired by John M. Murphy, a Democrat from Staten Island, New York, the Sundermans were highly critical of the CDC and the "flaws" in its investigation—flaws that they attributed to the "zeal" of public health authorities to see Congress enact legislation indemnifying vaccine manufacturers against prosecution arising from the swine flu immunization program. Sunderman Sr. was particularly critical, agreeing with a recent newspaper article in the *Washington Post* that had accused the CDC of "eagerness bordering on mania ... to find swine flu in Pennsylvania."[26] Indeed, in his congressional testimony, he went further than his son had been prepared to do, stating definitively that the outbreak was due to nickel carbonyl poisoning.[27] Congressman Murphy was similarly critical, stating it was "inconceivable" that no one could say with any certainty whether the outbreak had been "murder; a virus; accidental introduction of a toxic substance; or a ... convergence of factors yet to be determined."[28] In particular, he described the lack of coordination between the CDC and other agencies as a national "embarrassment," telling House committee members that "nothing was done to search for toxic evidence until it was almost too late." Pointing out that "many experts [had] recognized the toxicological symptoms very early," he argued that the possibility of "foul play" could not be excluded and that toxic substances may have been placed on telephones, food or the Legionnaires' ice cubes. "It is entirely possible that a terrorist group or single fanatic might possess the technology to distribute a deadly poison or bacteria among a large group," he concluded.[29]

It was not the first time Murphy had sought to stoke paranoia about the anti-war movement. In October, aides to his committee had leaked a story to the *Washington Post* saying that congressional investigators believed "a demented veteran or paranoid anti-military type" with some knowledge of chemistry may have been responsible for the Legionnaires' deaths.[30] Such stories played to the suspicion and anxiety that infected American society in the mid-1970s, which, arguably, has only become more pronounced with time. A decade earlier, historian Richard Hofstadter had coined the term "paranoid style" to describe "the sense of heated exaggeration, suspiciousness, and conspiratorial fantasy" he detected in extreme right-wing movements, such as the 1964 campaign for the White House by Barry Goldwater, the militantly anti-communist Republican senator from Arizona.[31] By the 1970s, this paranoid style was arguably no longer confined to the Right, but following the assassination of leading lights of the civil rights movement was also beginning to infect the Left, hence the popularity of theories blaming the deaths of Jack and Bobby Kennedy and Martin Luther King on the CIA, the Mafia, and the Ku Klux Klan, or some combination of all three.

The early 1970s was also a time of growing anxiety about nuclear energy and the dangers of environmental and chemical pollutants, such as Agent Orange, the highly toxic herbicide sprayed on the Vietnamese countryside, which was just beginning to give rise to cancers and other unexplained health problems among Vietnam vets and their children. As Laurie Garrett has argued, from the perspective of the Left, "events in Philadelphia fit neatly with the then vogue view that an unregulated chemical industry was raining toxic compounds upon the American people."[32] By contrast, the Right was more inclined to view the outbreak as an act of sabotage, or as the Philadelphia Veterans of Foreign Wars put it, "a sneak attack against the finest kind of Americans."[33] This sense of moral panic did not escape Bob Dylan, who incorporated some of the wilder speculation into "Legionnaires' Disease," a song written for his touring guitarist.[34]

In retrospect this panic seems irrational, laughable even. After all, unlike cholera and plague, Legionnaires' disease was not contagious. Nor was it a disfiguring disease like smallpox, or one freighted with metaphors of waste and decay, like cancer and tuberculosis. On the other hand, the fact that its identity was unknown made it ripe for the projection of society's worst fears. Like Jack the Ripper, the mysterious killer had descended suddenly and unexpectedly on the Bellevue, then vacated the scene just as mysteriously. In the process, it had left few clues—or at least, none that the CDC's disease detectives had been able to parse—turning what was usually considered a safe and secure location into dangerous ground. It was a blow from which the Bellevue, already in financial trouble before the outbreak, would never recover. With newspapers using phrases like "mysterious and terrifying disease" and "the Philadelphia killer" to describe the outbreak, guests cancelled their reservations one by one.[35] The result was that on 10 November, the management announced the Bellevue was no longer able "to withstand the economic impact of the worldwide, adverse publicity" and closed its doors to further business.[36]

Not long after, Fraser decided it was also time for him to close the book on the EIS investigation and begin the laborious process of drafting his final report, known as an EPI-2. Despite going over the hotel with a fine-tooth comb and many hours of interviews, he was still no closer to identifying the pathogen or means of transmission. Privately, he was dismissive of the nickel carbonyl theory as the metal usually has an incubation period of less than thirty-six hours and rarely causes fevers above 101°F. Nor did he think it was food poisoning: the Legionnaires had purchased food from many different sources, and EIS officers had been unable to implicate a common meal at the convention. Similarly, although the cross-connection between the AHU and the Bellevue's potable water supply suggested a waterborne illness, more than one-third of the ill delegates insisted they had never drunk water at the hotel. By contrast, almost all the hotel employees, none of whom had suffered Legionnaires' disease, said they frequently drank from a fountain in the lobby.

In October, Fraser discussed the case with his boss, John V. Bennett. Bennett had been the lead investigator of the 1965 outbreak at St. Elizabeth's Hospital. Based on the epidemiology of the outbreak (the cases were associated with proximity to open windows), Bennett had suspected airborne transmission. However, all attempts to identify the aetiological agent had failed, so at the end of the investigation Bennett had filed the blood from St. Elizabeth's patients in the CDC's serum banks in the hope that it might prove useful at a later date. "When you solve the Legionnaires' outbreak you will solve my outbreak at St. Elizabeth's," he told Fraser.[37]

Mulling over Bennett's words, Fraser thought an airborne agent might explain the sickness of both the Legionnaires and Broad Street pneumonia cases—individuals who had passed by the hotel without entering it. Fraser also noted the strong association between illness and time spent in the lobby, and the fact that after the convention a fault had been discovered in the AHU serving the lobby area, prompting the hotel's management to have the filters cleaned. This cleaning operation had taken place on 6 August and "may have inadvertently limited the ability of investigators to identify a toxic or microbiologic agent in the air handling system," Fraser wrote in his report. On the other hand, the relatively low attack rate "may rule against an airborne agent to some degree." All that Fraser could say with confidence was that the illness resembled an infectious disease and there had been no secondary spread. Unfortunately, despite exhaustive microbiological studies, all the tests had been negative. It was possible that as new tests and technologies became available, new toxins capable of causing pneumonitis might be discovered, but that lay in the future. At present, "no toxin is known that causes just this pattern of disease," he concluded, "and toxicological studies are also negative so far."[38]

In all his years as an outbreak investigator Fraser had never come across a case quite like it; it stuck in the craw, but he had to admit defeat. So did Langmuir. The Philadelphia outbreak, he informed the press, constituted "the greatest epidemiological puzzle of the century."[39]

5

LEGIONNAIRES' REDUX

"The discovery of the etiologic agent of Legionnaires' disease was accomplished in the face of overwhelming odds. All of the combined bacteriology and pathology experience accumulated since the beginning of the century pointed away from this agent being a bacterium."

William H. Foege, Director of the CDC, Senate Subcommittee on Health and Scientific Research, 9 November 1977

In a period when antibiotics and vaccines seemed to have closed the book on infectious disease, the Legionnaires' outbreak challenged medical confidence that America was on the brink of a germ-free era. Little wonder then that the CDC's failure to solve the puzzle of the century produced a lingering sense of insecurity and anxiety. However, outside of medical and public health circles, the same sense of anxiety did not attach to swine flu. This is odd when you consider that CDC officials had been warning of an epidemic since February. Indeed, in late March, President Ford had gone on television to drive home the concerns that an outbreak of swine flu was imminent. Flanked by the two godfathers of the polio vaccine, the scientists Albert Sabin and Jonas Salk, Ford told the American public that he had been advised that "there is a very real possibility that unless we take effective counteractions, there could be an epidemic of this dangerous disease next fall and winter." Accordingly, he was seeking a $135 million appropriation from Congress for sufficient vaccine "to inoculate every man, woman, and child in the United States."[1]

Congress approved the appropriation bill in April, and by the middle of August had also passed legislation waiving corporate liability for the immunization campaign. Ironically, Congress's willingness to indemnify vaccine manufacturers had little to do with its enthusiasm for the insurance business and everything to do with the fears raised by the Philadelphia outbreak. Even though on

5 August Sencer had told senators he did not think the outbreak was due to swine flu, politicians were petrified he might be wrong and that they would end up being branded obstructionists who had impeded the delivery of a life-saving vaccine.[2] Nonetheless, scientists' and politicians' enthusiasm for the flu immunization campaign was not shared by the public, with a Gallup poll in September indicating that only about half of all Americans were willing to be immunized.[3] In other words, faced with a repeat of an epidemic on the scale of 1918, the public's response was to shrug its shoulders. This indifference turned to resistance when at the beginning of October the campaign finally got under way. Within ten days, one million Americans had rolled up their sleeves and received the jab, but on 11 October the campaign suffered a disastrous blow when it was reported that three elderly people in Pittsburgh, Pennsylvania, had died hours after having the inoculation. The deaths prompted a media scare that led to nine states suspending their vaccination programs. To calm the public's nerves and restore confidence, President Ford and his family were photographed receiving jabs at the White House. CDC scientists, meanwhile, attempted to educate the public, explaining that the risk of temporally associated deaths within forty-eight hours of inoculation occurred at a rate of 5/100,000 a day. By comparison, the anticipated death rate per day for *all* causes among citizens in Pennsylvania was 17/100,000. In other words, it was to be expected that some people would die after receiving the flu shot, but that did not mean there was a causal connection.[4]

Unfortunately, by 1976 the public's unquestioning acceptance of scientific authority was beginning to wane, as were memories of life before vaccines against polio, measles, and other debilitating childhood diseases. Moreover, by now influenza experts in other countries were beginning to question the American scientific consensus that the swine flu isolated at Fort Dix was the harbinger of a new pandemic strain, a scepticism shared by WHO officials in Geneva who advocated a "wait and see" policy.[5] As October turned to November with no signs of the feared pandemic, scepticism hardened. Still, the campaign might have been saved were it not for reports of cases of Guillain-Barré syndrome (GBS). A rare and occasionally lethal neurological syndrome, GBS occurs at a steady rate in the general population and, if a pandemic had been occurring, would have been deemed an acceptable risk. However, in the absence of a pandemic, the reports in December that as many as thirty people had developed the syndrome within a month of receiving the flu jab sparked widespread alarm, prompting the government to suspend the campaign so that the association with the vaccine could be investigated. The program was never restarted, and as cases of the syndrome soared—by the end of December, 526 cases were being reported, of which 257 had received the flu jab—the press and politicians in Washington began looking for a fall guy. The *New York Times* was especially harsh, labelling the campaign a "fiasco" and, in view of the fact that the pandemic had never materialized, a waste of time and effort.[6] The result was that when Jimmy Carter moved into the White House in January, Joseph Califano Jr., the incoming secretary of Health, Education, and Welfare (HEW), demanded Sencer's resignation. Shamefully, Califano informed Sencer of his dismissal minutes before the pair were due to appear together at a meeting in Washington on the moratorium of the swine flu programme. Worse, the whispered conversation in an HEW hallway was captured by the TV cameras, deepening Sencer's humiliation. According to public health historian George Dehner, this was "shabby treatment" for someone who had given sixteen years of service to the CDC, eleven as its director. On the other hand, Dehner writes, in his efforts to convince administration officials of the vaccination campaign's necessity, Sencer had deliberately downplayed the scientific uncertainty so as to give "a distorted vision of the new virus." The result was that "only the most dire vision of a swine flu pandemic remained."[7]

Ironically, just three weeks before Sencer's very public firing, Shepard had rushed into his office to announce that he and McDade had solved the puzzle of the century. The culprit was a hitherto unknown Gram-negative bacterium. Other researchers had missed it because the bacterium was difficult to see using a conventional Gram stain. However, McDade had solved the problem using a different staining technique. According to Garrett, after all the pressure and frustration of the past year, Sencer was reluctant to accept what Shepard was telling him. "Shep, how sure are you?" "Better than 95 per cent," he replied, "but I'd like to run a few more experiments before we go public."[8]

There is an old saying in medical research: "fortune favours the prepared mind." The saying is usually attributed to Louis Pasteur, who famously stumbled on a vaccine against chicken cholera in 1880 when a colleague inoculated some chickens with an old culture of chicken cholera germs.[9] In McDade's case, however, it was because he was a novice to public health microbiology and therefore not schooled in the same thought processes as his colleagues that a chance observation led him to the answer that had eluded them. It also helped that McDade was a worrier and a perfectionist. To his way of thinking, the peculiar rod-shaped bacteria he had weakly glimpsed through his microscope in August represented a loose end, and he didn't like it. However, it was not until late December that he thought to return to the problem. The impetus was a conversation with a man who had cornered him at a party shortly before Christmas. "I don't know how he knew I was CDC but he did," recalled McDade. "He said, 'We know you scientists are a little weird but we count on you and we're very disappointed.' I stuttered because I didn't know what to say. But it bothered me and stuck in my mind."[10]

It had always been McDade's habit to use the week between Christmas and New Year's to resolve any outstanding paperwork in preparation for the new working year. While tidying his office he spotted the glass slides with the smears he had taken from the guinea pigs in a box on the shelf and decided to have another look. The exercise, he recalled, was like "searching for a missing contact lens on a basketball court with your eyes four inches away from the floor." Eventually, however, McDade spotted a cluster of organisms in the corner of one of the microscopic fields. To McDade's way of thinking, the fact that the organisms were clustered together "suggested that it wasn't just organisms that happened to be there but were actually growing there inside the guinea pig." It was at this point that McDade decided to have another go at culturing the organism. His thinking was, "if I can rule out that it has nothing to do with the disease my conscience will be salved and I can go about my business." It was at this point that McDade's expertise as a rickettsial specialist and his willingness to depart from conventional patterns of thought came into play. Going to the freezer drawers containing spleen tissue from suspect guinea pigs that had been put on ice in August, McDade thawed the samples and inoculated some of the tissue into embryonated eggs. However, this time he withheld antibiotics in order to allow whatever organisms were present in the guinea pig tissue to grow freely. Five to seven days later the eggs died and McDade took new smears. As before, he applied a Gimenez stain, a technique which had been developed specifically for rickettsial organisms, and, once again, spotted the same rod-shaped bacteria growing in clusters. Could these bacteria be responsible for the guinea pigs' deaths, and could the same bacteria be responsible for the Legionnaires' disease outbreak? To answer the question, McDade retrieved some preserved serum from the Legionnaires' cases and mixed it with the organism he had found in the eggs. If a patient's serum contained antibodies specific to the organism, an observable reaction would take place. It did. "They just lit up dramatically," he said. "My neck hair bristled. I wasn't sure what I'd got there but I knew it was something."

McDade immediately shared his findings with Shepard, and together they ran further tests using paired serum samples taken from Legionnaires two or more weeks apart. If it could be shown that the reaction took place at much higher dilution in the second serum sample than in the first, this would be strong evidence that the patient had recently recovered from the disease caused by the organism. At the same time, McDade and Shepard repeated the test using blinded samples from both Legionnaires' and non-Legionnaires' patients, some of whom had had other pneumonias or were healthy. Nearly fifty years later, McDade vividly recounted the moment of discovery:

> When we'd finished all the tests, later that evening, they brought down the paper and we broke the code. All the normal specimens from healthy people were negative, specimens from patients with other pneumonias were all negative. Then we looked at the Legionnaires' disease specimens. Specimens taken from Legionnaires early in the illness had little or no antibodies, and specimens taken later in illness had very high levels of antibody, which suggested they had been infected with this bacteria. So that was the moment when we knew we'd found the aetiologic agent.[11]

When Shepard informed Sencer of the breakthrough he could hardly contain his excitement and insisted that they issue an announcement in the next edition of the *Morbidity and Mortality Weekly Report*, the CDC's house journal, and schedule a press conference for the same day, 18 January 1977. This was earlier than Shepard and McDade had been anticipating—normally, scientific discoveries take several months to be written up before being submitted to a scientific journal. Because of the political pressure on Sencer, however, he could not wait for the usual peer review process. Worried that they would be laughing stocks if their methodology was subsequently found to be faulty, Shepard and McDade double-checked their results. Then, out of curiosity, McDade decided to look in the CDC's stores for serum from other unsolved outbreaks. That's when he came across the stored blood from the patients at St. Elizabeth's Hospital. McDade injected the blood into chicken eggs, then added the organism he had isolated in Philadelphia. The eggs lit up immediately, indicating that there was an antibody reaction and that the St. Elizabeth's patients had been infected with the same organism. Bennett's intuition had been correct: in solving the Philadelphia outbreak, Fraser and his team had also solved the mystery of the earlier outbreak in Washington, DC.

News of Shepard and McDade's discovery travelled around the world, prompting scientists at other research establishments in Europe and elsewhere to duplicate the CDC's results. As scientists exchanged information and examined old case files, it became apparent that St. Elizabeth's was not the only prior outbreak of Legionnaires' disease. Blood specimens from patients at the Oakland County Health Department in Pontiac, Michigan, in 1968 also tested positive for antibodies to *Legionella pneumophila*, as the organism was now known, suggesting that they had been infected by the same agent, though why there had been no pneumonia in the "Pontiac Fever" cases and why the outbreak had not resulted in any fatalities was unclear. That was not all: in May 1977, Marilyn Bozeman, a rickettsia specialist at the Walter Reed Army Institute of Research, in Bethesda, Maryland, informed McDade that she had seen very similar organisms in guinea pigs while investigating specimens taken from an outbreak in 1959. Like McDade, she had assumed these were contaminants and described them as "rickettsia-like."[12] It was only later, when she ran new tests, that she found they were actually two new species of legionella, *Legionella bozemanii* and *Legionella micdadei*. It was subsequently found that *L. micdadei* had also been responsible for an outbreak of "Fort Bragg fever" in 1943 and that Walter Reed also had an isolate of *L. pneumophila* dating from 1947.[13]

Then, in early summer, came news of an outbreak at a medical centre in Burlington, Vermont. EIS officers rushed to the scene, and by September they had documented sixty-nine cases of Legionnaires' disease. However, once again, the source of the exposure eluded them.[14] Soon, there were reports of other outbreaks in hospitals across the United States. The most notable was an outbreak that began at the Wadsworth Medical Center, a veterans' hospital in Los Angeles, in the summer and which by the end of the year had claimed sixteen lives. At around the same time, a smaller epidemic broke out at a hospital in Nottingham, England, sickening fifteen people. Once again, no common source was found, but two of the sera from patients sent to the CDC for analysis tested positive for antibodies to legionella.[15] That was not all: in 1978 CDC scientists confirmed that legionella had been responsible for a mysterious outbreak of pneumonia at the Rio Park hotel in Benidorm, Spain, that had been blamed for the deaths of three Scottish holidaymakers five years earlier.[16] The result was that when, in 1980, another outbreak occurred at the same hotel, epidemiologists took water samples and found the bacterium lurking in the shower heads. Apparently, an old water well had been brought back into use five days before the start of the outbreak and had fed water infected with *L. pneumophila* directly into the hotel. Investigators concluded that those who showered and washed first thing each morning were at most risk because the bacteria multiplied overnight in water standing in peripheral pipe work. In all, a total of fifty-eight people were sickened, and one woman died. Like the outbreak at the Bellevue, the Rio Park outbreak sparked considerable press interest and inspired the thriller writer Desmond Bagley to pen a novel, *Bahama Crisis* (1980), in which a Caribbean holiday resort's water system is deliberately seeded with Legionella bacteria in an act of industrial espionage.[17]

By now, it was becoming clear that Legionnaires' disease was closely associated with hotels, hospitals and other large buildings. But though it was suspected that cooling towers and modern air conditioning systems facilitated the spread of the organism, attempts to isolate *L. pneumophila* from the cooling towers of hospitals failed. Then, in 1978, came a breakthrough with the report of an outbreak in the heart of Manhattan's garment district. By September, the CDC had identified seventeen cases, the majority of them centred around a building on 35th Street between Seventh Avenue and Broadway. On the CDC's advice, the city ordered businesses in the immediate vicinity to switch off their air conditioners. The agency then collected epidemiological samples from nearby buildings, including the cooling tower on the roof of Macy's Department Store located directly opposite the building on 35th Street. The sample tested positive for legionella, but the CDC did not have sufficient epidemiological evidence to say the Macy's cooling tower was to blame.[18] However, earlier that year, investigators had attended another outbreak at the Indiana Memorial Union and recovered *L. pneumophila* from the Union's cooling tower, so it was pretty obvious that cooling towers were responsible for many of the outbreaks. In addition, scientists found a nearby stream teeming with other species of the same bacteria, suggesting that the organism was widespread in the environment.[19]

Currently, the genus *Legionella* comprises nearly forty different species[20] and sixty-one serogroups.* However, it is one species, *L. pneumophila*, that is responsible for 90 per cent of Legionnaires' disease cases. A facultative intracellular parasite, it is unable to grow outside of cells. Instead, it has evolved to live in natural aquatic environments, such as lakes, streams, ponds and ground water. These environments are teeming with amoebae and protozoa that routinely ingest other ubiquitous bacteria as food. However, legionellae are able to evade these microbial processes and "trick" the amoeba into ingesting them. Once inside an amoeba, the bacterium multiplies intracellularly before releasing dozens of newly formed legionellae into the water. The new organisms then try to trick other amoebae into ingesting them. In this way, legionellae are considered "Trojan horse" bacteria.[21]

Under natural conditions, water rarely reaches the temperatures necessary for the bacteria to multiply (legionellae grow best at temperatures of 72°F to 113°F), ensuring that populations are kept to safe levels. Man-made environments are different, however. Hotels, hospitals, and other large buildings are

---

* A serogroup is a group of bacteria that share a common antigen.

home to a number of devices that utilize water at ideal temperatures for the growth of legionella bacteria. These include showerheads, hot tubs, whirlpool spas, water fountains, humidifiers, misting equipment, and architectural fountains. Cooling towers are of particular concern because the pools of warm water are open to the atmosphere—indeed, legionella bacteria have been repeatedly isolated from the biofilms of slime and encrusted sludge on top of such towers, with some surveys indicating that as many as half of all cooling towers in the United States may be contaminated with the organisms.[22] If such towers are not regularly serviced, this contaminated water can be aerosolized into microscopic droplets containing legionella, enabling the organism to be drawn directly into a person's lungs. One way this may occur is during the cooling process, when warm water from the condenser or chiller unit is sprayed across the fill at the top of a cooling tower, splintering the water into tiny droplets. While most of the water returns to the collecting pan to be circulated to the heat source to cool refrigerant from the air conditioning unit, some of the water is aerosolized, resulting in the production of a fine mist at the top of the tower. If a drift eliminator is not fitted to the tower or the eliminator is inadequate, this mist may then be drawn into nearby air intake vents and air shafts.[23] Under certain temperature conditions, the mist can also cascade down the side of the building to ground level, from where it may be drawn in through open windows or inhaled by passing pedestrians. A third possible route of contamination is the pipework supplying potable water to showers and so forth, especially where hot water systems are run intermittently and water is left to stand for long periods in pipes. Finally, in theory, contamination can also occur if there is a direct link from the water tower to the chilled water supply of an air conditioning unit.

One reason legionella is so dangerous is that the same strategy that enables the organism to evade ingestion by amoebae also enables the organism to escape attack by the alveolar macrophages, the body's first line of defence against lung infections. Instead, legionellae multiply within the cells of the alveoli, before spilling out and colonizing other lung cells. If other host defence responses are not activated in time, the result is pneumonia and systemic illness.

In the United States, the incidence of Legionnaires' disease varies from state to state, with the highest incidence being recorded in the summer and autumn. Those aged sixty and over are at greatest risk, especially if they suffer from chronic lung disease or have other underlying medical conditions. The disease also occurs more frequently in men than women, though whether this is due to the higher prevalence of cigarette smoking and lung disease in men, or some other predisposing factor, is not known (cigarette smokers have a two- to fourfold higher risk of developing Legionnaires' disease than non-smokers). Hospitals present a particular risk because of inadequate servicing of hot water systems and the way that such settings bring together large numbers of immunocompromised patients. Confined to their beds for long periods in wards, these patients, many of whom may be suffering from other conditions and have compromised immune systems, present the organism with the ideal host. Surveys have also found that modern medical technologies such as immunosuppressive therapies, intubation, anaesthesia, and the placing of nasogastric tubes also increase the risk of pneumonias due to Legionnaires' disease.[24]

In 1978, the CDC held an international meeting to review what had been learned about legionella, its epidemiology and its ecology. By now, McDade had perfected a technique for visualizing the organism using a special silver stain that coloured the walls of the Gram-negative bacteria. Meanwhile, other researchers were learning how to cultivate it on charcoal yeast agar, a special medium supplemented with iron and cysteine. In addition, using a fluorescent-antibody staining technique, CDC researchers had demonstrated that organisms observed by pathologists in lung tissue recovered from Legionnaires in Philadelphia were in fact *L. pneumophila*.[25] Unfortunately, however, the final piece of evidence—legionella from the water tower on the roof of the Bellevue—eluded investigators as the hotel had now been closed and the tower and the air conditioning units thoroughly cleaned. Nevertheless, in light of the outbreaks seen at hospitals and other buildings in the United States, Fraser had little doubt that the hotel's water tower had been to blame. Noting that the convention had coincided with a marked temperature inversion in Philadelphia, he speculated that this inversion could have caused mist from the tower to come across the edge of the roof and "cascade down the side of the building."[26] In this way, the contaminated air could have enveloped people on the sidewalk and been sucked into the lobby through a vent near the ground floor, thus accounting for both the cases observed among delegates and the Broad Street pneumonias. There were two further pieces of evidence implicating the Bellevue. The first was the discovery of antibodies to legionella in eleven members of another convention group that had visited the hotel two years earlier and whose members had suffered similar fevers and pneumonias. The second was a survey of hotel staff who had been employed at the hotel at around the same time. They also had antibodies to legionella. This suggested that hotel staff had been exposed from time to time and had managed to acquire immunity, which was why so few of them had succumbed to the infection in 1976. By contrast, the Legionnaires had no such history of exposure.

* * *

The Legionnaires' disease outbreak is a classic example of how new technologies and changes to the built environment designed to improve hygiene and ameliorate the conditions of life are constantly giving rise to new threats to health and well-being. It also illustrates how, in certain political and cultural contexts, epidemics that might otherwise have gone unnoticed can command wide public attention and provoke considerable anxiety.

L. pneumophila has been around for millennia, but it was not until we began building cities and equipping buildings with indoor plumbing and hot water systems that we presented the bacterium with a new ecological niche in which to prosper. And it was not until we added other luxuries, such as air conditioning, showers, humidifiers and misters, that we gave the bacterium an efficient way to aerosolize and colonize the human respiratory tract. Even so, it took several years for doctors and public health experts to wake up to the pathogenic threat posed by the presence of this ancient organism in the heart of modern metropolises.

One reason is that prior to the invention of a method for culturing the bacterium and diagnosing legionella infections, Legionnaires' disease was indistinguishable from other atypical pneumonias for which a causative agent had yet to be identified. This made it largely invisible to physicians and respiratory disease experts who believed that pneumonia was largely a problem of the past. Even where outbreaks were sufficiently unusual to draw the attention of doctors and public health experts, as had been the case at St. Elizabeth's Hospital in 1965 and Pontiac, Michigan in 1968, investigations were inconclusive and had reached dead ends. This might also have been the fate of the CDC's inquiry into the outbreak at the Bellevue. That it was not is due, first, to its occurrence at a time of acute national anxiety about another epidemic disease, and second, to the intense media interest in the outbreak, sparked both by the focus on swine flu and by the fact that the victims were a venerated and vulnerable section of the American population. However, for all the resources at the CDC's disposal, in the final analysis these factors might have counted for nothing had it not been for the determination of one scientist and his willingness to set aside preconceived notions and patterns of thought.

By 1976, medical researchers were confident that they had identified all the leading causes of pneumonia and that, in any case, the condition responded to treatment with penicillin or one of the new generation of anti-biotics, such as erythromycin and rifampicin. What few realized was that only half of sporadic pneumonia cases could be determined with existing diagnos-tic tests, much less that there had been several outbreaks for which a causal agent had never been identified.[27] When examining pathology specimens and bacterial cultures, laboratory technicians had been taught to look, first, for the pneumococcus and, if that was absent, other known bacterial and myco-bacterial causes of the disease. Using long-established culturing and staining techniques, it was possible to grow these bacteria on laboratory media and then colour them with Gram stains or other common dyes. But what of an organism that could not be cultivated on the usual media and which, because it lacked a cell wall, could not be easily visualized with existing stains either? What, in other words, of an unknown unknown? This was the problem that confronted McDade when, using a stain developed for rickettsia, he peered through his microscope and spotted a faint rod-shaped organism growing in clusters. Because the organism did not conform to any of the known bacterial causes of pneumonia, McDade's colleagues insisted it must be a "contami-nant." That is what their experience of cultivating bacteria in guinea pigs and their microbiology training had taught them. By contrast, McDade's mind was unprepared by previous experience for such an observation, and the more he ruminated on it the more he became concerned. What if it was the stain and not experimental error that had brought the bacteria to light, and what if his observation was not an anomaly? Thus it was that a chance observation led McDade in the direction opposite to that of his colleagues and to an eventual resolution of the problem.

Legionnaires' disease also illustrates the role of medical technology and human behaviour in shaping our interactions with pathogens. It was not sim-ply that water towers and air conditioning systems afforded an old bacterium a new place in which to breed; to provoke an outbreak, the bacterium also had to meet a group of highly susceptible individuals. This happened first at hos-pitals and medical centres, where the expansion in intensive care beds in the 1960s and the growing number of elderly or mentally ill patients receiving institutional treatment increased the bacterium's chances of finding an appro-priate host. However, it also occurred at meatpacking plants and other large industrial premises with chiller units. And, of course, it also happened at luxury hotels and other large buildings with cooling towers and state-of-the-art air conditioning systems. The Bellevue was not alone in installing a Carrier refrigeration unit in the 1950s. In 1952, in preparation for that year's Republican and Democratic conventions, engineers from the Carrier

Company brought air conditioning to the International Amphitheatre in Chicago. Six years later, Carrier installed similar units in the Fidelity Building in Los Angeles, making it the first fully air-conditioned office building in California. By the end of the decade, air conditioning had also arrived in domestic homes, fuelling migration to Florida and other "Sun Belt" states. The result was that by 1969, when Carrier announced that the towers of New York's World Trade Center would be cooled and heated by its equipment, no American office or home, large or small, was considered complete without air conditioning.[28]

At the time, of course, no one realized that cooling towers and air conditioners presented an infectious disease risk. This only became significant after January 1977, when Joe McDade's isolation of *L. pneumophila* resulted in the discovery of the organism in other buildings across the United States. Once *L. pneumophila* had been identified, researchers were able to show it submitted to treatment with erythromycin and rifampicin, drugs that quickly became the standard therapy. The result is that today legionella is recognized around the world as an important cause of community-acquired pneumonia outbreaks, prompting routine checks on the cooling towers of hotels and hospitals. That is not to say the threat has disappeared: despite the wider availability of diagnostic tests, legionella is thought to be responsible for around 2 per cent of pneumonia cases in the United States annually (around 50,000 cases).[29] Moreover, outbreaks continue to occur with disturbing regularity wherever public water management standards or the inspection and cleaning of private water towers is found wanting. For instance, between 2014 and 2015, ninety people in Flint, Michigan, contracted Legionnaires' disease and twelve died after the town switched its water source from Detroit's system to the Flint River. And in 2015, New York City experienced the largest Legionnaires' outbreak in its history when the organism sickened 133 people living in apartment blocks in the South Bronx, killing sixteen. It later transpired that the source of the outbreak was a hotel water tower teeming with legionella bacteria. In the most recent period for which figures are available—2000 to 2014—the CDC recorded almost a threefold increase in cases of legionellosis, which comprises both Legionnaires' disease and Pontiac fever, across the United States. Of these, 5,000 cases a year were due to Legionnaires' alone and the mortality rate was 9 per cent.[30] Of course, not all these outbreaks were the result of poorly maintained water systems or aging plumbing. America's aging population, the wider availability of diagnostic tests, and more reliable reporting to local and state health departments and the CDC most likely also played a role. A further factor may be climate change: as summers become hotter and unseasonably warm temperatures continue into the autumn, the more likely it is that plumes of contaminated water will issue from water towers unless effective chlorination and other disinfectant measures are taken. Unfortunately, all too frequently, they are not.

To the extent that Legionnaires' disease tapped into Cold War fears about biological weapons and chemical toxins, it seemed to hark back to the preoccupations of the 1950s; hence, Congress's concern that it was a "missed alarm." But to the extent that it was a disease completely new to medical science, and one that could be traced to new technologies and alterations to the built environment, it seemed to represent a new paradigm of public health, one that would become increasingly relevant in the closing decades of the twentieth century. Indeed, by 1994, with the publication of Laurie Garrett's *The Coming Plague*, Legionnaires' disease was being seen as one of a series of "emerging infectious diseases" (EIDs), whose appearance was threatening to undo the medical advances of the post-war years and, with them, the certitude that advanced industrialized societies no longer needed to fear the plagues that had bedevilled previous eras. That the outbreak in Philadelphia in 1976 had coincided with the emergence the same year of a new viral haemorrhagic fever at a remote mission hospital in Yambuku, Zaire, close to the Ebola River, only served to underline these parallels; hence, the disease's inclusion in an iconic list of EIDs drawn up by the Institute of Medicine in 1992. The authors' biggest concern, however, was not Legionnaires' disease or Ebola, but HIV, a previously unknown virus that had first become visible to medical science in around 1981, and which by 1992 was recognized as the agent of one of the largest pandemics in history.

6

AIDS IN AMERICA, AIDS IN AFRICA

"This is a very, very dramatic illness. I think we can say, quite assuredly, that it is new."

James Curran, epidemiologist, 1982

In December 1980, Dr Michael Gottlieb was looking for an unusual teaching case to present to residents at the University of California Medical Center Los Angeles (UCLA) when one of his colleagues stumbled on a patient named Michael. A 33-year-old artist, Michael had been admitted to the emergency room suffering from extreme weight loss and looked like an anorexic. In addition, his mouth was full of thrush, or candidiasis, a yeast infection usually seen in patients with weakened immune systems. Intrigued, Gottlieb, then a young assistant professor specializing in immunology, led residents to Michael's bedside and afterwards discussed the case with them. "There was something medically interesting about him," Gottlieb recalled. "He *smelled* like an immune deficiency."[1]

Gottlieb's intuition was correct: Michael's antibody-producing capacity seemed to be intact, but when a colleague ran a specialized test using the latest monoclonal antibody technology he discovered that Michael had very few T cells.[2] In particular, he found that a subset of Michael's T cells, known as CD4 cells, were perilously low. The central controllers of the immune system, CD4 cells are required for every type of immune response—whether to signal CD8 "killer" cells, whose job it is to destroy virus-infected cells; activate macrophages, a type of white blood cell that patrols for pathogens; or alert B lymphocytes, which produce antibodies against foreign invaders. Once these CD4 cells have been eliminated, sooner or later the entire immune system crashes. Their absence almost certainly explained the thrush. According to Gottlieb, the yeast infection was so extensive that Michael's mouth looked as if it was full of "cottage cheese." But it was impossible to arrive at a definitive diagnosis, so Michael was discharged. However, within a week he had developed pneumonia and had to be readmitted.

Concerned that Michael might have contracted an opportunistic lung infection, Gottlieb convinced a pulmonary specialist to perform a bronchoscopy and send a sample of his lung tissue to the laboratory. To Gottlieb's surprise, the tissue came back positive for *Pneumocystis carinii pneumonia*, or PCP, a rare fungal infection seen almost exclusively in malnourished newborns and infants in intensive care, terminally ill cancer patients, or the recipients of organ transplants.[3] What such patients shared in common was compromised immune systems. For a young man to develop PCP was practically unheard of. "It was a distinctly unusual thing for someone previously healthy to walk into a hospital so significantly ill. It just didn't fit any recognized disease or syndrome that we were aware of."[4] By March, Michael had been hospitalized, but no amount of drugs or experimental therapies would arrest the progress of the infection, and in May 1981 he died. The autopsy found *Pneumocystis* throughout his lungs. Later, trying to figure out what could have caused Michael's immune system to give up on him, Gottlieb reviewed the artist's medical charts and saw that he had a cornucopia of sexually transmitted diseases (STDs). He also recalled a conversation in which Michael had mentioned that he was gay, but then Los Angeles had long boasted a sizable gay community, so it was difficult to see what bearing this could have on the matter.

Gottlieb was not the only doctor in Los Angeles to spot an unusual constellation of symptoms in gay men that autumn and winter. The previous October, Joel Weisman, a local physician with a largely gay practice, had also treated two men for thrush. In addition, the men had chronic fevers and suffered from diarrhoea and lymphadenopathy—swollen lymph nodes. In February one of the men's symptoms worsened and he was admitted to UCLA, where Gottlieb tested his blood and found the same abnormality that Michael had: a lower than expected number of CD4 cells. Soon after, he also developed PCP, as did the second patient in Weisman's care. In addition, both men had active cytomegalovirus (CMV), a type of herpes virus which is spread in bodily fluids, typically through kissing and sex, and which is usually quiescent in healthy adults.[5] By April Gottlieb was becoming sufficiently concerned to call a former student, Wayne Shandera, now a member of the CDC's Epidemic Intelligence Service in Los Angeles. Gottlieb told Shandera of his suspicion that there was a new disease circulating in Los Angeles and asked him to check the LA County health records for other reports of PCP and/or CMV. Shandera quickly located a report about a man in Santa Monica who had recently been diagnosed with *Pneumocystis* and was deathly ill in the hospital. Soon after Shandera's visit, the man died and, on autopsy, CMV was found in his lungs.[6]

Unbeknownst to Gottlieb and Weisman, by now physicians in New York were also seeing similar cases of swollen lymph nodes, low CD4 cell counts, and PCP in gay men in their care. At autopsy many were also found to be infected with CMV. Observing these patients up close was a shocking experience. Donna Mildvan, chief of infectious disease at Beth Israel Hospital, New York, recorded how in one case involving a German man who had formerly worked as a chef in Haiti and who had died in December, she had cultured CMV directly from his eyeball. "We were totally bewildered. ... I can't even begin to tell you what an awful experience it was." Dr Alvin Friedman-Kien, a dermatologist and virologist at New York University's Medical Center, was similarly disturbed to find that many of the patients also had Kaposi's sarcoma (KS), an extremely rare type of skin cancer typically seen in elderly Jewish men or men of eastern European and Mediterranean descent. Most dermatologists might go their whole career and see only one case of KS, but by February Friedman-Kien was aware of twenty cases of KS in the New York area alone. One of the most heart-breaking involved a young Shakespearean actor who presented at Friedman-Kien's practice in January with pink-purple spots on his face. The spots were so extensive, Friedman-Kien recalled, "he couldn't cover them up anymore."[7]

In medicine, as in other professions, being first is everything—no one remembers the second person to describe a new disease—and by June Gottlieb was ready to go into print, informing the editor of the *New England Journal of Medicine* that he had "possibly a bigger story than Legionnaires' Disease."[8] By now Gottlieb had five severe pneumonia cases (the fifth had come to him via a Beverly Hills physician). All were gay men between the ages of twenty-nine and thirty-six, all had PCP, candidiasis and CMV, and three had low CD4 cell counts (in the two others, immune deficiency had not been studied). In addition, Gottlieb and Weisman noted, all five had also used "poppers"—amyl nitrate or butyl nitrate inhalers so named for the noise the ampules make when broken.[9] However, their leading hypothesis at this stage was that the disease was due to CMV and, perhaps, some other virus, such as Epstein-Barr, interacting with one another so as to compromise the immune system. From a public health point of view this was worrying. Sexual health clinics across the United States had recently seen a marked increase in CMV cases which, along with other sexually transmitted diseases, such as hepatitis B and gonorrhoea, were running at epidemic levels in the gay community.

Given the interest in getting the announcement out quickly, the editor of the *New England Journal of Medicine* advised Gottlieb to submit a brief article to the CDC's Sexually Transmitted Diseases division for publication in the agency's house journal, *Morbidity and Mortality Weekly Report*, on the understanding that the *New England Journal of Medicine* would consider a longer article at a later date. Jim Curran, the official who headed the STD division, immediately recognized the article's significance, not least because he was concerned about the recent increase in STDs in gay men and had been working closely with the homosexual community to evaluate the risk factors for hepatitis B. Before publishing the article, however, he asked a female colleague to check whether there had been any other reports of PCP in people without cancer, or who had not received organ transplants and had been taking drugs to suppress their immune systems. Looking back over fifteen years, she could find only one such case. Alarmingly, however, orders for pentamidine, an anti-PCP drug that was no longer in commercial production and of which the CDC had a small emergency stock, had jumped from the usual fifteen requests a year to thirty in the first five months of 1981.[10] Curran did not require further convincing, and on 5 June 1981, he published Gottlieb's article in the *Morbidity and Mortality Weekly Report* together with an accompanying editorial. Noting that PCP was almost exclusively limited to severely immunosuppressed patients, Curran commented that its occurrence in previously healthy individuals was "unsettling," and the fact that all five individuals were gay suggested "an association between some aspect of a homosexual lifestyle or disease acquired through sexual contact and *Pneumocystis* pneumonia in this population." Although no definite conclusion could be reached about the role of CMV infections, Curran also noted recent surveys showing that many homosexual men carried CMV in their semen and that "seminal fluid may be an important vehicle of CMV transmission." In other words, there was no evidence that CMV was the cause of the mysterious new syndrome, but sexual transmission was suspected. Though hedged with qualifications, Curran's conclusion was prophetic: "All the above observations suggest the possibility of a cellular-immune dysfunction related to a common exposure that predisposes individuals to opportunistic infections such as pneumocystis and candidiasis."[11] No one could have imagined that within months of that article appearing, these strange symptoms would be the talk of Hollywood, and by the following summer the world would have learned a terrifying new acronym. Curran may not have realized it but he had just described AIDS, Acquired Immunodeficiency Syndrome.

* * *

In the forty years since—the CDC settled on the acronym in 1982—public attitudes toward AIDS have gone from indifference, to horror and dread, to seeing it as just another infectious disease, one that can be treated with an arsenal of drugs that suppress but never quite eliminate the Human Immunodeficiency Virus (HIV), which is the cause of the immune deficiency that allows the opportunistic infections with which AIDS is associated to occur. In this transition from fear to familiarity, it is easy to forget the shocking sight of the first AIDS patients and the dismay they provoked in doctors powerless to help them. As David Ho, a physician at the Cedars-Sinai Medical Center, recalled, those early patients "looked like concentration camp survivors." Adding to the dismay was the fact that the causes were "completely unknown."[12] As the true extent of the epidemic became evident—in 1982 the number of AIDS cases in the United States totalled 593; two years later there were nearly 7,000 cases and there had been over 4,000 deaths—AIDS came to be regarded as a plague (the "gay plague" to be specific) and the signal of a disastrous return to a former historical epoch when "the" plague and other epidemic diseases had routinely ravaged human communities. If Legionnaires' disease had been a warning to an overly complacent public health profession, then AIDS was the epidemic that drove home the lesson: despite vaccines, antibiotics and other medical technologies, infectious disease had not been banished but posed a continuing and present threat to technologically advanced societies. Worse, as scientists learned more about the disease and its origins, it soon became apparent that sex and medical technologies—in particular, the wide provision of hypodermic needles and reusable syringes via public health programmes and other humanitarian medical initiatives in Africa, plus blood banks and blood transfusion services—had greatly amplified transmission of the virus, transforming what had been scattered, isolated cases in Africa into a widely dispersed infection which eventually became a pandemic. Even so, no one could have imagined that by the end of the twentieth century 14 million people would have died of AIDS globally and 33 million more would be living with the virus. Or that by 2015, a further 36 million people around the world would have contracted HIV, and some 40 million would be dead, a figure that approaches the mortality of the Spanish flu.[13]

As we shall see, the AIDS pandemic was not only the result of technological interventions; as with psittacosis, economic, social and cultural factors also likely played a part. In particular, the emergence of AIDS appears to have been connected to the construction in the colonial period of new railways and roads in equatorial regions of Central Africa, projects that fuelled the influx of male labourers into rural areas, destabilizing gender relations and fostering a culture of prostitution in Léopoldville (Kinshasa) and other large towns and cities. The loosening of sexual taboos following gay liberation was a similarly important factor in the spread of AIDS in the United States, particularly in cities like New York and San Francisco where bathhouses became venues for unprotected anal sex between men boasting multiple sexual partners. However, it would appear that such practices only contributed to the explosion of AIDS in America after HIV had been imported to the United States from Haiti in the late 1960s.

In many respects, AIDS is the exception to the epidemics and pandemics canvassed in this book. Unlike the examples of influenza or Legionnaires' disease, medical researchers could hardly be accused of being blinded by overconfidence in 1981. Nor could the CDC be accused of being complacent about the threat posed by sexually transmitted diseases in the early 1980s, or of failing to recognize AIDS's peculiar constellation of symptoms sooner. On the contrary, AIDS might have continued its slow, stealth-like spread for several more years had it not been for key conceptual advances in oncology and new laboratory technologies that, for the first time, gave clinicians the possibility of identifying the depletion of CD4 cells that is the signature of advanced HIV infection, and medical researchers the ability to continuously grow T cells in culture. Indeed, reflecting on the history of AIDS, Robert Gallo, the NIH cancer specialist who would share credit for the discovery of HIV with Luc Montagnier of the Pasteur Institute, argued that had AIDS struck in 1955, scientists would have been "in a dark box," so limited was the contemporary understanding of retroviruses and scientists' ability to study them. "No one would have believed in this kind of virus. They did not even know what this kind of virus was," he told an interviewer in 1994.[14] Even in the 1960s and early 1970s, he argued, scientists would have struggled to comprehend HIV.[15] Or, to put it another way, the AIDS epidemic broke out at precisely the moment when, for the first time in history, scientists working in oncology and the specialized area of human retrovirology were inclined to believe that a retrovirus might be the cause of the peculiar new syndrome and possessed the tools and technology to test the hypothesis. Even so, from the beginning of the hunt for the virus of AIDS, research was clouded by presumptions about what sort of retrovirus HIV would turn out to be, and nowhere more so than in the mind of Gallo.

* * *

Today, in an era of antiretroviral drugs, when a diagnosis of AIDS is no longer an automatic death sentence, it is easy to forget the panic, hysteria and stigma of the early days of the pandemic. For conservative politicians such as Jesse Helms, the former Republican senator from North Carolina, and Moral Majority leader Jerry Falwell, AIDS was nothing less than "God's judgment" and divine retribution for homosexuals' "perverted" lifestyles.[16] Others argued that the virus had something to do with voodoo; hence, the way it appeared to target Haitians. Still others thought it had been transported to Earth on the tail of a comet from outer space, or that the virus had been incubated in a bioweapons lab by the CIA with the connivance of the Pentagon and Big Pharma.[17]

In fact, HIV is a special type of virus called a retrovirus. Due to its long latency and gradual onset, it is also classed as a lentivirus (from the Latin term for slow). When a person is first infected with HIV, the immune system produces antibodies to fight off the virus. This process of acute infection can take anywhere from two weeks to three months. During this period, virus levels in the blood are very high and patients are extremely infectious. Victims may also experience flu-like symptoms such as fever, rash, muscle aches, and joint pains, but frequently the symptoms are so mild they pass unnoticed. After seroconversion, HIV usually betrays no further outward sign of its presence for several years.[18] Instead, it works by stealth, silently parasitizing CD4 cells and colonizing the lymphatic system. During the silent phase of infection, HIV uses the machinery of CD4 cells to make copies of itself and spread throughout the body. At each stage, CD4 cells are repeatedly activated and die off. This cycle of activation followed by cell death continues until the body's capacity for replenishing CD4 cells is exhausted, a process that takes around ten years, but can be shorter or longer. Eventually, without an adequate supply of CD4 cells, the immune system can no longer signal B cells to produce antibodies, or CD8 cells—also known as T cells—to kill infected cells. It is at this point that a victim becomes susceptible to opportunistic infections and develops prominent signs of illness. Until then, however, HIV is quiescent: it lies hidden from view inside CD4 and other immune cells.

Measuring CD4 cells is the most important laboratory indicator of a person's immune status and how well their immune system is coping with the virus.[19] Viral load shows the amount of virus in the blood and gives an indication of the risk of progression and transmission, but without the ability to count Michael's CD4 cells, Gottlieb would have had no idea that his immune system was compromised and that he might be the victim of a new condition. In retrospect, it is astonishing to think that this technology became available at precisely the moment when AIDS first emerged in Los Angeles and other US cities. That the technology was available at UCLA and other hospital immunology departments could largely be attributed to the work of an Argentine émigré, César Millstein, and a German biologist, Georges Köhler. In 1975, these scientists found a way to produce an immortal cell line capable of producing endless quantities of antibodies that targeted specific antigens. Known as monoclonal antibodies—or Mabs for short—the technology removed the need to laboriously isolate and purify antibodies from laboratory cultures, and was soon being used in everything from the rapid typing of blood and tissue, to the development of new drugs against infectious diseases. Soon, Mabs were also aiding the study of leukaemia, and by 1981 commercial Mabs technologies also became available to distinguish one population of T cells from another. Thus it was that in the winter of 1981 Gottlieb's colleague found a virtual absence of CD4 cells in Michael's blood, suggesting that his symptoms were the result of an immune deficiency.[20]

If it is impossible to imagine AIDS being diagnosed without new Mabs technologies, it is also inconceivable that the virus would have been isolated without conceptual advances in oncology and knowledge of lentiviruses. The first lentivirus was described in 1954 by an Icelandic researcher investigating an outbreak of visna, a slow disease of sheep characterized by pneumonia and brain plaques similar to the demyelination of the central nervous system seen in multiple sclerosis. This was followed, three years later, by the description of kuru among members of the Fore tribe of Papua New Guinea highlands. A neurodegenerative disorder, kuru produces a steady deterioration of brain tissue similar to Bovine Spongiform Encephalopathy (BSE), also known as "mad cow disease." Like BSE, kuru is thought to be due to the transmission of an infectious protein called a prion. The difference is that whereas BSE is caused by eating food contaminated with prions from the brains and spinal cords of infected cattle, kuru most likely resulted from funerary cannibalism practices in which the Fore consumed the brains of dead relatives.

In parallel with discoveries of new lentiviruses, in the 1950s scientists were also describing new oncoviruses.* These viruses included mouse leukaemia and Burkitt's lymphoma, a rare jaw tumour especially prevalent in children in Uganda and other parts of East Africa with high rates of malaria, which was later found to be due to the Epstein-Barr virus, a close cousin of herpes.[21] Until the 1960s, it was thought that all viruses, including oncoviruses, replicated by inserting their DNA into animal cells and co-opting the cell's machinery to make multiple copies. The only difference in the case of

---

* Oncovirus is the term for any virus that causes cancers or tumours.

oncoviruses was that, instead of being lytic and killing infected cells, they entered into a state of symbiosis with cells and caused them to replicate. However, this theory hit a major roadblock with the finding that the oncovirus of feline leukaemia contained the "messenger" molecule, ribonucleic acid (RNA), rather than DNA, thereby violating one of the central tenets of molecular biology: namely, that genetic information flows from DNA to RNA to protein, not in the opposite direction.

The first breakthrough came with the demonstration in 1970 by David Baltimore of the Massachusetts Institute of Technology and Howard Temin of the University of Wisconsin that certain RNA viruses could achieve integration into cellular genomes with the help of an enzyme, reverse transcriptase. This was an enzyme that they alone, among all RNA viruses, carried, and which enabled them to form DNA from the genes of viral RNA. At first, Baltimore and Temin's discovery of reverse transcriptase was regarded as "heresy," but it was eventually accepted and led to them being awarded the Nobel Prize in 1975. It also led to the coining of the term retroviruses for viruses that possessed this special ability, removing an epistemological obstacle to the understanding of how viral genes could cause cancerous transformations of cells. When a retrovirus infects a cell, the reverse transcriptase takes the clockwise RNA helix and re-transcribes it in the reverse direction, rendering it into double-stranded DNA. This DNA "provirus" is then inserted into the host chromosomal DNA with the help of another viral enzyme, integrase. Because the integration site of the provirus is random, it frequently triggers disruptions of adjacent genes, causing cancer. At the same time, integrated into the cell, the virus is protected from attack by the immune system and is effectively invisible to detection with scientific instruments. The virus remains there for the life of the cell, being replicated along with cellular DNA and passed on to daughter cells.[22]

In 1975 only retroviruses causing cancer in animals were known (the classic examples being chicken sarcoma and feline leukaemia) and many cancer researchers, discouraged by the contamination of cell lines with infectious viruses of other species, had given up hope of ever finding a human oncogenic retrovirus. Robert Gallo, an ambitious young researcher at the National Cancer Institute, a branch of the NIH, in Bethesda, Maryland, thought otherwise. The son of a metallurgist from Waterbury, Connecticut, with unkempt crinkly hair that betrayed his Italian heritage, Gallo understood right away that reverse transcriptase could add an important dimension to cancer research. He began searching for the enzyme in white blood cells from human leukaemia patients. Gallo had two things going for him: a fierce competitive streak—he made no secret of the fact that he hankered after the Nobel Prize—and a novel technology that enabled him to continuously grow T cells in culture—the T cell growth factor, interleukin-2. Prior to the late 1970s, oncologists investigating leukaemia had to laboriously culture malignant white blood cells on agar media in order to produce sufficient numbers for the detection of reverse transcriptase. However, the leukaemia cells frequently refused to cooperate, resulting in frustration and wasted effort. But in 1976 all that changed when two of Gallo's colleagues at his Laboratory of Tumor and Cell Biology discovered that a plant derivative stimulated certain T-lymphocytes and caused them to release a growth factor. This was interleukin-2, and soon Gallo's lab had demonstrated that it could be used to prompt leukaemia cells to grow and multiply, thereby perpetuating cell lines indefinitely.[23] Nevertheless, even with this method it took nearly three years of trial and error before Gallo's group hit paydirt, detecting reverse transcriptase in 1979 in the lymphocytes of a 28-year-old African American man from Alabama who had been diagnosed with *mycosis fungoides*, a type of T-cell lymphoma. Soon after, both Gallo's laboratory and a group of Japanese researchers found the same virus in other patients with leukaemia and in 1980 named it HTLV, short for Human T-cell Leukaemia Virus.[24] This discovery made headlines around the world, earning Gallo the prestigious Lasker Prize, and was followed, in 1982, by the isolation of a second human retrovirus in the same family, designated HTLV-II by Gallo.[25]

In his book on the discovery of AIDS, *Virus Hunting: AIDS, Cancer & The Human Retrovirus*, Gallo acknowledges that his interest in HTLV was partly inspired by the finding, a decade earlier, that the feline leukaemia virus more often caused an AIDS-like immune deficiency in cats than it did leukaemia. He was also inspired by research by his Harvard colleague, Myron "Max" Essex, showing that Japanese infectious disease wards were full of people who had tested positive for HTLV-I.[26] Nevertheless, there is no doubt that the discovery of HTLV-I paved the way for the isolation in 1983 at the Pasteur Institute in Paris of the lymphadenopathy virus (LAV), the virus now known as HIV, by the French researchers Françoise Barré-Sinoussi and Luc Montagnier.

HTLV infects CD4 cells and spreads by blood and sexual contact, often producing leukaemias several decades after the originating infection. The difference is that HTLV is oncogenic; for reasons which are not fully understood but which involve a protein called Tax, it causes cells to replicate rather than killing them. However, similar techniques are required to grow the virus continuously in cell cultures, and had Gallo not demonstrated that HTLV depended on reverse transcriptase and was associated with a depletion of

CD4 cells, it is unlikely that Barré-Sinoussi and Montagnier would have thought that the retrovirus they were studying might possess similar properties. However, it is also clear that Gallo's conviction that the virus of AIDS was an oncogenic virus, similar to the feline leukaemia virus, blinded him to other research avenues that might have seen him isolate HIV before the French.[27] Instead, in May 1983, in a note published in the *Morbidity and Mortality Weekly Report* and followed by a series of articles in *Science*, Gallo announced that a variant of HTLV-I, or its near relative HTLV-II, was most likely the pathogen of AIDS.[28] Unfortunately for Gallo, in the same issue of *Science*, Barré-Sinoussi and Montagnier announced their discovery of LAV. As the virus showed little or weak cross-reactivity with HTLV-I, it was clear that theirs was a different virus.[29] Despite this, at the request of the editors, Montagnier agreed to an abstract, written by Gallo, stating that the French had discovered "a retrovirus belonging to the same family of recently discovered human T-cell leukaemia viruses (HTLV), but clearly distinct from each previous isolate."[30] That sentence would leave the Pasteur Institute researchers with a nasty aftertaste, one that would provoke a bitter international dispute over the correct nomenclature of the virus and who had discovered it—a dispute that in turn would engender misunderstandings about HIV's identity and its precise relationship to AIDS, fuelling conspiracy theories that persist to this day.

The dispute between Gallo and Montagnier, and the scientific and commercial stakes that lay behind it (one of the fiercest issues was who should collect royalties for the development of an HIV diagnostic test), has been the subject of books by both of the principals and has also been analyzed extensively by other writers.[31] The bad feeling between the French and American scientists was exacerbated by an ill-considered press conference in April 1984 at the US Department of Health and Human Sciences at which Gallo announced that he had isolated the virus of AIDS[32] and followed up that announcement with four further papers in *Science* in which he named the virus HTLV-III.[*] In 1986, the dispute appeared to have been settled when the International Committee on the Taxonomy of Viruses renamed the virus HIV and, soon afterwards, Ronald Reagan and François Mitterrand, who was then the president of France, announced that both groups of scientists deserved equal credit for the discovery, only for the dispute to be reopened in 1990 by new genetic tests suggesting, wrongly as it turned out, that Gallo had

---

[*] It subsequently emerged that HTLV-III was identical to LAV and was almost certainly a contaminant from a virus that Montagnier had shared with Gallo's lab.

misappropriated samples forwarded to his laboratory from the Pasteur Institute in 1983. This is not the time or place to revisit that fraught history or whether in naming the virus HTLV-III Gallo intended to suggest it was related to other viruses in the HTLV family or even that it was the cause of AIDS (he would subsequently say he had never made this claim).[33] However, it is worth dwelling on one aspect of the dispute because it goes to the heart of the question as to what both groups of scientists knew, or thought they knew, about the virus at the time they first posited its aetiological role in AIDS, and the extent to which Gallo was blinded by his belief that the AIDS virus belonged to the cancer family of retroviruses.

In the second set of papers published in *Science*, Gallo described how he had isolated HTLV-III from forty-eight patients and spelled out how to grow the virus continually in laboratory cultures. This was a critical feat. HIV routinely kills the cells it infects, making it difficult to grow the virus in the quantities needed to study its properties and develop a blood test, let alone a vaccine. Indeed, using the new cell line, Gallo's group was already well on the way to developing a prototype screening test (or ELISA), as well as a confirmatory test (known as the "Western blot"). However, in his earlier 1983 paper Gallo had made no mention of the virus's cell-destroying properties, merely observing that it could be immunosuppressive in vitro: that is, it could harm the function of T cells in laboratory cultures. This left open the question of how precisely HTLV, a virus that was known to cause lymphocytes to divide, also resulted in them becoming depleted.

By contrast, the French started from the premise that because the virus reduced and destroyed the numbers of circulating T cells, it would be difficult to isolate in peripheral blood. At this stage, Montagnier's group accepted that it was most likely a retrovirus closely related to, or identical to, HTLV. However, rather than look for it in blood they decided to look for it in fluid taken from the lymph nodes of a presumed AIDS patient, reasoning that there might be higher levels of the virus present in people who were at an earlier stage of illness before most of their T cells had been killed off. Thus it was that on 3 January 1983, a researcher at the Pitié-Salpêtrière Hospital in Paris removed a lymph node from the neck of a 33-year-old man* with "lymphadenopathy syndrome"—a condition of chronically swollen lymph

---

* The patient was identified in Montagnier's laboratory notes by the first three letters of his name, BRU. He was later named by newspapers as Frédéric Brugière, a homosexual who had allegedly had relations with fifty partners a year and who had visited New York City in 1979.

glands increasingly prevalent in gay men—and added interleukin-2 to encourage cell-line growth.[34] If the virus had been a species of HTLV, the addition of interleukin-2 should have maintained the culture and its population of T cells, but that is not what happened. Instead, no sooner had Barré-Sinoussi observed the production of reverse transcriptase by the cultured lymphocytes on 25 January, than production of the enzyme reached a peak, before falling back. The virus seemed to be killing the T cells rather than causing them to replicate. Fearing that without a new supply of lymphocytes she would lose the virus, she asked a member of the team to obtain fresh blood from a nearby blood bank. Adding the new source of lymphocytes to the culture, she saw that cell death correlated once again with the detection of reverse transcriptase activity. It was as if the addition of the plasma containing fresh lymphocytes caused the elusive virus to begin gobbling up T cells again, leaving an unmistakable trail of reverse transcriptase, much as a shark leaves a blood trail after attacking its prey. It was at that moment that Barré-Sinoussi realized that the virus was killing the T cells, that it was a new retrovirus and that it was almost certainly not Gallo's HTLV. As she later recalled: "It was very easy. We received the first sample at the beginning of 1983 and, fifteen days later, we had the first sign of the virus in the culture."[35]

If Barré-Sinoussi thought the wider world would immediately grasp the significance of her experiment she was wrong, however. The publication of her paper on LAV in the May 1983 edition of *Science* was completely overshadowed by the papers by Gallo and Essex. Not only that, but when in the fall of 1983 Montagnier travelled to an international virology conference held each September in Cold Spring Harbor, New York, and reported finding LAV in about 60 per cent of patients with lymphadenopathy syndrome and 20 per cent of those with AIDS, and that none of these patients appeared to be infected with HTLV, his findings were fiercely disputed by Gallo. In his book, Gallo would later write of his "regret" about his aggressive questioning of Montagnier and acknowledge his failure to spot LAV's cell-killing properties earlier—a failure that he attributed to the "distortion" of his laboratory's measurement of reverse transcriptase activity due to the fact that tests usually began later in the course of infection, by which time most of the T cells were already damaged or dying, as well as to inconclusive immunofluorescent assays that were sometimes positive for HTLV-I and sometimes not (perhaps because some of the subjects were infected with both HIV and HTLV simultaneously, or one or other of the viruses separately).[36] However, in his account of his own investigation Montagnier argues persuasively that, with the superior financial resources available to the Americans, had Gallo believed in the

French virus from the very beginning, he "would have rapidly left us far behind." That is a conclusion with which Gallo reluctantly concurred, acknowledging that his "overconfidence" that AIDS could not be a type of retrovirus different from HTLV probably cost him six months and that he should have solved the problem before Montagnier's group embarked on their first experiment. "AIDS being identified right after the discovery of the first and second human retroviruses ... misled me," Gallo admitted. "As well as leading me right, it also led me wrong."[37] Or as the historian of science, Mirko Grmek, put it rather more directly, "If Gallo had not discovered HTLV-I, he might well have been the discoverer of HIV."[38]

* * *

In her book *Illness as Metaphor*, the cultural critic Susan Sontag draws attention to the way in which any disease whose causality is murky and for which treatment is ineffectual tends to be awash with significance. "First, the subjects of deepest dread (corruption, decay, pollution, anomie, weakness) are identified with the disease. The disease itself becomes a metaphor. Then, in the name of the disease (that is, using it as a metaphor), that horror is imposed on other things."[39] Those words were written in 1978 and were originally inspired by Sontag's experiences as a cancer patient, when she had been made to feel that the disease was shameful and somehow her fault, but as she recognized when she revisited her thesis in the wake of the AIDS epidemic, her comments applied even more to AIDS. Indeed, by 1989 she argued that the secrecy, shame and feelings of culpability experienced by cancer patients in the 1970s had to a large extent been replaced by those of AIDS patients. This was particularly the case for homosexual men and other designated at-risk groups, such as intravenous drug users, whose dangerous behaviours were thought to have somehow invited the affliction. Such groups, she argued, had been made to feel like "a community of pariahs." Worse, whereas in the case of cancer, culpability for illness had been linked to unhealthy habits such as cigarette smoking and excessive drinking, the unsafe behaviour that produced AIDS was viewed as something more than weakness of will. "It is indulgence, delinquency—addictions to chemicals that are illegal and to sex regarded as deviant." The result was that what should have been considered an individual "calamity" that invited sympathy for the afflicted was judged harshly "as a disease not only of sexual excess but of perversity," resulting in the widespread stigmatization of people with AIDS.[40]

At what point this stigmatization morphed into hysteria and panic about the threat that such patients posed to wider society is harder to say. Initially, the public responded with indifference to news of the outbreak, perhaps taking their cue from White House press spokesman Larry Speakes who, when asked by a reporter in October 1982 whether the Reagan administration had any reaction to the CDC's announcement of over six hundred cases of the mysterious new disease, famously responded, "I don't know anything about it." This indifference was due partly to ignorance and partly to prejudice about a disease that was thought to affect only homosexuals. As long as AIDS was framed as a disease of gay lifestyles, and therefore not a problem for "straight" society, it could be safely ignored by mainstream politicians. Instead, Ronald Reagan's administration, backed by the Republican-controlled Senate, starved AIDS researchers of funds, forcing scientists at the NIH and CDC to beg and steal money from other programmes. Indeed, for the first three years of the epidemic, Reagan refused to mention the "A"-word, only referring to AIDS in public for the first time in the fall of 1985. By then, of course, the actor Rock Hudson had been forced to admit that he had the dreaded disease, issuing a press release from his sickbed at the American Hospital in Paris, and the CDC was reporting that more than 10,000 people had been diagnosed with AIDS, many of them children and haemophiliacs. According to David France, a contributor to the New York *Native* who would go on to make an Oscar-nominated film telling the story of how AIDS activists took on the scientific establishment in the quest for medications that would prolong their lives, Hudson's announcement was a game changer. "We prayed for a day when the disease struck someone who mattered," he wrote.[41] In particular, it prompted reporters to ask embarrassing questions about why the Hollywood icon had been forced to seek treatment in Paris, unleashing a wave of publicity that finally broke the administration's murderous silence around AIDS and persuaded the White House to release much needed funds for research into experimental treatments, such as AZT. What France and other activists did not foresee is that it would also unleash a wave of fear and hysteria.

This hysteria can be traced to three factors: the first was the discovery that AIDS was a blood-borne disease that could also be spread by intravenous drug use and the sharing of needles and that it was in the nation's blood supply; the second was poor public health messaging and the use of vague terms such as "bodily fluids," which gave the impression that you could contract AIDS from saliva and sneezes, or even from touching an object that had been handled by someone with AIDS; and the third was the realization that the disease was due to a deadly new type of virus that might also be capable of heterosexual spread, and there were no drugs available to treat it, making diagnosis equivalent to a death sentence. Suddenly, it seemed, there was no safe ground, no place that was secure from the virus. Instead, AIDS rapidly took on the aspect of a contagion, sparking what the journalist Randy Shilts called an "epidemic of fear."[42]

Looking back, Shilts had little doubt that scientists and medical experts—not the media—were largely responsible for this new framing of AIDS. In March 1983 the CDC had named the principal risk groups as homosexual men with multiple sexual partners, heroin addicts who injected drugs, Haitians, and haemophiliacs—the so-called "four Hs." However, two months later, the *Journal of the American Medical Association* gave a completely different impression, publishing an article about eight cases of unexplained immune deficiency among children in Newark, New Jersey, four of whom had died, and stated that "sexual contact, drug abuse or exposure to blood products is not necessary for disease transmission." Worse, in an accompanying editorial, Anthony Fauci, the head of the National Institute of Allergy and Infectious Diseases (NIAID) and the leading federal AIDS researcher, compounded the offense by stating there was a "possibility that routine close contact, as within a family household" could spread the disease.[43] In case the press failed to get the message, the American Medical Association also issued a press release headlined, "Evidence Suggests Household Contact May Transmit AIDS," in which it quoted Fauci as saying that the possibility of "non-sexual, non-blood borne transmission" had "enormous implications" and that "If routine close contact can spread the disease, AIDS takes on an entirely new dimension." The release was immediately taken up by the Associated Press, who interpreted it to mean that the general population was at greater risk of AIDS than had previously been thought, and flawed versions of the AP story were soon running in *USA Today* and other newspapers. Within days, officials in San Francisco began distributing face masks and rubber gloves to police and fire officers, and an image of an officer trying on one of the masks appeared in several metropolitan dailies, becoming what Shilts calls "a virtual emblem of the AIDS hysteria" sweeping the nation. Not long after, other police departments began agitating for the same masks, and California dentists were advised to take similar precautions.[44]

Although Fauci would subsequently accuse the media of taking his comments out of context and of failing to appreciate the nuances of his editorial, his comments were compounded by the language employed by health officials who, nervous about offending public sensibilities by specifying that AIDS was spread through "semen" and blood, adopted the euphemism "bodily fluids." The result was that it was a year before Fauci corrected the misunderstanding by clarifying in an article for another peer-reviewed journal that there was no evidence that AIDS could be transmitted by routine household or social contact.[45]

The capacity of this new framing of AIDS to provoke panic and hysteria was driven home by the news in July 1985 that a middle school in Kokomo, Indiana, was refusing to readmit a 14-year-old haemophiliac, Ryan White, who had been infected with AIDS following a routine blood transfusion a year earlier. Even though White had been declared fit by doctors, the local school corporation had bowed to pressure from hysterical parents worried about their children sharing a classroom with an AIDS "carrier." The hysteria spread rapidly to other school districts, including New York, where, in an article headlined "The New Untouchables," *Time* reported that some nine hundred parents at an elementary school in Queens were refusing to let their children attend classes because of one AIDS-infected second grader.[46] Soon, newspapers in other countries were carrying stories of similarly hysterical overreactions. In England, the *Sun* newspaper reported that AIDS was "spreading like wildfire" and that a victim of the disease had been entombed in concrete in a cemetery in North Yorkshire "as a precaution." In Brussels, according to the *Daily Mirror*, a court had been emptied in seconds after a prisoner declared that he was infected with the virus, prompting the judge, clerks, and several prison officers to flee in terror.[47] Meanwhile, back in the United States, researchers William H. Masters and Virginia E. Johnson warned that AIDS could lurk on toilet seats, while in Chicago a worried motorist who had just run over a gay pedestrian telephoned an AIDS hotline wanting to know whether he should decontaminate his car.[48] Even family physicians, whose Hippocratic oath meant they owed a duty of care to all patients, found excuses not to treat people with AIDS or to refer them to specialist colleagues.

In the early months of the epidemic, it was common for both network news anchors and gay men to refer to AIDS as a lifestyle disease associated with homosexuality and living in the "fast lane." In retrospect, it can be seen that this construction was a product of the initial case descriptions used by CDC epidemiologists to identity the main risk groups. Thus in the first report about the new syndrome in the *Morbidity and Mortality Weekly Report*, Curran had floated the hypothesis that the incidence of PCP in Gottlieb's UCLA patients suggested an association with "some aspect of a homosexual lifestyle or disease acquired through sexual contact." This was followed in July 1981 by a second report in the same journal, detailing how KS had been diagnosed in twenty-six male patients in New York.[49] Coinciding with an article in the *New York Times*, in which Friedman-Kien, himself a gay man, provided fifteen more cases of KS to a reporter, it was at this point that the wider medical community and the media began to talk about a "rare cancer" and, afterwards, a "gay plague."[50]

Perhaps the CDC's most significant contribution to the stigmatization of homosexuals was the publication in 1982 of a study of patients with KS and other opportunistic infections in Los Angeles and Orange Counties. Known as the Los Angeles cluster study, it was this that introduced the public to perhaps the most notorious patient in the history of infectious disease after Typhoid Mary: French Canadian flight attendant Gaetan Dugas.[51] Subsequently immortalized as "patient zero" by the journalist Randy Shilts in his popular history of AIDS, *And the Band Played On*, Dugas was ready-made for demonization as the epidemic's "bad guy." A complex character who boasted hundreds of casual sexual partners, Dugas refused to give up his addiction to bathhouses even as his body was ravaged by KS and evidence mounted that AIDS might be sexually transmitted. After Dugas's death in March 1984, Friedman-Kien and other physicians were quick to label him a "sociopath." But such judgments tend to ignore the extent to which, in the early years of the epidemic, knowledge about AIDS's aetiology and its routes of transmission were uncertain and subject to conjecture. They also obscured the fact that, though sceptical of medical claims about gay lifestyles contributing to the epidemic, Dugas was very helpful to William Darrow, the CDC sociologist who led the study, providing him with the names of 72 of the roughly 750 men he had slept with in the previous three years. Ironically, it was this frankness about his sexual history, and his willingness to assist epidemiologists in reconstructing the pathways of transmission, that would result in Dugas being accorded a starring role in Darrow's study and Shilts's book, leading to what the historian of medicine Richard McKay calls Dugas's "posthumous notoriety."[52]

In contrast to microbiologists and other laboratory-based investigators, epidemiologists tend to privilege multifactorial models of disease: that is, they believe a given disease may have a number of causes or antecedents, a combination of which may be required to produce the disorder. By investigating this "web of causes," the aim is to identify the disorder's most vulnerable point and intervene, thereby curtailing further spread of the pathogen before its identity is known. Prior to the identification of the virus in 1983, this was the situation that confronted Curran and his colleagues in the STD division of the CDC. At that point no one realized that the epidemic was due to a new virus unknown to medical science, let alone that it could be transmitted in blood as well as semen. However, as discussed above, new medical technologies had already made the depletion of CD4 cells visible to medical researchers, alerting physicians and epidemiologists to the immune deficiency that is one of AIDS's hallmarks. Moreover, the CDC had just completed a multi-year, multi-site study of hepatitis B, a disease which is often sexually transmitted and whose prevalence was known to be very high among homosexual men. In analyzing the data, the researchers found that blood markers for the disease were significantly associated with, among other factors, having a large number of male sexual partners and engaging in sexual practices involving anal contact. At the same time, researchers at the NIH and elsewhere were growing concerned about the increase in CMV transmission among homosexuals—a phenomenon that had never been seen on such a scale before among adults, homosexual or otherwise.[53] The analysts who read these studies were mostly heterosexual and middle-aged and had little understanding of gay lifestyles, so it is not surprising that they were quick to link the epidemic in STDs to the gay liberation movement and its attendant world of bathhouses and anonymous hook-ups. In addition, as Garrett reports, many researchers began to worry that these same gay lifestyles might be altering the "ecology" of STDs.[54] In this way, the same factors that made the new syndrome visible to epidemiologists for the first time also contributed to the stigmatization of gay men and their supposed behaviours, and it was not long before the CDC was referring to the disorder as Gay-Related Immune Deficiency (GRID).

This stigmatization of gay men's lifestyles was almost certainly inadvertent. Curran, who headed the CDC's new Task Force on Kaposi's Sarcoma and Opportunistic Infections, had previously worked closely with the gay community to evaluate the hepatitis B vaccine, so he was well aware of the community's sensitivities. However, as an STD specialist he also could not help but favour the sexual transmission theory. This bias deepened when Curran ordered a "quick and dirty" survey of 420 males attending venereal disease clinics in San Francisco, New York and Atlanta, and then selected thirty-five for interview. Two patterns of behaviour caught the task force's attention: first, the men had had many sexual partners in the past year (the median was eighty-seven), and second, they had frequently used marijuana, cocaine and amyl nitrate poppers. In particular, there was a close association with the number of sexual partners and the use of poppers.[55] This soon led to the suggestion that it might be exposure to amyl nitrate, rather than the sexual behaviour of the subjects, which caused the immune deficiency. The theory received a boost with a study showing that exposure to amyl nitrate was associated with an increased risk of KS in New York, and an investigation of eleven immunocompromised men with PCP, also from New York, seven of whom were identified as drug "abusers" (what received rather less attention was the fact that five of the men had described themselves as heterosexual).[56] However, with the publication of the first instalment of the Los Angeles cluster study, and even more so with the publication of Darrow's expanded study linking forty homosexual male AIDS patients in ten US cities, this theory gradually gave way to the sexual transmission hypothesis, prompting news networks to talk about the "gay plague." In particular, Darrow reported that the linked men were more likely than nonlinked controls to have met sexual partners in bathhouses and to have participated in "fisting" (manual-rectal intercourse). Darrow also pointed out that the index patient in the cluster study diagram had had approximately 250 different male sexual partners each year from 1979 through 1981, and that eight of his named partners were AIDS patients, four from Southern California and four from New York.[57] Darrow would later claim that the "O" indicating the index patient in the cluster diagram stood for "Out[side]-of California," not zero. However, Shilts reports that when he visited the CDC to speak to members of the task force, officials were already using the term "Patient Zero"* and he immediately thought, "Ooh, that's catchy."[58]

Whether or not Darrow meant to brand Dugas Patient Zero by designating him the index case, the LA Cluster Study gave the impression that this was where AIDS in America had begun. This impression was reinforced by Shilts's unmasking of Dugas and the revelation that the air steward had made frequent trips to France and, perhaps, to Africa, a continent long feared as a seat of plagues. The result was that in the hands of Shilts and other journalists, Dugas rapidly became a "super spreader" and the prime suspect in the mass murder of hundreds of young men. Thus it was that on 6 October 1987, shortly after the publication of *And The Band Played On*, the tabloid *New York Post* published a front-page story with the headline, "The Man Who Gave Us AIDS." Even supposedly serious news outlets embraced Shilts's partial narrative, with CBS's *60 Minutes* describing Dugas as both the "central victim and victimizer" of the epidemic, and the *National Review* dubbing the Canadian flight attendant "the Columbus of AIDS."[59] Perhaps the most shameful moment came at the end of the year when *People* magazine published an article naming Dugas as one of the "25 most intriguing people of '87" and speculating that it was his "fierce sexual drive" that had given impetus to the epidemic. The article prompted one reader to scrawl "Pervert" and an arrow in a red pen next to Dugas's picture and mail the article to the San Francisco AIDS Foundation.[60]

---

* Patient zero is a trope that crops up time and again in narrative accounts of epidemics. In epidemiological terms, patient zero is simply the index case; but in nonfiction and novelistic accounts, patient zero is the embodiment of the pathogen and the personification of the infection about to burst forth in society.

The perception that Dugas was the main culprit for America's AIDS epidemic was only finally debunked in 2016 when scientists examined stored blood taken from gay and bisexual men in the late 1970s in San Francisco and New York City and found that they already carried antibodies to the main pandemic strain of HIV, suggesting that the index case had probably arrived in New York in around 1970. Not only that, but when scientists examined the genetic sequences in detail, they found them to be similar to HIV strains found in the Caribbean, particularly Haiti, but with enough differences to suggest the virus had already been circulating and mutating on both coasts of America since 1970. When scientists compared these with blood taken from Dugas, they found that Dugas's HIV genome fell right in the middle of the phylogenetic tree of these strains, proof not only that Dugas had not introduced HIV to the US but that his sexual activity had not been a significant factor in the spread of AIDS in the United States.[61]

What makes the stigmatization of Dugas all the more unfortunate is that by early 1982 the CDC had good reason to believe that homosexuals were not the only victims of AIDS and that sexual intercourse was not the only means of transmission, but it took them some time to revise their blinkered view. The first clue had come in September 1981 when infectious disease specialists at Miami's Jackson Memorial Hospital noticed similar symptoms in men and women of Haitian origin. The same month, paediatricians in Miami and New York recognized the same syndrome in children born to Haitian mothers, but when they brought the cases to the attention of the CDC, agency officials were reluctant to believe them. However, by the following summer the CDC task force was hearing of more and more cases of PCP in heterosexuals who were injecting drug users, leading them to believe that GRID might also be transmitted intravenously. At around the same time, the CDC received the first reports of severe PCP in haemophiliacs. The cases involved three men from Denver, Colorado and Westchester, New York—parts of the country not yet known to be affected by the epidemic. Ominously, none of the men had a history of homosexuality or needle sharing, but all three had been given multiple injections of Factor VIII, a blood coagulant concentrate pooled from the plasma of thousands of donors across the United States. This was followed, in July 1982, by a report that a disease identical to GRID had broken out among thirty-four Haitian emigrants to the United States, most of them heterosexual men who had arrived in the country in the previous two years. In addition, eleven cases of KS were discovered in the Haitian capital, Port-au-Prince. However, it was only in September 1982, after the agency learned that a paediatrician at the University of California Medical Center was treating an infant with PCP and that the two-year-old had received multiple blood transfusions at birth, that the CDC finally dropped the term GRID and in September 1982 began referring to the disease as AIDS.[62]

* * *

By the late 1980s, with half of America's haemophiliacs infected with HIV—70 per cent in the case of those with the most severe form of the disorder—few experts doubted that AIDS was also a blood-borne disease. But that still left open the question of where the virus had come from and how it had infected such a diverse range of social and ethnic groups—homosexuals, Haitians, heroin addicts, haemophiliacs—before anyone in the medical community had noticed. By now every region of the world had reported at least one case of HIV, leading the WHO to suggest that the pandemic had emerged simultaneously on three continents. However, few people accepted this theory, not least because it was in Africa that AIDS appeared to be spreading most quickly. Moreover, by the close of the decade, tests on historical serum samples had demonstrated that HIV had already been present in Zaire and Uganda in the 1970s. That these HIV-infected patients included women and children suggested that HIV might have been seeded in heterosexual populations in Central Africa several decades before it arrived in America. Coupled with the growing awareness of AIDS infections among Haitians, this suggested an African point of origin.

The first evidence for this hypothesis had come in 1983 when serum collected from a woman in the obstetrics ward of Mama Yemo Hospital in Kinshasa tested positive for LAV.[63] The findings prompted Montagnier to conduct further tests on archived blood samples from Zaire dating back to 1970, many of which also turned out to be positive for the virus. At the same time, using the ELISA test, Gallo began examining stored blood samples that had been collected by the National Cancer Institute in 1972 and 1973 from schoolchildren in Uganda as part of a study of Burkitt's Lymphoma. To his astonishment, these showed that two-thirds of the Ugandan children were infected with HTLV-III.[64]

In 1983 Peter Piot, a Belgian microbiologist who had become concerned about the number of wealthy Zairians presenting with symptoms of immune deficiency at his tropical diseases clinic in Antwerp, decided to investigate the full extent of the problem in Zaire.[65] Focussing on Mama Yemo Hospital, where doctors had first noted AIDS-like wasting symptoms in the late 1970s, he found that during a three-week period scores of patients on the wards were infected with AIDS.[66] Subsequently he was joined by Jonathan Mann, a former CDC epidemiologist who would go on to become director of the WHO Global Program on AIDS, and the pair began gathering further epidemiological data as part of *Project SIDA*, the first and largest AIDS research project in Africa. By 1986, they had established that AIDS was an escalating problem in Zaire and Rwanda, with up to 18 per cent of blood donors and pregnant women infected with HIV. They also noted that the syndrome affected men and women more or less equally, and that most of the men surveyed considered themselves heterosexuals. If this was not enough to dispel the canard that AIDS was a predominantly homosexual disease, researchers went on to report that up to 88 per cent of commercial sex workers in Kinshasa and the Rwandan capital Kigali were also infected with the virus, with a similarly high frequency of HIV infections in their clients.[67]

However, perhaps the best evidence that the virus had been present in Africa for some time came from retrospective tests of stored serum samples collected during the Ebola outbreak in Yambuku in 1976. Of the 659 samples drawn from patients in villages close to the Catholic mission hospital, 0.8 per cent tested positive for HIV. But while the shocking symptoms of Ebola and the high mortality rate had immediately attracted the attention of investigators from the CDC and elsewhere, no one had noticed these HIV infections at the time. If evidence were ever needed of HIV's cunning, this was it. Unlike Ebola, and other animal-origin viruses that are new to humans, HIV does not draw attention to itself by killing its host suddenly or violently. Instead, the virus has evolved a slow-but-sure strategy that enables it to infect human cells and replicate unnoticed. The result is that people parasitized by HIV can live and quietly pass on the virus for ten years or more before showing any signs of illness. Indeed, it was only in 1985–86 when three of the villagers in Yambuku developed illnesses suggestive of AIDS that scientists thought to screen the local population for HIV. Interestingly, this survey turned up similar levels of HIV infection as a decade earlier, suggesting that, in rural areas of Africa at least, the virus had made little progress in ten years. This would be an important clue to its epidemiology.

As scientists began screening other collections of archived sera, so other missed alarms came to light, this time in Europeans. One of the most interesting was that of the Danish surgeon, Grethe Rask, who had died in Copenhagen in 1977, after suffering a range of AIDS-like opportunistic infections, including PCP. At the time she became ill, in 1975, Rask had been working in Kinshasa, but prior to that, between 1972 and 1975, she had been based in Abumonbazi, a rural hospital sixty miles north of Yambuku. Initial tests in 1985 using an early version of ELISA were negative for HIV, but when the tests were repeated two years later with more sophisticated assays they were positive for the virus.[68] Another case was that of a Norwegian family— father, mother and nine-year-old daughter—all of whom had died of AIDS-like symptoms in 1976. In 1988, retrospective tests showed they all had HIV, and since the daughter had been born in 1967, this suggested the mother had already been infected by that date. Intriguingly, the father had been a sailor who had visited a number of ports in West Africa in the early 1960s, including Nigeria and Cameroon in 1961–62. The hypothesis was that at one of these ports he may have slept with a prostitute and contracted the virus.[69]

By the mid-1980s, evidence of similarly early cases of AIDS were also coming to light in Africa. The first HIV-positive specimen was isolated from a Bantu man who had given blood in 1959 in Léopoldville, the old Belgian colonial name for Kinshasa. The blood specimen had lain in a refrigerator for twenty-seven years.[70] At the time, it was not possible to identify to which HIV group the specimen belonged, but in the 1990s it became possible to amplify genetic material using a new technique called polymerase chain reaction (PCR), and in 1998 scientists established that it belonged to the same group responsible for the vast majority of pandemic infections. Then, in 2008, a group of scientists writing in *Nature* announced they had sequenced HIV from another specimen, also from Léopoldville. This specimen had been taken from the lymph gland of a woman in 1960, after which it had been stored in the pathology department of the University of Kinshasa. Although the material was badly fragmented, using PCR the team, led by Michael Worobey, an evolutionary biologist at the University of Arizona, were able to sequence a few strands of DNA and RNA. After amplifying the genetic material, Worobey then compared the virus to the earlier isolate from Léopoldville and established that it was a closely related subtype. The next stage was to use a molecular clock to calculate how long it would have taken the two viruses to have diverged from one another. This produced a date for the common ancestor virus between 1908 and 1933 (with a median of 1921).[71] Given the uncertainty of molecular clock calculations (RNA does not mutate at the same rate as DNA), these measures should be viewed with a degree of scepticism. However, there is little doubt that HIV was present in Léopoldville by 1959, and, if Worobey's calculations are correct, very possibly as early as 1921.[72]

Using the same PCR techniques, scientists have also gone on to study current circulating strains of HIV. To date, these studies have shown that there are two main types of HIV: HIV-1, which is highly transmissible and is responsible for the vast majority of infections worldwide, and HIV-2, which circulates mainly in West Africa and is associated with comparatively low levels of virus in the blood. To complicate the picture further, HIV-1 has been divided into four groups and one of these groups, group M, has been subdivided into ten subtypes. In addition, if individuals are infected with more than one subtype, the subtypes can swap genes and form new recombinant strains. The result is an alphabet soup highly confusing to the layman.

Nevertheless, today few scientists doubt that AIDS originated in Africa. This is not only because the two oldest isolates of HIV come from Kinshasa, but because nowhere else in the world does the virus show such diversity. HIV evolves only in one direction, from a single model of a virus to an increasingly complex differentiation into subtypes and recombinants, so viral diversity is strong evidence of point of origin. So far, so uncontroversial. But almost everything else about the origins of HIV and its association with AIDS has been contested. For instance, some retrovirus experts, such as Peter Duesberg, a biologist at the University of California, continue to deny that HIV is the cause of AIDS, even though the virus's aetiological role has long been accepted by all competent scientific authorities. Similarly, the British writer and journalist Edward Hooper maintains that AIDS can be traced to mass polio vaccination campaigns conducted in Central Africa in the late 1950s (Hooper argues that the inhabitants of the Belgian Congo, Rwanda and Burundi were given an oral polio vaccine, known as CHAT, contaminated with a simian immune-deficiency virus [SIV] as a result of the chimpanzee cells used in the production of the vaccine). Hooper's thesis is described in exhaustive detail in his 1999 book, *The River: A Journey Back to the Source of HIV and AIDS*, and on his website, where he continues to wage an increasingly lonely campaign against his scientific critics, the vast majority of whom consider the weight of evidence against his theory overwhelming.[73] Whether or not Hooper or his critics will ultimately be proved right, one of the consequences of his and Duesberg's critiques has been to fuel conspiracy theories about the role of medical science in spreading AIDS, and to undermine faith in AZT and other potentially life-saving drug treatments. This is particularly true of South Africa where Thabo Mbeki, who was president from 1999 to 2008 and who had taken advice from Duesberg, refused people access to antiretroviral drugs, thereby resulting in 330,000 unnecessary deaths from AIDS between 2000 and 2005, according to one study.[74] Similarly, there is evidence that Hooper's vaccine contamination theory may have contributed to the distrust of modern polio vaccines, particularly in countries such as Nigeria, Afghanistan, and Pakistan where suspicions about the vaccines and the motivations of international health workers have fuelled resistance to mass immunization campaigns, jeopardizing the WHO's attempts to eradicate the disease from its last endemic centres.[75]

Regardless of the truth or otherwise of these theories, no one disputes that both HIV-1 and HIV-2 are descended from Simian Immune-deficiency Viruses (SIVs) that parasitize, respectively, chimpanzees and sooty mangabeys indigenous to Central and West Africa, and which cause simian versions of AIDS.[76] The question is, how did these viruses jump species or "spillover" from monkeys and become widely amplified in human populations?

A leading spillover mechanism is thought to be the hunting and butchering of monkeys captured in the tropical rain forests of Cameroon, Gabon and the Congo—the region that is home to *Pan troglodytes troglodytes* chimpanzees.[77] When hunters are cut or bitten in the course of capturing the monkeys or when the animals are butchered for the table, their viruses can readily be transferred to humans. Both Simian Foamy Virus (SFV) and the Ebola and Marburg viruses have been acquired from monkeys in this way. Serological tests of pygmies and Bantu huntsmen show that many carry antibodies to SIVs, suggesting that exposure is a common occurrence in nature. Furthermore, from analysis of the genomes of HIV-1 and 2, as well as their various groups and subtypes, it is known that modern HIV viruses are more closely related to their nearest ancestral SIVs than they are to one another.[78] This is evidence that the simian progenitors of human HIVs must have jumped to humans several times in the course of their evolution. However, as only one group of HIV-1— the M group—is responsible for 99 per cent of HIV-1 infections worldwide, this also suggests that the AIDS pandemic started not because a lot of people were infected directly from chimpanzees, but because a rare case of infection managed to spread and multiply in humans, something that all the other simian-origin infections that came before and after it had not managed to do.[79] Fortunately, as the isolate taken from the Bantu man in Léopoldville in 1959 belongs to the HIV-1 M group, and it is there that the virus shows the greatest genetic diversity, when and where this event occurred is no longer a matter of conjecture. The pandemic strain of HIV must have been up and running in 1959 in Léopoldville or else in a nearby town in the Belgian or French Congo. It is in answering the question of how this happened that the debate gets interesting.

Broadly speaking, there are two schools of ecological thought. The first is that a combination of bushmeat hunting and economic and social changes driven by colonialism, plus globalization—better road, rail and plane connections—are sufficient to account for the amplification of the HIV-1 M group in Africa and the subsequent international spread of the virus. The second is that, yes, all those factors are significant but insufficient to explain how this particular group came to be so widely dispersed, first in urban African populations, and later in rural Africa and the rest of the world. This is because, in practice, it is very difficult for a simian virus to establish itself in a new human host. Indeed, many SIVs that cause infection in the short term are rapidly eliminated by the host's immune response. Even if an infection establishes itself in one person, the virus may not spread easily to others. To explain that we need an additional amplifying effect, and the best candidate is provided by medicine. In particular, Jacques Pepin, the leading proponent of this school, points to the reuse of inadequately sterilized hypodermic needles and syringes in the administration of drugs against venereal diseases such as syphilis and tropical diseases such as malaria and yaws in clinics across Africa. As transmission of HIV-1 is ten times more effective through shared needles and syringes than via sexual intercourse, Pepin, a Canadian infectious disease specialist and epidemiologist with broad African experience, argues that these well-meaning medical interventions, many of which were launched during the colonial era, could have given the virus the boost it needed to go from a localized urban epidemic in Léopoldville/Kinshasa to one capable of infecting people as far away as Haiti, New York and San Francisco.[80]

Unfortunately, it is not possible to go back in time and test Pepin's theory by conducting serological tests of patients who attended clinics in the Congo and elsewhere in the colonial period. The only evidence available is historical serum samples containing surviving fragments of HIV, and inferences from analogous examples of the inadvertent transmission of other blood-borne viruses via needles and syringes used in humanitarian medical programs. A good example of the latter is the tragedy that occurred in Egypt during the government campaigns against schistosomiasis, a potentially fatal disease caused by a parasitic blood fluke spread by snails that live in irrigation channels along the River Nile and other watercourses. Between 1964 and 1982, more than two million injections of tartar emetic were administered each year to 250,000 Egyptians to combat schistosomiasis. On average patients received ten to twelve weekly IV injections with hastily sterilized syringes and needles. The result was a huge increase in hepatitis C, with half of the individuals aged forty and over testing positive for the virus in areas where the schistosomiasis treatment was administered.[81] Similar iatrogenic transmission of hepatitis B occurred in the 1950s during the administration of IV drug treatments for syphilis and gonorrhoea at STD clinics in Léopoldville. Of course, while such studies may lend support to Pepin's theory, the evidence, such as it is, must be considered circumstantial and speculative. Like a jury presented with a murderer but no clear-cut murder weapon, we must weigh the evidence and decide who—or, in this case, what—is the most likely culprit.

The first question a jury must address is why, given the fact that humans living in Cameroon, Gabon, Guinea and Congo-Brazzaville have been in contact with chimpanzees infected with the SIV progenitor of HIV-1 for at least 2,000 years, an epidemic of HIV did not occur sooner? One answer is that in the precolonial period the lack of firearms made it more difficult to hunt apes and the dearth of roads through densely forested areas of Central Africa would have reduced interactions between humans and chimps. Even if, as seems likely, a bushmeat hunter was occasionally infected with HIV and managed to transmit the virus to his wife—or conversely, a cook infected her husband—the worst that might happen is that both would die of AIDS ten years later. Even if the couple were not monogamous, it is highly unlikely that in a remote village setting the virus would have spread far beyond the immediate community. Thus, in the precolonial period such infections would have represented epidemiological dead ends for the virus. However, around the turn of the nineteenth century, these epidemiological conditions began to change, creating new opportunities for progenitor HIV viruses to passage between people and be amplified more widely. The first development was the inauguration in 1892 of a steamship service from Léopoldville to Stanleyville (Kisangani) in the heart of the Congo. By connecting populations that had previously been largely separated, the service created the potential for viruses that might have died out in isolated, rural populations to reach growing urban centres. The population of Léopoldville received another boost in 1898 with the opening of the Matadi-Leo railway, prompting an influx of economic migrants and Belgium administrators. The result was that by 1923 Léopoldville had become the capital of the Belgian Congo. At around the same time, the city began hosting domestic flights and in 1936 inaugurated a direct international service to Brussels. More significant perhaps was the construction of new roads and railways by the French, including the 511-kilometre Chemin de Fer Congo-Ocean railroad. Connecting Brazzaville, on the opposite bank of the Congo River from Léopoldville, with Pointe-Noire on the coast, the railroad required the conscription of some 127,000 male labourers, resulting in the influx in the 1920s and 1930s of adult men into precisely the rural areas that were home to the chimpanzees that carried the progenitor of HIV-1. It also resulted in a constant passage of Africans and Europeans to and from Brazzaville, the new capital of the French federation.

Once these rural-urban connections were up and running, it would not have taken very much to initiate a chain of sexual transmission in Brazzaville or Léopoldville. Pepin argues that one of the most important factors would have been the disruption of social relations that occurred during the colonial period. In particular, he points to the gender imbalances caused by the Belgian policy of conscripting large numbers of men into the labour force while discouraging their wives and families from leaving their villages. This was nowhere more pronounced than in Léopoldville, where by the 1920s men outnumbered women by 4 to 1—an imbalance that encouraged unmarried, working women known as "*femmes libres*" to turn to part-time prostitution to supplement their income. Perhaps a bushmeat hunter travelled to Léopoldville and slept with one of these women. Or perhaps a labourer on the railway alighted at Brazzaville and then caught a ferry to the opposite bank of the Congo River before making his way to a prostitute in Léopoldville. Or perhaps a migrant worker carried the virus to Brazzaville from higher up the Congo River, via one of its tributaries with Cameroon—the HIV-1 M group is most closely related to an SIV indigenous to chimpanzees from southeastern Cameroon; at the time of writing this is the favoured scenario.[82] The virus would have had an even greater chance of spreading if the person had earlier been treated for a tropical disease at one of the rudimentary hospitals near the railway and had contracted the virus from a contaminated syringe. This is not as far-fetched as it may sound. According to Pepin, the authorities were conducting campaigns against sleeping sickness and yaws along the railway in the 1930s, and in the same period southern Cameroon saw massive iatrogenic transmission of hepatitis C following the administration of intravenous quinine to treat malaria.[83] Alternatively, the amplification effect could have occurred when an infected hunter presented himself at an STD clinic in Léopoldville to receive treatment for syphilis, or a prostitute infected by one of her clients presented herself for IV drug treatment at the same clinic. The prostitute would then have transmitted the virus sexually to her clients, and they in turn would have infected other sex workers, leading to an expanding circle of onward transmission and the gradual spread of HIV to other cities and towns in the Congo. The next amplifying effect would have come with independence from Belgium in 1960. As political chaos and civil war engulfed the Congo, thousands of refugees made their way to Kinshasa, resulting in a further expansion of prostitution. According to Pepin, it was this that most likely transformed HIV into a generalized epidemic; hence, the cases of AIDS that physicians encountered at the Mama Yemo hospital in the late 1970s and early 1980s. From Kinshasa, the virus was most likely spread by truckers and business travellers to other African cities and, afterwards, via planes to other countries and continents.

But this is only one theory. Others put more emphasis on the rapid growth of African cities; the increased prevalence of STDs, including genital ulcers, which would have increased the transmissibility of HIV; and ecological and environmental factors such as the construction of roads through the Congo basin by corporations eager to harvest timber from equatorial Africa.[84] Such roads would have afforded the virus several opportunities to establish itself in human populations: first, by enabling hunters to venture deeper into the habitat of *Pt. troglodytes* in search of bushmeat; and second, by encouraging the growth of prostitution near camps supplying labour to the timber companies. In this respect, it is argued, HIV may be similar to other viruses, such as Ebola, that are thought to reside in discrete ecological niches and whose emergence can be traced to ecological degradation and environmental changes that bring humans into closer contact with wild animals. However, there is no doubt that phylogenetic analysis of HIV has revolutionized the understanding of AIDS's global spread, and this is nowhere more true than in the case of one isolate from Africa, known as subtype B.

The story begins in 2008, when Worobey studied six blood samples from Haitian AIDS sufferers who had been treated in Miami in the early 1980s. The isolates exhibited greater genetic diversity than subtype B isolates from any other part of the world except for Africa. This was proof that the subtype had jumped from Africa to Haiti before it had reached the United States. Using the same molecular clock technique he had used to date the common ancestor of the isolates from Léopoldville, Worobey calculated that the founder virus had reached Haiti in around 1966 and had spread to the United States around 1969. A possible source were Haitians who had travelled to Zaire in the early 1960s to work as teachers, doctors, and nurses for WHO and UNESCO programs, one of whom, on their return to Haiti, could have introduced the virus. Pepin further believes that the subtype may have been amplified by unsterile conditions at a private blood-collecting company, Hemo-Caribbean, run by a close ally of the then-Haitian president, François Duvalier. Pepin believes that after the virus spread to Haiti's heterosexual population, bisexuals communicated it to American sex tourists, including homosexuals from New York and San Francisco who holidayed on the island. Alternatively, since Hemo-Caribbean exported 1,600 gallons of plasma to the United States monthly, and plasma clotting factors were widely used by American haemophiliacs, many of whom died of AIDS, the B subtype could also have been introduced to homosexuals in New York and San Francisco via a haemophiliac.

What is not in dispute is that homosexuals in New York were already infected with the subtype B strain in 1976 and that the same strain was isolated from

Gaetan Dugas in 1983. In other words, not only could Dugas not have been patient zero but it is highly unlikely that homosexuals from New York or San Francisco introduced HIV to Haiti either. More likely, it was the other way around. Once gay men from New York and San Francisco were infected with the B strain of HIV from Africa via Haiti, however, the high numbers of sexual partners within this community, coupled with practices such as anal sex, triggered an exponential amplification of the virus, eventually bringing AIDS to the attention of Gottlieb and other American doctors in 1981.

* * *

Even more so than Legionnaires' disease, the AIDS pandemic forced scientists to confront the hubristic assumption that medicine was on the verge of conquering infectious disease. This was not only because AIDS patients presented with conditions—PCP, KS, thrush—that were thought to have been consigned to the medical curiosity chest, but because by the time experts woke up to the new syndrome, HIV was widely dispersed and spreading on several continents. As we have seen, this was not the fault of epidemiologists or cancer specialists. On the contrary, AIDS became a pandemic at precisely the moment when, for the first time in history, scientists had the technology and intellectual tools to identify a new retrovirus and devise tests and treatments for it. However, AIDS also underlined something that had been overlooked by scientists and public health officials in the wake of the celebrations that followed the eradication of smallpox in 1980. The first was that pathogens are constantly mutating in ways that are difficult to predict. The second is that humans, either through their changing social and cultural behaviours, or through their impact on the environment and animal and insect ecologies, exert powerful evolutionary pressures on microparasites.[85] Sometimes, these pressures select for a particularly virulent strain of the parasite. At other times, they present the parasite with an opportunity to colonize a new host and extend its ecologic range. This is a particular risk in the case of zoonotic diseases bridged by rodent and insect vectors, such as plague, yellow fever and dengue. However, it was realized that in an era of increasing globalization, it was also true of other zoonoses that were not nearly as mobile. In particular, it was argued, AIDS would not have been able to escape Africa had humans not changed the rules of "viral traffic."[86] According to the virologist Stephen Morse, who coined the phrase, these rules included not only environmental and social changes that afforded the simian progenitor of HIV new opportunities for interspecies transfer and amplification within human populations, but such factors as better road and rail connections and international jet travel. Morse's concerns were soon echoed by other scientists, including the bacterial geneticist and head of Rockefeller University, Joshua Lederberg. In 1989 Lederberg and Morse organized a conference in Washington, DC, then followed it up in 1991 with a scientific report looking at the threat posed by "EIDs." As defined by the Institute of Medicine report, EIDs included diseases such as AIDS and Ebola that were previously unknown as afflictions of human populations and whose "emergence may be due to the introduction of a new agent, to the recognition of an existing disease that has gone undetected, or to a change in the environment that provides an epidemiologic 'bridge.'"[87] Taking up a theme explored by René Dubos, Lederberg went on to argue that in an era of increasing "globalization," air travel and the rapid mass movements of goods and people from one part of the globe to another had tilted the balance in favour of microbes, "defining us as a very different species from what we were 100 years ago." The result, according to Lederberg, was that despite new medical technologies and the wider availability of vaccines and antibiotics, the human race was "intrinsically more vulnerable than before."[88]

Lederberg's warning was not lost on the journalist and science writer Laurie Garrett, who had witnessed the ravages of AIDS in Zaire first-hand. In her 1994 bestseller, *The Coming Plague*, Garrett explained that thanks to globalization "few habitats on the globe remain truly isolated or untouched," and because of rapid international jet travel, "a person harboring a life-threatening microbe can easily board a jet plane and be on another continent when the symptoms of illness strike." AIDS, she concluded bleakly, "does not stand alone," but was a harbinger of epidemics and pandemics to come.[89]

7

SARS

"SUPER SPREADER"

*"The island of Hong Kong is not only the most unhealthy spot in China ... but the site
selected for Victoria, the principal town and seat of government, is the most unhealthy
locality of the whole Island, situated as it is on the side of an arid rock, which reflects
the rays of a tropical burning sun in a fearful manner."*

Sir Henry Charles Sirr, *China and the Chinese*, 1849

It is hard to imagine a less promising site for a major international metropolis
than Hong Kong, much less one boasting seven million souls. Perched on the
southern edge of the Chinese mainland, sixty miles east of Macau, the Special
Administrative Area, as Hong Kong has been known since 1997 when the
British crown colony reverted to Chinese control, occupies an area of 400
square miles. But as most of that comprises scattered islands and rugged hills
rising steeply from a narrow shoreline, in practice most of the population is
crammed into a strip of land on the northern side of Hong Kong island overlooking Victoria Bay, plus the peninsula of Kowloon and the adjoining New
Territories. The result is one of the most densely populated cities on Earth and
an urban wonder.

Whether arriving by cruise ship or swooping through the clouds in a Boeing
747, one's first sight of Hong Kong takes the breath away. It is not just that
Hong Kong boasts more high rises than any other city on Earth, or that its
iconic skyscrapers, such as IM Pei's Bank of China building, once the tallest
office building in Asia, seem to defy gravity; it's the juxtaposition of all that
sharp-edged glass and steel with the soft verdancy of those vertiginous hillsides. No matter the depths of a bank's pockets or the ingenuity of its architects, no human construction can equal the majesty of Victoria Peak, let alone

the view from Tai Mo Shan, which at nearly 3,300 feet above sea level marks the highest point on the island. Looking up from the trading floor first thing in the morning, or sipping a cocktail in a luxury penthouse late at night, even a star bond trader cannot help but feel a sense of wonder and reflect on the limits that nature sets on man's ambitions.

It is not only Hong Kong's forbidding landscape that has made human settlement a challenge. The island's unusual topography and subtropical climate are also an ideal breeding ground for malaria and other mosquito-borne diseases, especially during the summer monsoons or the typhoons that batter Hong Kong in the autumn. Indeed, such was the island's reputation for insalubrity that the early British colonists preferred to sleep on board their ships in Victoria harbour rather than risk a bout of "Hong Kong fever" on land. In an era when such fevers were thought to be due to noxious gases emanating from the earth and rocks, such measures made sense. "The geological formation of Hong Kong," wrote Sir Henry Pottinger, the second colonial governor, in 1843, "is found to consist of strata which quickly absorb any quantity of rain, which it returns to the surface in the nature of a pestiferous mineral gas. The position of the town prevents the dissipation of this gas, while the geological formation favours the retention of the morbific poison on the surface." Other authorities agreed, arguing that "in the intervals of rain, a nearly vertical sun acts with an intense evaporating power and a noxious steam or vapor rises from the foetid soil, yielding a gas of a most sickly and deleterious nature." This gas, the writer continued, "produces a depressing effect on mind and body which undermines and destroys the strongest constitutions."[1]

One of the most feared areas was the harbour and the predominantly Chinese Tai Ping Shan district, a warren of poorly constructed wooden shacks running with raw sewerage in which people, pigs and rats mingled freely. Even before bubonic plague forced the authorities to level Tai Ping Shan in 1894, the area had a reputation for disease: cholera, typhoid and smallpox were rife. To escape the successive waves of infection, Hong Kong's wealthier residents built their homes as far from the waterfront as possible, inching up the slopes of Mount Victoria to about the midpoint of the mountain. One of the first residents of the Mid-Levels, as the area became known, was George Bonham, the governor of Hong Kong from 1848 to 1854. His gated mansion set a precedent, and soon others with names like "Rose Hill," "Cringleford," and "Idlewild" followed (one resident was Sara Roosevelt, the mother of Franklin D. Roosevelt, who took up residence here with her family during the American Civil War).

Of course, not everyone could afford such views or such commodious quarters. Instead, as workers from the Chinese mainland poured into Hong

Kong in the early 1980s, drawn by its booming economy and liberal political climate, so architects devised ever more ingenious solutions to accommodate the city's growing population. These public housing projects frequently took the form of multiple occupancy tower blocks rising to forty stories or more. With upwards of twenty apartments per floor, and as many as ten blocks occupying sites of five acres or less, these complexes were practically cities in themselves. Typically, whole families were crammed into single occupancy apartments, reducing the average adult living area in Hong Kong to under two square metres.[2]

With no air conditioning, the apartments were stiflingly hot in summer, the only solution being to throw open a window and risk a lungful of smog from the traffic-clogged streets below, or to install high-powered fans adjacent to the light wells that ran through the centre of the blocks. Most families who could afford it opted for the latter, but there was little that could be done about the creaking plumbing and, with so many people showering and flushing at the same time, backups and breakdowns were frequent.

Little wonder, then, that on weekends many sought the fresh air and open spaces of Shek O Country Park or the paved paths and trails that encircle Victoria Peak. But even here, above the mosquito line, comfort was not guaranteed and the island could still spring a surprise. Indeed, long-time residents know that for all that Hong Kong boasts its own subway system, at heart it is still a jungle. Those inviting hillsides, for instance, teem with wild boar and venomous snakes, and hikers are advised to keep a wary eye on the undergrowth for hungry pythons.

It is not pythons that pose the principal threat to Hong Kong's residents, however. Nor is it mosquitoes: malaria and dengue are no longer endemic to Hong Kong, though on occasion doctors see imported cases. The principal ecological danger comes from Hong Kong's giant neighbour to the north and the modernizing and urbanizing processes that have intensified the microbial traffic between animals and humans. From Kowloon, on the opposite side of Victoria Bay, it is just ninety minutes by train to Shenzhen and the gateway to Guangdong, the most populous province in China, which is home to some 80 million people. Since the market liberalization measures introduced by China's leadership in the late 1970s, Shenzhen and the provincial capital, Guangzhou, have witnessed astonishing rates of economic growth. Spurred by the production of sports trainers, cheap toys and electronics, between 1978 and 2002 Guangdong's GDP grew by an average of 13.4 per cent per annum, while the urban population of the Pearl River Delta region, which encompasses Guangzhou, expanded to the point where it now accounts for

70 per cent of the province's total population. This manufacturing boom has had two major ecological effects. First, to feed the vast labour force in its factories, Guangdong raises millions of chickens on industrial-scale poultry farms (in 1997, the province was home to an estimated 700 million chickens and by 2008 it was producing one billion "high quality" broiler chickens a year).[3] At the same time, rice farmers and smaller livestock producers fatten domestic chickens and ducks in their backyards, hawking the birds in "wet markets" on the edge of urban areas when they are plump and ready for the pot. The result, according to the sociologist and urban historian Mike Davis, is a "fractal pattern of garden plots next to dormitories and factories [that] has brought urban populations and livestock together in more intimate contact." As many smallholders also keep pigs close to chicken pens, these farming patterns also increase the chances that bacteria and viruses harboured by chickens will inadvertently be communicated to the swine in faecal deposits and that, in turn, pigs will communicate the pathogens to humans. In short, Guangdong has become the potential source of a viral Armageddon and what Davis calls the ecological "monster at our door."[4]

To cater to Guangdong's newly affluent entrepreneurial classes, in the early 2000s chefs also began offering ever more exotic fare on restaurant menus, including game animals that had previously been considered rare seasonal delicacies. Animal traders responded to this increased demand by sourcing exotic game from countries such as Laos and Vietnam, or breeding game animals on small, unregulated farms, from where they were transferred to animal markets in Guangzhou and Shenzhen when they were ready to be eaten. The result was a mixing of multiple species in animal markets that would rarely, if ever, encounter one another in nature, and certainly not in such crowded conditions.

Fortunately, Hong Kong, unlike Guangzhou and other provincial towns and cities in Guangdong, benefits from world-class medical facilities and teaching hospitals equipped with the latest diagnostic technologies. Because of the greater political freedoms enjoyed in Hong Kong, Kowloon and the New Territories under China's "one country, two systems" policy, Hong Kong is also not subject to the cloying regulations and fear of authority that make potentially embarrassing disclosures anathema to the communist authorities on the Chinese mainland. Rather, Hong Kong health officials, many of whom were trained overseas in American and European universities, seek to apply the same clinical and public health standards as they would anywhere else in the world. This reputation for medical rigour, combined with Hong Kong's unique political and geographical position, make it something of a "sentinel" for the health of the rest of the world. In short, when a new epidemic or pandemic virus emerges somewhere in China, it is in Hong Kong that the alarm is likely to sound first.

* * *

From his sixth floor office at Hong Kong University's School of Public Health, Malik Peiris has a perfect view of Pok Fu Lam country park and Queen Mary Hospital. For the soft-spoken microbiologist with a passion for epidemiology and viruses that cross the species barrier, it is the perfect situation. In the winter, geese, teal and other wild migratory birds swoop past his window en route to the Mai Po Nature Reserve, a protected wetland on the edge of the Inner Deep Bay that is an important waystation for birds migrating south from Siberia to New Zealand during the northern winter. And when an unusual respiratory case presents itself in the emergency room of Queen Mary Hospital, Peiris's laboratory is well placed to perform a viral assay. So when in November 2002 public health officials began hearing rumours of an unusual respiratory outbreak in Guangzhou, it was only natural that Peiris's lab should be placed on alert in the expectation that similar cases would soon be presenting themselves at Queen Mary and other public hospitals in Hong Kong.

Peiris's interest in viral ecology dates from 1987 when, shortly after obtaining his PhD in microbiology at Oxford University, he was asked to investigate an outbreak of Japanese encephalitis in his native Sri Lanka. A viral disease spread by mosquitoes that breed in rice paddies, Japanese encephalitis had broken out in Anuradhapura, an historic city in northern Sri Lanka famous for its architectural ruins. Some 360 people fell ill, the majority of them rice farmers. This was puzzling; although the virus can be transmitted to humans, it usually cycles between birds, mosquitoes and pigs. Moreover, although outbreaks of Japanese encephalitis in humans had previously been documented in Japan and other parts of Asia, large human outbreaks had not occurred in Sri Lanka before. Clearly something had changed; the question was what?

At first, Peiris and his colleagues thought that the outbreak might be due to a sudden change in the virulence of the virus, but when they looked at the virus in the lab they could see it had not mutated. Next, they trapped mosquitoes in and around farmers' fields to see if there had been a change in the transmission dynamics of the disease. Perhaps a species other than *Culex*, the usual vector, was now transmitting the virus, or there had been a sudden increase in mosquito numbers. But, once again, in both cases the answer was negative. Then they looked at pigs. To diversify the agricultural base and supplement farmers' incomes, the Sri Lankan provincial authorities had handed each farmer twenty pigs free of charge. These pigs now grazed freely in the farmers' backyards beside the rice paddies. In so doing, Peiris discovered, the pigs not only provided mosquitoes with a ready blood meal, but greatly increased the chances of transmission of Japanese encephalitis to humans. "It was like putting a match to dynamite," he said. "Pigs turned out to be perfect amplifiers. With the best intentions, somebody puts this in and, boom, you have this huge explosion." The investigation peaked Peiris's interest in veterinary epidemiology and the interface of animal and human diseases, and set him wondering about other human interventions that might alter the balance of microbial ecologies.

Peiris's next big opportunity came in 1997 soon after he joined Hong Kong University's medical faculty as a senior lecturer in microbiology. His appointment coincided with the first documented transmission of avian influenza from birds to humans. An influenza virus, known as H5N1, had been isolated from the throat washings of a three-year-old boy. He had been admitted to Queen Elizabeth Hospital in Kowloon in early May with what appeared to be a run-of-the-mill upper respiratory tract infection.[5] Initially, the boy was given aspirin to relieve his fever and sore throat, but within days his condition had deteriorated and he was transferred to intensive care. Soon, his tiny body was being racked by an unusual cluster of conditions, including viral pneumonia, Acute Respiratory Distress Syndrome (ARDS) and Reye's syndrome. He died on 21 May, the cause being recorded as multi-organ failure.[6]

H5 influenza viruses were not entirely unknown to flu researchers in 1997—the virus had first been isolated nearly four decades earlier in Scotland. However, since then, veterinary virologists had seen it on only two other occasions: during a devastating outbreak of "fowl plague" in Pennsylvania in 1984 that had forced the authorities to cull 20 million chickens, and on an English turkey farm in 1991.[7] The point is that until 1997 no one had imagined that H5N1, or any other bird flu virus, might be capable of jumping the species barrier and sickening humans, much less killing them.

Working backward, a team from the CDC, headed by Keiji Fukuda, a Japanese-American clinical epidemiologist and the future coordinator of the WHO's Global Influenza Program, learned that a few months earlier chickens on farms near Yuen Long, in rural northwest Hong Kong, and the Mai Po Marshes close to Kowloon, had been struck by a mysterious plague. The culprit also seemed to be H5N1. Alarmingly, one of the farms was only fifteen miles from the boy's home. Not only that but several weeks before he had fallen ill, teachers at his nursery school had brought in three baby chicks and two ducklings for the children to play with. By the time Fukuda arrived at the school in August both ducklings had died, as had two of the chicks.[8]

To flu ecologists the latter findings were especially worrying. Ducks are considered "silent reservoirs" of bird flu viruses—silent, because they harbour and excrete the virus without exhibiting symptoms of illness or other obvious signs of infection. Not so chickens, which are highly susceptible. When they come into contact with diseased ducks and are exposed to the virus for the first time—typically through excreted faecal matter—they fall violently ill. One moment they are clucking contentedly, the next they are staggering from side to side as their brains, stomachs, lungs and eyes leak bloody haemorrhagic fluids. It is for this reason that poultry farmers describe such infections as a "plague" and that Robert Webster, the world's preeminent avian influenza expert, has dubbed mallards and teals "Trojan ducks."[9]

Both chickens and ducks can also transmit bird flu to pigs, and because swine can simultaneously be infected with human strains of influenza this makes them the perfect vessel for the reassortment of avian and human flu viruses. Indeed, scientists hypothesize that it is when these avian and human strains exchange genes, reconfiguring their surface proteins and generating a new, hybrid virus, that you get pandemics. This is what appears to have caused both the 1957 "Asian flu" pandemic and the 1968 "Hong Kong" flu pandemic, triggered respectively by H2N2 and H3N2 hybrid viruses containing both bird and mammalian influenza genes.

In addition, scientists suspect that pandemics may also be triggered by spontaneous mutations of avian viruses. Viruses are continuously making copying errors, and avian viruses are no exception. The theory is that some of these mutations could result in subtle changes to the molecules on the surface of the virus, enabling it to bind deeper into the human respiratory tract. As people are not ordinarily infected with bird flus, once such a virus found a way of transmitting efficiently to humans, runs the theory, there would be little to stop it because our immune systems would be powerless to mount an antibody response. Instead, the infection might trigger a catastrophic cascade similar to the syndrome that killed the three-year-old Hong Kong boy. Indeed, when scientists looked more closely at the genome of H5N1 they discovered that its surface proteins had the ability to bind to both avian receptor sites and human cells deep in the lungs. That discovery sparked renewed interest in the natural history of influenza and the ecological conditions driving adaptations of wild viruses circulating in aquatic bird populations. It also led to speculation that similar processes may have triggered the emergence in 1918 of the Spanish flu—a virus that a leading flu expert has described as "the most bird-like of all mammalian flu viruses" and which was associated with a similarly unusual pathology in young adults.[10]

As spring turned to summer then autumn, Hong Kong held its breath. By now teals and other migratory waterfowl had begun to gather in the city's Deep Bay and Mai Po Marshes en route from their Siberian breeding grounds, adding to anxieties that the birds might communicate H5N1 to local ducks and chickens. Then in November there were two further human cases, followed in December by several more. Panicked, the Hong Kong authorities closed the city's wet markets and ordered the culling of 1.5 million of the territory's chickens. That seemed to do the trick. Although the virus continued to turn up every now and again in samples collected from wild birds, no more cases were reported in domestic chickens. Nevertheless, by the time the outbreak ended in 1998, eighteen people had been infected and six had died, five of them adults.

For Peiris, the outbreak was a wake-up call. Together with his Hong Kong University colleagues Yi Guan and Ken Shortridge, he warned that the H5N1 virus had been "possibly one or two mutational events from achieving pandemicity." The good news was that because of Hong Kong's geographical position and the territory's concentration of microbiological expertise, it was well positioned to act as an "influenza sentinel"—an early warning post for avian flu viruses that might suddenly emerge from their aquatic reservoirs.[11] By 2002 these included not only H5N1, but another bird virus, H9N2, that was widely seeded in pigeons, pheasants, quail, and guinea fowl in southern China.[12] More alarming still was the fact that the H9N2 virus had also infected two children in Hong Kong, though without sickening them, and shared several of the same internal proteins as H5N1. Indeed, the more Peiris, Guan and Shortridge looked at the range of viruses circulating in live poultry markets, the more they realized that genetic reassortment was a common occurrence in nature, and that, far from being in evolutionary stasis in aquatic birds, avian flu viruses were constantly transiting between ducks and poultry and back again, generating "multiple reassortants."[13]

The result was that when, in December 2002, ducks, geese, flamingos, swans, egrets and herons suddenly started dying in two popular Hong Kong parks, and soon after Peiris began hearing rumours of an unusual respiratory outbreak in Guangzhou, he naturally assumed that bird flu had returned in a more virulent form. Two months later, at the beginning of February 2003, using web-crawling software to scan the internet for reports of unusual respiratory outbreaks, the WHO picked up an item about an outbreak of "atypical pneumonia" in three hospitals in Guangzhou. Soon after, the WHO intercepted text messages saying there had also been a major outbreak at a fourth Guangzhou hospital and that there was panic-buying of gauze masks, antibiotics and white vinegar, a traditional Chinese remedy for warding off respiratory infections. This was followed by an advertisement by the Chinese subsidiary of the Swiss drug company Roche that its antiviral medication Tamiflu was effective against bird flu. According to Klaus Stohr, the head of WHO's influenza vaccination program, "that put in the minds of people that a bird flu epidemic had started."[14] However, the clincher came when a seven-year-old girl from Hong Kong suddenly died of respiratory disease while visiting her family in Fujian. Although she was buried before the cause of death could be ascertained, nine days later her father was stricken with what appeared to be the same disease, dying in mid-February in Hong Kong. His son also developed symptoms of respiratory distress but recovered. Laboratory tests subsequently showed that both had been infected with the same strain of H5N1 that had been killing ducks and other birds in Hong Kong's parks. By now Peiris was convinced he was seeing the start of a new bird flu outbreak, possibly far bigger than the one that had visited Hong Kong in 1997. He was sceptical of the official line being peddled by the communist authorities in Guangdong that the respiratory outbreaks were due to a form of chlamydia, so he asked two Chinese colleagues who had previously worked at the Institute of Respiratory Diseases in Guangzhou to make discreet inquiries. Ignoring the usual diplomatic channels, the medics travelled to Guangzhou independently and returned with throat washings from twenty Chinese respiratory patients. Peiris and Yi had expected the washings to light up when they added the samples to sera infected with H5N1, but to their surprise nothing happened. Next, they looked for reactions for other common respiratory viruses, but once again the serological tests were negative so they began testing for more exotic viruses, such as Hanta. Finally, Peiris and Yi added the washings to various off-the-shelf cell cultures to see if they could persuade anything to grow in them. But whatever was lurking in the throat washings did not replicate in the usual laboratory growth media. All they could be sure of was that it was not bird flu or other commonly known causes of respiratory illness.

* * *

Like other Hong Kong streets commemorating important events in British history, Waterloo Road seems to belong to a bygone era. Named after the

Belgium battleground at which the Duke of Wellington bested Napoleon Bonaparte, the road is one of Kowloon's principal thoroughfares, running east past Ferry and Nathan Roads, before turning sharply in the direction of Logan's Rock to the north. It is not a pretty road. Clogged with traffic and hemmed in by ugly high-rises, it is for passing through rather than lingering in. Indeed, were it not for Kwong Wah Hospital at one end and the 487-room Metropark Kowloon—a mid-priced hotel formerly known as the Metropole—at the other, there would be little reason for stopping here.

On 21 February, Liu Jianlun, a 64-year-old professor of nephrology, checked into room 911 on the ninth floor of the Metropole. A doctor at the Second Affiliated Hospital of Zhongshan Medical University in Guangzhou, Liu was feeling a little under the weather. A few weeks earlier, a Guangdong seafood trader had presented at his hospital with peculiar respiratory symptoms. Although the trader spent only eighteen hours in the emergency room, in that time he infected twenty-eight hospital staff. He was then transferred to the Third Affiliated Hospital, where he set off further respiratory clusters among health care workers, earning himself the nickname "poison king."[15] On 15 February, Liu had developed similar respiratory symptoms. But after dosing himself with antibiotics he felt well enough to travel and boarded a bus in Guangzhou for the three-hour ride south to Kowloon. After checking in to the Metropole, Liu had mustered the energy to go shopping, but the following morning he woke with a high fever. Instead of attending his nephew's wedding he turned right outside the hotel and walked to Kwong Wah Hospital. Once there Liu asked to be admitted, informing medical staff that Guangzhou had many patients with atypical pneumonia and that it was "a very virulent disease."[16] He also said that he had treated some of the patients in the hospital's outpatient clinic, but as he had been wearing a mask and gloves he was confident he had not contracted anything. He was wrong.[17]

On 4 March Liu died of what would later be called SARS—short for Severe Acute Respiratory Syndrome. Not only that, but during his stay at the Metropole, via a mechanism that was never identified, he managed to transmit the disease to sixteen other guests on the same floor plus a visitor to the hotel, though not, miraculously, to the hotel's staff. Within seventy-two hours, sixteen of those guests, who included airline crew members, had introduced the disease to seven other countries, including Vietnam, Singapore, and Canada, sparking similar respiratory outbreaks in hospitals in Hanoi and Toronto. At this juncture, no one connected those outbreaks to Liu or to room 911 of the Metropole—that would come later. Instead, convinced that this was the start of the long-feared bird flu pandemic, on 12 March the

WHO issued a global travel alert. As images of nervous Hong Kong commuters in face masks flashed around the globe, air travel to Southeast Asia ground to a halt and financial markets went into a tailspin. On a China Airlines flight from Hong Kong to Beijing, a 72-year-old man who, unknown to him or anyone else on board, had been infected with SARS while visiting Hong Kong, communicated the disease to twenty-two passengers on the same flight, as well as two crew members. Meanwhile, in Thailand, at the end of March the mysterious pathogen claimed the life of one of Asia's most respected doctors, Carlo Urbani. The head of WHO's infectious disease division in Vietnam, the Italian parasitologist and clinician had contracted the infection while tending to a young Chinese American businessman who had presented with severe respiratory symptoms at the French Hospital in Hanoi on 26 February. A few nights before, the businessman, Johnny Chen, had been staying on the ninth floor of the Metropole, though it was only later that the significance of that fact would be appreciated.

Urbani's death at the age of forty-six, heavily sedated on morphine and hooked up to a ventilator in a makeshift isolation room in a Bangkok hospital (after treating Chen, Urbani had flown to the Thai capital, not realizing he was incubating the infection), sent shock waves through Southeast Asia's expatriate medical community. How was it possible that at the dawn of the twenty-first century a physician familiar with the measures for treating highly infectious patients had contracted such a severe respiratory disease? And why had the pneumonic ailment resisted treatment with antibiotics and antiviral drugs? Once again the question was asked: was it H5N1 or some other strain of avian influenza?

In March 2003 no one knew the answers to those questions and, except for Peiris and other specialists in viral ecology, few people appreciated the threat posed by SARS. This was understandable given that, at the time, the world's attention was focused on the Middle East, where British and American troops were massing on the Iraqi border in preparation for a ground war prompted by "intelligence" that the Iraqi dictator Saddam Hussein was harbouring weapons of mass destruction in breach of United Nations Security Council resolutions. It had been less than two years since Islamist terrorists had seized the controls of four commercial airliners and piloted three of them into the World Trade Center and the Pentagon in a shocking act of international terrorism. The Bush administration was eager for revenge, and it had decided Iraq was the place to exact it. In fact, there was no evidence of Saddam's involvement in 9/11 and, it subsequently emerged, the Iraqi dictator had destroyed his deadly weapons arsenal several years earlier. Instead, the real weapon of mass destruction had been incubating in Guangdong and was now, seemingly, in the process of spreading worldwide through the simple expedient of hitching rides on buses, trains and airplanes.

Solving the mystery of SARS involved the mobilization of hundreds of scientists and laboratories all over the world. It would also require microbiologists to challenge their assumptions about a pathogen that had long been considered uninteresting and a "Cinderella" of the microbial world. As with the Legionnaires' disease outbreak nearly thirty years earlier, unravelling the mystery hinged on epidemiologists and microbiologists working hand-in-hand. And their efforts would lead to a deeper appreciation of the importance of urban ecologies, medical technologies, and human-made surroundings—particularly hotels, hospitals, and apartment blocks—in the spread of respiratory infections. But on 12 March, when WHO issued its alert, and as Peiris experimented with yet another cell culture in an effort to grow the virus—or whatever organism was lurking in the throat washings—all this lay in the future. By now, with the help of Dr Wilimina Lim, chief virologist at Hong Kong's Department of Health and the head of Queen Mary's public health laboratory, Peiris had set up a surveillance system for people presenting with atypical pneumonias at Hong Kong outpatient departments. Specimens were pouring into his laboratory (Peiris had wanted to include recent travel to Guangdong in the case definition, but his request was overruled out of concern that it might offend the Chinese authorities).

The urgent need for a reliable diagnostic test, so as to distinguish true cases of SARS from run-of-the-mill pneumonias and respiratory infections, was underlined by the horror stories reaching Peiris from clinicians and health workers on the front line. At the Prince of Wales Hospital in Sha Tin, in the New Territories, some fifty doctors, nurses, and medical orderlies appeared to have contracted the infection, prompting the hospital's management to quarantine them in a special isolation room with its own air conditioning system. However, the measures were ineffective. Over the following days and weeks nearly one hundred more health workers and patients succumbed, followed by friends and relatives who had visited them in the hospital. As at the Second Affiliated Hospital in Guangzhou, the outbreak appeared to have begun with a single case—what would later be dubbed a "super spreader" event.[18]

* * *

On 4 March, a 26-year-old airport worker, identified only as "Mr CT," presented at Hong Kong's Prince of Wales Hospital complaining of fever, body aches, and breathlessness—typical symptoms of community-acquired pneumonia. Accordingly he was admitted to the hospital's eighth-floor medical ward and given a course of antibiotics. The drugs appeared to do the trick, and over the next few days his fever abated and the patches on his lungs faded. However, the scratch in his throat would not go away and he coughed incessantly. Finding his airways choked with phlegm, doctors decided he needed a nebulizer—a device that delivers drugs to the lungs in the form of a fine mist. It was a big mistake. A nebulizer is an excellent way to deliver drugs to the lungs. Unfortunately, it is also a highly efficient way for viruses and bacteria lingering in the respiratory tract to be diffused more widely as after each inhalation comes an exhalation. In the case of Mr CT, it is thought the nebulizer aerosolized the virus-laden droplets in his breath, turning them into a mist that scattered the particles throughout the Prince of Wales's medical ward. Four times a day, for seven days in a row, Mr CT sucked on the nebulizer, then exhaled, releasing a fine mist of viral particles that drifted over the beds of other patients and infected passing health care workers. Although Mr CT was eventually isolated in a private room with negative-pressure ventilation and medical staff were instructed to wear disposable gloves and N95 masks, the measures came too late. The result was a mini-epidemic that very nearly closed the hospital.[19]

By the second week of March there were also several reports of cases occurring outside of hospitals, fuelling rumours that the pathogen was spreading freely in the community and that no one was safe. At first, Dr Yeoh Eng-kiong, Hong Kong's secretary for Health, Welfare, and Food, tried to make light of the rumours, but on 18 March he was forced to acknowledge the reports were true and convened a "war council" at health department headquarters in Queen's Road East. There, using a computer program loaned from the police, Yeoh and his director of health, Dr Margaret Chan, the future director-general of the WHO, pored over the latest reports as they tried to predict the pathogen's next move. "Every day we asked, 'What are we dealing with? What do we know?'" Chan recalled.[20]

In an office on the eighteenth floor of the same building, Thomas Tsang Ho-fai, a consultant in the communicable disease unit, was asking similar questions. A slightly built man, Tsang was a graduate of the CDC's elite Epidemic Investigation Service. Tipped for higher things (he would eventually be appointed controller of Hong Kong's Centre for Health Protection), Tsang had first come to prominence during the 1997 bird flu outbreak, but it was during SARS that he got a chance to demonstrate his sleuthing skills and was dubbed "detective Fai" by the Hong Kong media. Since the first week of

March, Tsang had been working around the clock, tracking SARS patients and their contacts. On 26 March he noticed that one hospital had reported fifteen SARS cases in a single day and that all the patients had given their address as Amoy Gardens, a nearby housing complex overlooking Kowloon Bay. That was unusual, so Tsang decided to take a closer look.

When he arrived at the complex he found that cases were increasing at an alarming rate: thirty-four people hospitalized on 28 March, thirty-six more the following day, and sixty-four more on 31 March. With the outbreak threatening to overwhelm the public hospital system, and his bosses considering quarantines, Tsang was under pressure to locate the source of the outbreak as quickly as possible. The problem was how. Without knowing whether SARS was a virus or a bacterium, and whether it was an aerosol or droplet infection, it was difficult to determine how it was transmitted and how best to halt its progression. However, Tsang reasoned that since most of the SARS cases had come from block E, that was the logical place to start.[21]

Built in 1981, Amoy Gardens is typical of many of the middle-income housing projects that blight Hong Kong. The complex consists of fourteen hideous beige tower blocks laid out in a cruciform shape. Each block has thirty-three floors and each floor has eight units arranged in pairs. In all, the blocks are home to some 19,000 residents. As a solution to Hong Kong's housing shortage, Amoy Gardens must at one time have seemed elegant. Unfortunately, the complex also presented the ideal environment for the spread of SARS.

Tsang noted that most of those who had fallen ill lived in the corner units, numbered seven and eight on each floor, suggesting that the disease had spread vertically between each floor.[22] Tsang also noted that while there had been cases in other blocks, those who lived in Block E had fallen ill about three days earlier, indicating that this was probably the seat of the outbreak. But what was the mechanism? Was it contamination from the water tanks, as had occurred during the Legionnaires' disease outbreak? Or could it have something to do with the high-powered exhaust fans that many of the residents had installed in their bathrooms? Tsang set up a classic epidemiological study, comparing rates of infection among residents who owned exhaust fans with those who did not. The results showed that those who used exhaust fans while taking showers had a five times greater chance of contracting SARS, suggesting that the pathogen may have been sucked into their bathrooms via sewerage leaking into the drains fitted to the floors of showers. However, when Tsang took samples from the sewer pipes and the building's water tanks, the tests were negative. Next, he examined the rubbish for signs of cockroaches and rodents. Also negative. Finally, he considered the possibility that, like the anthrax letter mailings that had followed the 9/11 terrorist attacks in the United States, the residents of Amoy Gardens had been deliberately targeted by a foreign power or a terrorist organization.[23] "We thought it might be a biological attack because of the vertical arrangement of cases," Tsang explained.[24] However, this theory was also soon ruled out.

Amoy Gardens was not the only building to attract Tsang's attention. By now epidemiologists from the Department of Health were also scouring the Metropole Hotel. The first indication that the hotel might be implicated in the outbreak came on 12 March when the Singaporean authorities notified Hong Kong's health department that three young women who had recently been hospitalized with SARS in Singapore had stayed at the Metropole. It subsequently transpired that one of the women, Esther Mok, a 23-year-old former airline stewardess who had been in Hong Kong on a shopping expedition, had stayed in a room on the same floor as Liu. On 28 February she had been admitted to Singapore's Tan Tock Seng Hospital, sparking an outbreak that infected twenty-one of the hospital's medical staff. One of the people she infected was a prominent infectious disease physician, Leong Hoe Nam, who subsequently had to be hauled off a flight that was returning to Singapore from New York, where he had been attending a conference. Deplaned at Frankfurt airport, Leong, who was traveling with his pregnant wife and mother-in-law, became Europe's first official SARS patient.[25]

By 18 March, Tsang had learned of two further cases who had stayed at the Metropole: a 72-year-old Canadian man who had been hospitalized in Vancouver, and a 78-year-old Chinese-Canadian woman, Kwan Sui Chu. Mrs Kwan and her husband had been visiting their sons in Hong Kong over the new year and had taken a room at the Metropole as part of an airline package deal, their stay overlapping with Liu's. Two days after returning to Toronto, Mrs Kwan fell ill and by 5 March she was dead. In the interim, she transmitted SARS to four family members, including her 44-year-old son, who in turn introduced SARS to Scarborough Grace Hospital, in Toronto, sparking the worst disease outbreak in the hospital's history.[26]

The information prompted the Hong Kong health department to review all its files on severe community-acquired pneumonia, and by 19 March Tsang knew of seven SARS cases linked to the ninth floor of the Metropole, including Johnny Chen, the Chinese American businessman who had introduced SARS to Hanoi, infecting Carlo Urbani. Tsang and his colleagues spent days combing the Metropole for clues, taking samples from the carpets, furniture, elevators, air vents, and toilets. Perhaps Liu had sneezed on Chen when he walked by him in the corridor of the ninth floor, or perhaps Chen had been infected when they shared an elevator. Or perhaps, the bug had been communicated to Chen and other guests via the hotel's air conditioning system, as had occurred with Legionnaires' disease at the Bellevue-Stratford in Philadelphia. These were all plausible hypotheses, but without knowing what they were looking for and being able to test for it, Tsang and his team could make little progress.

* * *

The discovery that the Metropole was the common denominator in the spread of SARS to other countries shook senior WHO officials. Unlike on 9/11 when the Pentagon's inability to imagine that terrorists might weaponize commercial airliners had caught America's security apparatus by surprise, in 2002 the WHO felt sure it had a system in place for detecting novel biological threats before they could cause widespread epidemics or pandemics. The name of that system was GOARN, short for Global Outbreak Alert and Response Network. The brainchild of David Heymann, the head of WHO's Communicable Diseases Division and a former CDC epidemiologist who was a veteran of the Legionnaires' and Ebola outbreaks, GOARN routinely trawled the internet for electronic "chatter" about outbreaks occurring in remote regions of the world. It used systems developed by Canada's Global Public Health Intelligence Network (GPHIN) and the Program for Monitoring Emerging Diseases (ProMED). The idea was that once alerted to a suspicious event, WHO officials could make discreet inquiries with the relevant health authorities and dispatch a team to investigate. Essentially, the electronic eavesdropping network was WHO's version of 999 and GOARN its fire and ambulance service. Indeed, it was the WHO's interception in November 2002 of the report about an unusual respiratory outbreak in Guangdong that had first prompted officials to make inquiries. But of course, in 2002 the pathogen that WHO officials had in mind was bird flu. The result was that when officials persuaded the Chinese to forward samples from Guangdong to a WHO laboratory for testing and it was found that those samples contained only routine strains of flu, no one thought to check for other pathogens and the samples were discarded.

Initially, Peiris had also assumed that the respiratory outbreaks in Guangdong and Hong Kong were due to a mutant strain of bird flu. "It was not at all clear at that stage that we were looking at something unknown," he said. "The only unusual thing about the disease was that health care workers seemed to get affected disproportionately, but a particularly severe influenza could conceivably have produced the same effect."[27] What changed Peiris's view and swept away the assumptions clouding experts' view of the SARS outbreak were two samples that arrived at Peiris's laboratory in the second week of March. As it happened, one of those samples came from Liu's brother-in-law, Chan Ying-pui, who had also been hospitalized in Hong Kong and who had died shortly after the 64-year-old professor of nephrology. Unlike other samples arriving at Peiris's laboratory, many of which only broadly fitted the WHO's case definition and may not have been true cases of SARS, Chan's clearly was.[28] Moreover, as the biopsy had been taken while he had been alive, there was a good chance that live virus might still be present in the tissue.

Once again, Peiris instructed technicians at his laboratory and at Queen Mary's to run tests using the usual cell cultures for growing respiratory viruses. It was only when these failed, as they had before, that Peiris suggested using other cell lines, including foetal kidney cells from rhesus monkeys that had proved useful for growing hepatitis and the human metapneumovirus, a common cause of severe bronchitis in children. Thus it was that on 13 March, Dr Chan Kwok Hung, a senior scientist in the microbiology laboratory at Queen Mary's, introduced Chan's lung biopsy into a monkey cell culture. Two days later, examining the culture through a microscope, he spotted a sheet of cells that appeared shinier and rounder than the others. However, the change in the culture was extremely subtle so he asked Peiris for a second opinion. Peiris agreed the culture looked "a bit unusual," but two days later there had been no further change, as one would expect if a virus were growing, so Peiris suggested scraping a bit off and transferring the material to a fresh cell line.[29] This time, they could see more of the rounded bodies, suggesting that something was definitely growing in the monkey cells. However, the same effect might be produced by a contaminant, such as a mycoplasma, or a drug that had been administered to the patient in hospital. To be certain Peiris asked a pathologist colleague, John Nicholls, to examine the cells through a high-powered electron microscope. Gathering in a room in the hospital's pathology department, Nicholls and Peiris could clearly see the particles. Peiris now had no doubt that a virus was growing in the cell culture, but what kind of virus was it and how could he be certain it was the cause of SARS?

Microbiologists tend to be a cautious lot and Peiris is no exception. To be sure he had isolated the agent of SARS he needed to confirm that the virus was also present in other SARS cases. The simplest way to do that was to use a serology test—the same test McDade had used to demonstrate that legionella was the cause of Legionnaires' disease in 1977. If the virus they had isolated was SARS, then serum from SARS patients would contain antibodies that would react with it. The strongest evidence of all would be if the virus reacted with serum taken from patients at an advanced stage of infection. Accordingly, to make the test as rigorous as possible, Peiris asked Lim at the public health laboratory to send him "paired" serum samples from patients with suspected SARS, i.e., samples collected from patients in the early and late stages of infection. In addition, he asked for serum from patients who did not have SARS and instructed Dr Lim not to tell him which was which. As they added the serum samples to the virus, they noted a marked antibody reaction. Importantly, the sera from the patients who did not have SARS gave no reaction. Moreover, using an indirect immunofluorescence assay to demonstrate seroconversion, they could see the reaction was stronger in the later serum samples—a strong indication of rising antibody levels in the SARS patients.

Peiris was now confident he had found the virus of SARS, and on 21 March he emailed Klaus Stohr at the WHO to tell him the news. However, as Peiris still did not know the classification of the virus, he asked Stohr to keep the finding confidential to give him time to complete the identification. Unfortunately, at this point scores of suspect cases were being reported in Canada, Hong Kong, Vietnam and Singapore, many of them among health workers, and the WHO was desperate for positive news. Somehow or other the news leaked out, forcing Peiris to go public on 22 March.

By now, researchers at several WHO collaborating laboratories were claiming they had also isolated the pathogen of SARS and that it resembled a paramyxovirus, the same type of virus that causes mumps and measles. However, none of these researchers had grown the virus in cell culture or tested it against serum from known SARS patients, so their statements were premature. To know what sort of virus it was, Peiris needed to match it to sequences stored on GenBank, a database managed by the National Institutes of Health that contains a repository of all known viruses. "But you can only do this if you know the sequence of the virus you are looking for and in this case we didn't know this," Peiris explained.[30]

That just left one option: to fish out bits of the viral genome from the infected cells using a random primer. Peiris had asked his colleague Leo Poon to set up this technique to directly test specimens. Now Poon applied the technique to the virus-infected cells in the hope of finding a match with sequences on GenBank. Thirty-five times Poon got fragments of genetic information, but each time the result came back as monkey cell DNA or some other "junk." By the thirty-eighth attempt Poon was losing hope. Then, on the thirty-ninth attempt, there was a partial match. "It was not perfect, but it seemed to be a coronavirus," said Peiris. If accurate, this was astonishing news. Coronaviruses are typically the concern of veterinarians. First isolated in 1937, coronaviruses had long been associated with fatal enteric and respiratory infections in pigs, rodents, chickens, and other animals. However, in humans they usually resulted in nothing worse than a sniffle and mild respiratory illness. In short, coronaviruses were considered the "Cinderellas" of the virus world, beautiful to look at after work but too insignificant to take up microbiologists' daylight hours.

To be sure there had not been an error, Peiris also spun the fluid containing the virus in a high-speed centrifuge and asked Lim to look at the concentrated virus particles under an electron microscope. Each virus particle was ringed by a halo of tiny spikes as if it were wearing a crown—that, too, strongly suggested a coronavirus. Peiris was now confident that SARS was indeed a coronavirus. He speculated that the reason the homology was not perfect was that it was very likely a new type of coronavirus that had emerged recently from an animal reservoir and therefore had yet to be typed by GenBank.[31] Using the partial genetic sequence of the virus, Peiris and his colleagues set up a PCR test to detect the virus, and on 28 March made the test available to hospitals in Hong Kong and to the WHO. "It is not the way we would normally set about it but time was of the essence," he explained.[32]

Events now moved rapidly. Within three days of the WHO's receiving this information, two other laboratories also reported finding the coronavirus, and by 25 March the CDC had uploaded images of the virus to a secure WHO website, prompting Peiris's group to do the same. Nonetheless, some researchers continued to insist that SARS was caused by a paramyxovirus or perhaps the human metapneumovirus. This prompted speculation that the viruses worked synergistically, with the coronavirus weakening the immune system to the point where the other viruses colonized the respiratory tract, triggering SARS's distinctive pathology. However, the patients with SARS that Peiris had investigated showed no evidence of metapneumovirus, only the coronavirus. Nor were the coronavirus or antibodies to the coronavirus found in other patients who did not have SARS. Peiris was therefore sure that the new coronavirus was the cause of SARS and that it had been newly introduced to humans, and he submitted a paper to this effect to the British medical journal *The Lancet*.[33] Researchers at Erasmus University in Rotterdam eventually resolved the dispute by performing an experiment on macaques, one group of which was infected with the coronavirus, a second with the human metapneumovirus, and a third with both viruses. Only the animals infected with the coronavirus developed full-blown SARS. By contrast, the metapneu-movirus resulted in only a mild rhinitis, while animals infected with both viruses did not develop worse symptoms than the first group. Ergo, the coro-navirus was both a sufficient and necessary cause of SARS.[34]

It had taken scientists more than two years to discover the cause of AIDS and develop a diagnostic test for HIV, and five months to demonstrate that Legionnaires' disease was due to legionella. By identifying the SARS virus so quickly and having a rough-and-ready test at hand, Peiris and other microbiolo-gists were now in a position to say who had the disease and who did not, and hence who presented a risk to the community and ought to be isolated to prevent wider spread.* At a time of growing panic in Hong Kong this was a significant achievement, one that would help health authorities gain the public's support for quarantines and other vigorous public health measures. Unfortunately, with hundreds of specimens pouring into Peiris's laboratory every day, he did not have enough staff to run the tests, and when he advertised for additional technicians hardly anyone responded. "Basically, people were scared to work with SARS in case they were accidentally contaminated. It really was a nightmarish situation. It was all we could do to keep our heads above water."[35]

If laboratory technicians were wary of the virus, so were other medical workers. Nowhere was the danger of SARS more acute than at the Scarborough Grace Hospital in Toronto. Following his arrival on 7 March, Mrs Kwan's son had waited twenty hours in the emergency department with only a thin cur-tain separating him from other patients. When, the following day, he was finally admitted he was so sick that he had to be rushed to intensive care for intuba-tion. Suspecting tuberculosis, the attending physician isolated him. Unfortu-nately, during his stay in the emergency room he had been given oxygen and vaporized medications. The result was that a week later a patient who had been in a nearby bed returned to Scarborough Grace complaining of similar symp-toms. The patient was immediately isolated and moved to the ICU, where he was intubated by a physician wearing a surgical mask, eye protection, gown and gloves. But the infection control measures failed and a few days later the physician developed full-blown SARS, followed by three nurses who had been present in the room when the doctor had inserted the tube into the man's

---

* One of the first samples Peiris tested came from Amoy Gardens; it was positive for antibodies to the coronavirus, confirming that the outbreak in the apartment complex was due to SARS.

trachea. Worse, the man's wife had not been asked about her exposure risk and was allowed to wander freely through the hospital's corridors even though, by then, she was incubating the disease and would also soon fall sick. During her visit to Scarborough Grace she infected six health care workers, two patients, two paramedics, a firefighter and a housekeeper.

In the meantime, in mid-March another patient who had been in contact with her husband, and who later presented with symptoms of a heart attack, plus a mild fever, was transferred to York Central Hospital, Toronto, where he became the source of another SARS cluster. Some fifty individuals were eventually infected, forcing the authorities to close the hospital. On 23 March Scarborough Grace followed suit, and anyone who had entered the hospital after 16 March was asked to observe a ten-day home quarantine. By now, guards had been posted at the entrance of the hospital and the city was running out of negative pressure rooms. In an effort to care for patients safely, West Park Hospital recommissioned twenty-five beds in a facility that had previously been used to house tuberculosis patients. Having worked out that SARS was a droplet infection, medical workers were told to apply stringent infection controls, such as handwashing, and wearing gowns, gloves and N95 masks. Despite these precautions, by 26 March some forty-eight people in Ontario had been hospitalized with "presumptive" SARS and eighteen were confirmed to have the disease, leading to the quarantining of hospitals across the province and the declaration of a "code orange" emergency. All but essential hospital services were suspended in Toronto.[36]

By now, SARS was dominating the news feeds, with press and TV competing to report every aspect of the outbreak. Toronto was gripped by hysteria. Panicked producers, concerned about their health and the expense of caring for sick crew members should they contract SARS, cancelled film and TV shoots. Chinatown became a ghost town as diners, spooked by rumours of the disease's Chinese origins, avoided dim sum restaurants and noodle shops. Anyone presenting with suspicious respiratory symptoms was advised to quarantine themselves at home, and when the child of a nurse from Scarborough Grace exhibited symptoms of SARS, her school shut its gates rather than take the risk of her infecting other children. Yet still, SARS continued to spread.

Public health officials had no choice but to assume the worst. As James Young, Ontario's provincial coroner and commissioner of public safety and security, recalled: "We did not know the duration of the incubation period. We did not know whether it was spread by droplet or by air. We had no reliable diagnostic test, no vaccine, no treatment." Indeed, wandering around

Toronto, Young was reminded of a "bioterrorist" attack, the difference being that when a bomb detonated you could see the carnage on the streets, but with SARS there was no "obvious destruction." Other colleagues feared it might be the harbinger of a pandemic, but "we realized that we simply didn't know enough about it to tell whether or not this was 'the big one.'"[37] For all the supposed medical progress that had been made since 1918, officials resorted to the quarantine measures that had proved effective in stemming plague and other outbreaks of infectious disease in the eighteenth and nineteenth centuries.

By April, officials were hopeful the crisis had passed, but shortly before Easter a new cluster of cases emerged among a Catholic sect in Toronto. In response, Ontario's health department asked clergy to place communion wafers in the hands of congregants, rather than their mouths, and advised priests not to enter confessional booths to take confessions. Then, on Easter weekend, healthcare workers at Sunnybrook Hospital contracted SARS while performing an intubation on a patient. Three days later, WHO issued a second travel advisory, warning tourists not to visit Toronto unless absolutely necessary. Ontario's minister of health was outraged and flew to Geneva to try to persuade WHO officials to change their minds, but it was to no avail. Instead, after lifting the travel advisory at the end of April, the WHO reinstituted it in May when a further twenty-six cases unexpectedly emerged at four Toronto hospitals. The result was that it was not until 3 July that the travel advisory was finally lifted. In all, SARS had resulted in 250 infections and 44 deaths in Toronto and Vancouver. That was not a lot when set against the annual death toll from cancer and chronic lung infections. However, in psychological and economic terms, the impact was dramatic. At the height of the crisis, one member of Ontario's SARS advisory scientific committee recalled waking up drenched in sweat, convinced that "Toronto and Kingston had been consumed by SARS and were desolate."[38] The hotel industry suffered a 14 per cent drop in bookings. Toronto's film industry, which had enjoyed a record year in 2001, taking nearly one billion Canadian dollars in production money, saw a similar dip in its fortunes. It would not be until 2010 that Toronto's film industry would rebound to 2001 levels boosted by the remake of the Arnold Schwarzenegger film *Total Recall* and the depreciation of the Canadian dollar that had occurred in the meantime.[39]

If SARS was a calamity for Toronto, for Hong Kong it was disaster. Public anxiety had been mounting steadily since the end of March when government officials descended on Amoy Gardens. As officers secured the housing complex with metal barricades and tape, TV viewers were treated to pictures of health workers in biohazard suits guarding the entrance to the high rises as health officials went door-to-door to issue residents with notices informing them that Amoy Gardens was being quarantined and they would not be able to step outside their apartments for the next ten days. The eerie images relayed around the world were the first that many people knew of SARS. The following day, 1 April, a 14-year-old boy decided to play an April Fool's prank by posting a bogus message on the website of a local newspaper. The message stated that Hong Kong was about to be declared an "infected port," that the Hang Seng Index had collapsed, and that its chief executive had resigned. Terrified, people rushed to grocery stores to stock up on rice and other essential commodities, then bolted the doors of their apartments and telephoned and texted those who had not yet heard the "news." That afternoon Margaret Chan held an emergency press conference in an attempt to reassure the public, but the following day her efforts were undone by the WHO's declaration that it had issued an advisory warning against unnecessary travel to Hong Kong. Prior to 2 April, Hong Kong's airport had been one of the busiest in the world, processing nearly 100,000 inbound passengers a day. Within weeks passenger numbers had fallen by two-thirds, and by the end of the month Hong Kong was seeing just 15,000 arrivals a day. "Hong Kong is a city gripped by fear," reported CNN. "A place that markets itself as 'The City of Life' and whose lifeblood is travel, trade and international business, is acquiring a reputation as a place of disease."[40]

The effects of this fear were far-reaching. In Britain, Hong Kong children attending a boarding school on the Isle of Wight were informed that they would be quarantined on the island following the Easter vacation. At the University of California, Berkeley, Hong Kong students and their families were asked to stay away from graduation ceremonies. Meanwhile, in Switzerland, health officials issued a decree banning anyone who had been in Hong Kong, Singapore, China or Vietnam since 1 March from attending the World Jewellery and Watch Fair in Basel and Zurich. Hong Kong, which usually mustered the second biggest delegation after the Swiss, threatened to sue, but the Swiss refused to budge, prompting one Hong Kong company to erect a sign over an empty booth that read: "Due to our fear of Swiss Aggravated Respiratory Syndrome we are going home."[41]

From an economic perspective, SARS could not have come at a worse time for Hong Kong as the territory was only just beginning to recover from the 1998 Asian financial crisis. The previous year Hong Kong had seen its real GDP grow by 2 per cent, and in 2003 the government had been forecasting 3 per cent real GDP growth. Within weeks of the WHO's travel advisory, those forecasts were revised downward as shops reported a halving of retail sales and hotels saw their occupancy rates plunge by 60 per cent.[42] As malls emptied and banks like HSBC ordered bond traders to stay home, the only people seen to be doing a brisk trade on the formerly packed streets were salesmen of N95 masks. The sense of panic was palpable. As a lawyer and filmmaker recently arrived in Hong Kong recalled, "It was no longer an animal flu, but 'Severe Acute Respiratory Syndrome'—an altogether more urban-sounding virus."[43]

By now there was little doubt that SARS was spread by respiratory droplets, but could it also be communicated in other ways, through contaminated faecal matter, for instance? And why, if the disease was so infectious, had none of the hotel staff at the Metropole contracted it? The questions recalled the epidemiological puzzle that had confronted CDC investigators at the Bellevue-Stratford in Philadelphia nearly thirty years earlier. Until Peiris identified the coronavirus and diagnostic tests became available, investigators had no way of checking these intuitions. Now, they were in a position to gather samples from different locations of the Metropole and at Amoy Gardens and send them to Peiris's laboratory to be analyzed. In late April a team of environmental health experts from Health Canada arrived in Hong Kong to assist the Department of Health with its investigation, and on 16 May they reported their findings. The investigators had concentrated their efforts on the ninth floor of the Metropole as this was where most of those who had fallen ill had been staying. In all, genetic material of the SARS virus had been found in 8 of 154 samples. The interior of Liu's room, 911, had yielded no traces of the virus. However, four positive samples had been collected from the carpet and door sills outside his room and the rooms on either side, suggesting that he may have thrown up when he stepped out of his room or else spread the virus when he coughed in the corridor. In addition, four positive samples were collected from the air inlet fan of the elevator that served the ninth floor. That suggested that Liu's body fluids had been aerosolized when he entered the elevator, meaning that anyone who stepped out of the ninth-floor lift shortly afterward would have been exposed. However, the investigators dismissed the theory that the virus was transmitted through contact with elevator buttons, door handles, or handrails, pointing out that, if that had been the case, then other guests in the hotel, as well as staff, would also have been infected.

Disappointingly, despite collecting and testing 143 samples from Amoy Gardens, the investigators were unable to recover any genetic material from the SARS virus at the housing complex. However, they noted that the outbreak had begun after a kidney patient who had been receiving dialysis treatment at Prince of Wales Hospital, and who had later developed what the hospital thought was influenza, was discharged and spent several nights at his brother-in-law's apartment at Amoy Gardens. As well as a fever and a cough, the man had suffered from diarrhoea, a symptom that Peiris's group would later discover occurs in about 10 per cent of SARS patients. As the virus had been found in stools for at least two days and the investigators suspected the man had had a high viral load, they speculated that his faeces could have been the cause of the outbreak. Noting that many of the drain taps in the bathrooms had dried out or been removed, and that many residents had bought exhaust fans that were six to ten times more powerful than were needed for such a small space, the investigators suggested that contaminated faecal matter could have been sucked into the bathrooms via the sewerage system when people showered. Alternatively, contaminated air from nearby bathroom vents could have carried droplets from adjoining bathrooms via the light well, releasing contaminants through the open windows of apartments above and below. Another factor that may have contributed to the spread of the virus was a sixteen-hour water shutdown that occurred in Block E on the evening of 21 March in order to allow a broken pipe to be fixed. During that period, many residents flushed their toilets with buckets of water, a practice that may have resulted in splashing, increasing the risk of contamination.[44] Overall, the epidemiological evidence suggested that SARS was primarily a droplet infection and that the risk was greatest when an infectious patient coughed or sneezed, propelling infectious particles over distances of about three feet. In many ways, that was good news as it meant that, unlike influenza, SARS did not linger in the atmosphere for long periods, making it an unlikely vehicle for a pandemic. Nor, despite the fears generated by the reports of hospital super spreaders, was it an efficient aerosol, meaning it was unlikely to recommend itself to terrorists. Having said that, at the point when patients develop symptoms—typically two to seven days after infection—they are highly infectious and one person can infect as many as three other people, possibly more if infection controls are inadequate and there is frequent contact between patients and nurses, as occurred in hospitals. Not only that, but SARS had spread efficiently in large buildings, such as the Metropole and Amoy Gardens. Clearly, the virus was a particular threat in urban settings.

* * *

Once scientists had cracked SARS's genetic code and established it was a coronavirus, the next obvious question was to ask where it had come from.

The two types of coronavirus previously known to infect humans belonged to groups that typically infected mammals and birds. SARS, however, did not appear to belong to either of these groups. Still, it was likely that SARS had zoonotic origins and that its animal host was located in Guangdong, where the earliest cases had occurred. As several of those cases had been traced to chefs and seafood merchants, the obvious places to look were the markets where restaurants bought exotic animals for their clientele.

In May 2003 Peiris's colleague Yi Guan packed a satchel with syringes, swabs and sample vials and set off by train for Shenzhen's Dongmen Market. There, working with the Shenzhen Centers for Disease Control, Guan approached animal traders and asked to take nasal samples and faecal swabs. Those who demurred were reassured that if any animal died they would be compensated up to the sum of 10,000 Hong Kong dollars (about $6), but more often than not Guan was able to anaesthetize the animals and take samples on the spot. As you might expect, there was a wide array of animals on sale: raccoon dogs, Chinese ferret badgers, beavers, Chinese hares and Himalayan palm civets. At the end of two days, Guan had collected twenty-five samples. They showed that four out of six of the palm civets carried a coronavirus that was 99.8 per cent genetically identical to the human coronavirus. In addition, one of the raccoon dogs carried the same virus as the civet cats, while one ferret badger had antibodies to the virus. When the animal viruses were sequenced, they were found to have a short section of twenty-eight nucleotides that were missing in the human virus, leading Guan and his colleagues to conclude that it was the absence of this sequence, or perhaps a random mutation, that had enabled the virus to transmit easily between humans. Moreover, 40 per cent of the animal traders whose blood was tested and 20 per cent of those involved in slaughtering the animals had antibodies to the virus carried by the civet cats, indicating that the virus had probably been circulating between animals and market traders for some time without causing disease. Even though other researchers were not immediately able to replicate Guan's findings, the Chinese halted sales of fifty-four species of wild animals while further tests were conducted in other markets. Those tests also found evidence of SARS antibodies in traders who dealt in palm civets, suggesting that the virus was regularly passing from animals to humans in southern China. However, it did not resolve the question of where the virus normally resided in nature. Nor did it explain why the SARS viruses carried by some of the civet cats at the market in Shenzhen had subtle differences when compared to human variants. One explanation was that the civets had been infected by some other animal in the wild, or on the farms where they bred.

"It is conceivable that civets, raccoon dogs, and ferret badgers were all infected from another, as yet unknown, animal source, which is in fact the true reservoir in nature," wrote Guan and his colleagues. In other words, civet cats and other animals popular in Chinese markets might be "intermediate hosts that increase the opportunity for transmission of infection to humans."[45]

Since then, further evidence has emerged to support this hypothesis. In 2005 researchers found that Chinese horseshoe bats harboured SARS viruses that were 88 per cent to 92 per cent identical to isolates from humans. However, those viruses were missing a crucial protein that binds to a receptor on the surface of human cells, meaning that the bat viruses could not infect humans directly—they would have to pass through an intermediary animal host first. Then, in 2013, scientists from China, Australia and the United States announced another discovery: after visiting a cave inhabited by horseshoe bats in Kunming, in southern China, they identified two new strains of coronavirus. Unlike previous strains isolated from bats, these did contain the crucial protein enabling them to infect mammalian cells, including cells lining the human lung.[46] Although this was not definitive evidence that SARS could move directly from bats to humans, it suggested that, as with other bat viruses, such as Nipah and Hendra, that also cause disease in humans, it had the potential to do so. "I think people should stop hunting bats and stop eating bats," commented one of the report's authors, Peter Daszak, the president of EcoHealth Alliance.[47]

They should probably also stop eating civets. To the credit of the Chinese, following the identification of civets infected with SARS, the animals were banned from wet markets and strict infection controls were introduced on civet farms. However, it seems that nothing could sate the Chinese appetite for the exotic mammals, and soon customer demand had driven up the price for civets to $200, making it likely they would find their way onto restaurant menus whatever action the authorities took.[48] The reason? Roasted whole, braised or added to soups, civets are considered a delicacy by the Chinese. They are also said to be full of *yang*, a heat-giving energy source that, according to traditional beliefs, helps people stay warm in cold weather.

* * *

If AIDS had given the world a preview of how the consumption of bushmeat and faster international communications were presenting animal pathogens with new opportunities to infect human populations and spread around the globe, SARS underlined the risks that the demand for exotic sources of protein and faster international air travel presented in the twenty-first century. Dubbed the "millennium's first jetset disease," SARS managed to infect thirty countries worldwide by the simple expedient of hitching lifts on airplanes.[49] All it required were unwitting dupes to carry it onto flights bound for Singapore, Hanoi, Toronto and other international destinations. That it found these human vessels at the Metropole Hotel was bad luck for the hotel's owners, but it could just as easily have been any Hong Kong hotel catering to international business travellers and package tourists. Once it was airborne, the virus ensnared the globe in a web of interconnecting lines, like a Lufthansa map iterated to the power of ten. This was something new and scary, serving as a reminder that unlike the physical borders between countries, international airspace is highly porous and vulnerable to interflows of people and pathogens. Coming in the wake of 9/11 and the anthrax letter mailings, it was also a reminder that, in the words of Peiris and Guan, "nature' remains the greatest bioterrorist threat of all."[50]

There were other lessons, too. Perhaps the biggest was that for all that the internet and new web-crawling technologies had given the WHO the ability to monitor disease outbreaks occurring far from the eyes of prying international health officials, governments still had considerable powers to cover up outbreaks and spread disinformation within their own borders, especially where it was felt that transparency might be detrimental to their economic and political interests. Indeed, it was not until mid-April, when a Chinese whistleblower revealed the true numbers of SARS infections in Beijing, that the authorities owned up to the full extent of the outbreak and mobilized resources on a scale necessary to quell it. Previously, the Communist Party had insisted there were just thirty-seven cases in the Chinese capital. In fact, by 19 April, Beijing had already seen 339 cases, including eighteen deaths, and SARS had also spread to Shanxi province, inner Mongolia, Guangxi and Fujian. Thanks to the institution of mass quarantines and the construction of new treatment facilities—a feat the Chinese accomplished virtually overnight— disaster was averted, but it was a close call. In all, China reported 5,327 SARS cases, more than any other country. Luckily, the vast majority were confined to Beijing and Guangzhou. However, had the virus become seeded in poorer, rural areas lacking sophisticated medical facilities, it could have been a different story.[51]

Chinese secrecy during the first three months of the outbreak, when SARS was spreading in Guangdong, had sown considerable confusion. Fed misleading information and with incomplete knowledge, WHO officials assumed the outbreak was due to bird flu. On the other hand, once the WHO triggered an international alert and named SARS as the culprit, screening measures at airports were sufficient to prevent further importations of the disease. And for the most part SARS was also controlled in hospitals once the risk of super spreaders was recognized and managers instituted rigorous infection controls. The result was that although there were 8,422 cases of SARS and 916 deaths globally, the disease was contained without the need for vaccines or specific therapies. Unfortunately, the same thing could not be said for the fear propagated by the WHO alerts. In an era of global news and the internet, news of SARS spread far faster than the virus, amplifying anxiety about the outbreak. As airports shut and pictures of nervous Hong Kong commuters flashed around the globe, the tourism, aviation and service sectors took a massive financial hit, resulting in an estimated $50 billion in losses to the global economy.[52]

On the other hand, the WHO could take encouragement from the way that GOARN had operated. SARS had been the first opportunity to test whether scientists and clinicians could set aside academic rivalries and work together for the public good by sharing information about the virus and the most effective treatment strategies. Within a month of establishing an international laboratory network, scientists had identified a coronavirus as the cause of SARS. Not long after, they completed the sequencing of its DNA and were on the trail of its animal reservoir. SARS, concluded Heymann, was "proof of the effectiveness of GOARN." At the same time, he recognized the WHO was also "aided by good fortune" in that the outbreak had occurred in Hong Kong. "Had SARS established a foothold in countries where health systems are less well developed cases might still be occurring," he observed, "with global containment much more difficult, if not impossible."[53]

* * *

At a post-mortem at the Royal Society in London, Roy Anderson, the rector of Imperial College and an internationally renowned epidemiologist, was similarly cautious. Although the WHO's handling of SARS had restored faith in the UN, the world had also been "very lucky," he wrote. It was only thanks to the low transmissibility of SARS and the fact that China and other Asian countries had been able to introduce "fairly draconian" public health measures, such as home isolations and mass quarantines, that disaster had been averted. He predicted such measures would have met greater resistance in North America, where people tended to be more litigious, and to a lesser extent in western Europe. The persistence of SARS in animal reservoirs meant that further outbreaks were inevitable. In the meantime, the real global threat came from the emergence of an antigenically novel influenza virus. "One of the major dangers arising from the effective control of SARS is complacency," Anderson concluded. "Sentiments of the type, 'we have been successful once——we will be again,' may be far from the truth."[54]

8

EBOLA AT THE BORDERS

"The outbreak ... delivered some horrific shocks and surprises. The world, including WHO, was too slow to see what was unfolding before us."

Dr Margaret Chan, Special Session of the Executive Board on Ebola, Geneva,
25 January 2015

In December 2013 a group of children gathered around the stump of a hollowed-out tree in Meliandou, a remote farming village in south-eastern Guinea, and began probing the hollow with a stick. The tree was a well-known roosting spot for *lolibelo*—a species of insectivorous, long-tailed bats—and the children liked nothing better than coaxing the tiny grey mammals from their hiding places. This was not merely idle sport. In a region where chimpanzees and other sources of bushmeat are scarce, the Angolan free-tailed bat *Mops condylurus* was an important source of protein. Indeed, for the children of Meliandou the tree stump en route to the village watering hole was the nearest thing to a hamburger stand and *Mops condylurus* was the equivalent of a Big Mac.[1]

It is not known how many bats the children caught and cooked that morning. In recent years, as more and more forested areas around Meliandou were cleared for palm oil cultivation, the *lolibelo* had taken to nesting under the roofs of the villagers' simple mud-and-wattle dwellings and had become a familiar sight. What is known is that shortly after visiting the tree stump, one of the children, a two-year-old boy named Emile Ouamouno, developed a high fever, with vomiting and bloody stools. His father gave him soup in the hope of calming his stomach, but nothing would halt the progress of his illness and on 6 December Emile died. Not long after, Emile's mother, who was seven months' pregnant, also fell ill, followed by Emile's three-year-old sister. This time there was even more blood, and on 13 December Emile's mother died together with her stillborn baby, followed soon after by Emile's sister.[2]

Like other villages in the forested region of south-eastern Guinea, Meliandou is an endemic area for malaria and Lassa Fever, a haemorrhagic infection spread by rats. Emile's symptoms and those of his mother and sister resembled both diseases, so at this point no one had any reason to suspect a new pathogen, much less that the *lolibelo* might be responsible. Had Meliandou lain deep within the forest that might have been the end of the matter, but the village is just six miles along a dirt track from Guéckédou, a busy trading town close to the borders of both Sierra Leone and Liberia. From Guéckédou, a poorly paved highway also leads north to Kissidougou, after which it joins the N1, the road to Guinea's coastal capital, Conakry.

For the main local ethnic groups, the Kissi and the Gola, trade is their lifeblood. Indeed, the ethnonym "Gola" is said to derive from the word for a nut, commonly known as *kola*, with stimulant properties revered throughout West Africa. It is thought that both groups settled the upper Guinea forest in around the fourteenth century, emigrating west from modern-day Côte d'Ivoire. Of the two, the Kissi are the largest, numbering some 220,000. As they are cut off from the Muslim majority in Conakry, census figures are hard to come by, but it is thought that as many as 80,000 live in the forest on the Guinean side of the border, and a further 140,000 in Liberia and Sierra Leone (by contrast, the Gola are concentrated in western Liberia). Linked by blood, traditions and a common language, the Kissi have little regard for the colonial-era borders that separate the countries, and extended families travel easily from one to another either by motorcycle along unpaved roads, or, just as frequently, by dugout canoes along the Mano River, which forms a natural boundary between Liberia and Sierra Leone.[3] Little wonder then that within weeks of the mysterious illness appearing in Guéckédou, it had spread beyond the town limits, radiating west to Macenta, east to Kissidougou, and south to Foya in Liberia.

The first person to fall ill outside the family was a midwife who had been summoned by Emile's grandmother to try to save her pregnant daughter and baby. She was admitted to a hospital in Guéckédou on 25 January and died eight days later on 2 February. Unfortunately, before being hospitalized she transmitted the disease to a relative, setting off a new chain of infections in the Guinean border town. By now Emile's grandmother had also died and at her funeral her sister and several mourners were likewise infected, probably because they prepared her body for burial in accordance with traditional funerary practices. This was followed, on 10 February, by an outbreak at a hospital in Macenta. The infection, which was introduced by a health worker from Guéckédou, sparked fifteen further deaths, including that of a local doctor, prompting Guinea's Ministry of Health to issue an alert on 10 March.[4]

One of the first to respond was the private medical charity Médecins Sans Frontières (MSF). In 2010, MSF had established a sentinel facility in Guéckédou to monitor the incidence of malaria; it was only natural that they would assume that the deadly mosquito-borne disease was to blame. But when MSF staff interviewed health workers about the outbreak they discovered that while many of the victims had exhibited symptoms typical of malaria, such as severe headaches and muscle and joint pains, they had also reported profuse bleeding, vomiting and violent diarrhoea, symptoms not at all typical of malaria. In addition, many complained of hiccups. The MSF medics initially suspected Lassa, but when they forwarded their report to Dr Michel Van Herp, a senior viral haemorrhagic fever expert at the organization's Brussels headquarters, it was the hiccups that caught his attention. They reminded him of a patient he had previously seen with the same symptoms. That patient had had Ebola.[5]

* * *

Ebola haemorrhagic fever is one of the most virulent diseases known to man. It is also one of the most terrifying. One moment, victims are complaining of fever, headache and a sore throat; the next, they are doubled up with abdominal pain, vomiting and diarrhoea. As the symptoms worsen, many also develop a dazed, glassy expression and a purple rash, accompanied by hiccups—caused, most likely, by irritation to the nerves that control the diaphragm. The most alarming symptoms occur several days into the illness when cells infected by the Ebola virus attach themselves to the insides of blood vessels, causing bloody fluids to leak from the mouth, nose, anus and vagina—even, on occasion, from the eyes. Ebola is especially damaging to the liver, where the virus wipes out cells required to produce coagulation proteins and other important components of plasma. Eventually, this damage reaches a point of no return and patients suffer a fatal drop in blood pressure, terminating in shock and multiple organ failure.[6] Little wonder, then, that one writer has described Ebola as "a perfect parasite ... [that] transforms virtually every part of the body into a digested slime of virus particles."[7]

Perhaps the only disease that compares to Ebola for visual shock value is yellow fever, which in acute cases can also cause bleeding of the mouth, eyes and the lining of the gastrointestinal tract, as well as the production of a viscous black vomit from the stomach. However, while Ebola is sometimes horrifying to behold, bleeding only occurs in around half of the cases; diarrhoea is a far more common symptom. Compared to HIV and SARS, it is also not that contagious. Ebola patients only become infectious when they develop symptoms—typically two to twenty-one days after exposure—and on average one Ebola patient will infect just two other people. By contrast, with HIV and SARS, the reproduction rate rises to four, and for truly catchy diseases such as measles, that number is eighteen.

Nevertheless, in previous outbreaks in the Democratic Republic of the Congo (DRC) and other countries in Central Africa, Van Herp knew that Ebola had been associated with mortality rates as high as 90 per cent. Then, as in 2014, there had been no vaccine, nor were there any approved treatment drugs. Instead, doctors' only option was to connect patients to an intravenous drip and keep them hydrated with fluids until such time as their immune system managed to defeat the virus. The problem is, while Ebola is not all that communicable, the disease is highly infectious—a cubic centimetre of blood contains one billion copies of the virus—and the attachment of an IV-line can result in blood leaking uncontrollably from the site of a puncture. If the outbreak in Guinée Forestière was due to Ebola—and the hiccups strongly suggested to Van Herp that it was—it was imperative to immediately isolate patients and their contacts, as well as anyone handling infectious cadavers, and introduce strict barrier nursing controls in hospitals. The problem was that as soon as news got out that MSF suspected Ebola, there would be panic across the region, not least among the organization's staff in Guéckédou, none of whom had experience with the pathogen. On the other hand, Van Herp knew that, other from a case in Côte d'Ivoire in 1995 involving a Swiss zoologist, Ebola had never been detected in West Africa before. Nevertheless, until such time as diagnostic tests could be conducted, Van Herp thought it best to err on the side of caution. "After further examination, I said to my colleagues, 'We're definitely dealing with viral haemorrhagic fever, and we should be prepared for Ebola, even if never seen in this region before."[8]

Van Herp was right to say that Ebola had never been seen in Guinea, but wrong to think that no one had previously suspected its presence in West Africa. In 1982, German scientists examined blood from hundreds of Liberians in Lassa-endemic rural areas of the country. Rather than simply testing for Lassa, however, they also looked for Ebola and a related filovirus called Marburg—so called because it was first isolated in the German town of Marburg in 1967—using a fast and inexpensive microscopic test known as indirect immunofluorescence.* They found antibodies to Ebola in 6 per cent

---

* Filoviruses belong to the family Filoviridae and take their name from the Latin word *filum*, meaning filamentous, a reference to their elongated filamentous structure.

of the samples. Similar rates were also found in samples from Guinea and Sierra Leone. However, because the test depended on skilled interpretation and sometimes resulted in false positives, few experts took much notice.[9] This was followed in 1994 by the infection of the Swiss zoologist. The zoologist most likely contracted Ebola when she performed a necropsy on a chimpanzee that had been found dead in Tai National Park, near Côte d'Ivoire's border with Liberia, but there was no further transmission and, after being flown to Switzerland for treatment, she recovered. Then, in 2006, a group of medical researchers made a further intriguing discovery at Kenema General Hospital, in eastern Sierra Leone, not far from the Guinean border. As in Liberia, the researchers had decided to run a quick antibody test on blood from patients who had presented at the hospital for Lassa Fever. Previously, one-third of these patients had tested negative for Lassa, leading the researchers to suspect they were infected with another type of haemorrhagic fever, or possibly a mosquito-borne virus, such as dengue or yellow fever. To their surprise, of four hundred samples taken between 2006 and 2008, nearly 9 per cent tested positive for Ebola. Not only that, but when they ran a more sophisticated assay, the researchers also saw that most of the antibodies were against *Zaire ebolavirus*, the most virulent of the five strains of Ebola. *Zaire ebolavirus* had previously been found in only three countries: the DRC, the Republic of the Congo, and Gabon. How the Zairean strain had come to be in Sierra Leone, 3,000 miles northwest of its endemic centre of transmission, was a mystery. Nevertheless, the researchers thought the findings worth publishing and in August 2013 submitted a paper to the CDC's journal, *Emerging Infectious Diseases*. As the research was a collaborative effort between the US Army Medical Research Institute of Infectious Diseases (USAMRIID) and Tulane University, the lead investigator, Ronald J. Schoepp, was reasonably confident the paper would be accepted. But after waiting nearly a year for a reply he was told it had been rejected; the final reviewer informed Schoepp, "I don't believe there is Ebola virus in West Africa."[10]

By the middle of March, MSF's senior leadership in Geneva was sufficiently alarmed by the reports from Guéckédou to dispatch three medical teams to the area. One was a team from Sierra Leone trained in the containment of viral haemorrhagic fevers. They arrived in Guéckédou on 18 March and immediately set about securing the area. Van Herp joined them soon after and began touring nearby communities to track the infection and raise awareness. Unfortunately, there was no laboratory in Guinea equipped to handle Ebola, much less to run sophisticated tests for detection of a filovirus, so blood samples were shipped all the way to the Institut Pasteur in Lyon. There, in a secure biosafety level 4 laboratory, Sylvain Baize, a specialist in haemorrhagic fevers who had previously worked in Africa, ran the critical assays that, on 21 March, confirmed the presence of Ebola in several of the blood samples. It was too early to say which strain of Ebola was responsible—that would require more sophisticated tests using specific assays for each of the five strains—but the Pasteur Institute's finding was sufficient to convince the Guinean government it had a problem.[11] On 22 March, Guinea's Ministry of Health made the news public and the following day the WHO followed suit, declaring that it had been notified of a "rapidly evolving outbreak of Ebola virus disease in forested areas of south-eastern Guinea."[12]

The announcement could not have come at a worse time for the WHO. After its success containing SARS, the United Nations organization suffered deep budget cuts due to the global recession that had begun in 2008. The result was that by 2014, 130 members of GOARN had been laid off, leaving the WHO with a skeleton crew in the event of an emergency. The WHO's management was already monitoring concurrent outbreaks of bird flu in China, the MERS coronavirus in Saudi Arabia, and polio in war-torn Syria. In addition, there were ongoing military and humanitarian crises in the Horn of Africa and the Sahel region of Africa. Set against these problems, an outbreak of Ebola in a remote forested region of Guinea that had so far triggered just twenty-three deaths struck officials in Geneva as small beer. Besides, as the WHO's press spokesman Gregory Hartl tweeted on 23 March: "There has never been an Ebola outbreak larger than a couple of hundred cases." Two days later Hartl went further, insisting that "Ebola has always remained a localised event."[13]

Not everyone shared Hartl's complacency. The following day in an emergency teleconference involving officials in the WHO's Africa office (AFRO) and emergency directors in Geneva headquarters, WHO personnel warned that the outbreak in Guinée Forestière was spreading faster than anyone had anticipated and there was a "high possibility of cross-border transmission." Worried that the deaths of health workers were an indication that barrier nursing controls in hospitals were inadequate and that there was a risk of the outbreak being amplified, the officials recommended raising the WHO's alert to Grade 2, the second highest level possible. Instead, senior officials in Geneva decided to keep the alert at Grade 1 and deploy a multidisciplinary team, comprising thirty-eight individuals, to Guinea to supervise infection control measures and help with surveillance and case tracking. By now, MSF was also hearing of suspected cases across the border in Foya, in northern Liberia. Then came reports of a case in Conakry. For Van Herp, the appearance of Ebola in Guinea's coastal capital, four hundred miles to the west of Guéckédou, was clear evidence of the "unprecedented" geographic spread of the virus.[14] His statement infuriated Guinea's minister of health, Colonel Rémy Lamah, who responded by instructing officials to record only laboratory-confirmed cases of the disease, thereby allowing suspected cases and contacts of suspected cases to go unreported. This policy would come back to haunt the WHO when official figures from Guinea showed a fall in case numbers in the last week of April, leading observers to believe that the worst was over.[15]

* * *

No one knows for sure if bats are the natural reservoir of the Ebola virus. To date the only live filovirus that has been recovered from bats is Marburg. However, in surveys conducted in Ebola-stricken areas of Gabon and the Republic of the Congo, Ebola antibodies and fragments of Ebola RNA have been recovered from three species of fruit bat. One of these, the hammer-headed bat, *Hypsignathus monstrosus*, is routinely hunted as a source of protein. Coupled with the isolation of Marburg from the Egyptian fruit bat, *Rousettus aegyptiacus*, this lends support to the theory that bats are the virus's natural reservoir and the main source of human infections. However, gorillas and chimpanzees are also known to be infected with Ebola and Marburg from time to time, and on occasion, they suffer dramatic die-offs, so it is possible they could also transmit the viruses to humans. In 1967 an outbreak of Marburg in a consignment of African green monkeys shipped from Uganda to vaccine research laboratories in Germany and the former Yugoslavia sparked thirty-seven infections leading to the deaths of seven laboratory workers. In 1994 the Swiss zoologist in Côte d'Ivoire almost certainly contracted Ebola from a monkey that had died in the forest. Then, in 1996, nineteen people in Mayibout, Gabon, were infected with Ebola after butchering and eating a chimpanzee they had discovered on the forest floor. Similar outbreaks in humans following extensive deaths of chimpanzees and gorillas have been documented in the Republic of the Congo. On the other hand, the high case fatality rates recorded in apes, combined with their declining geographic range, indicate that they are likely dead-end hosts for the virus and therefore not the primary reservoir for Ebola.

To date, five strains of Ebola have been identified, each name corresponding to the place where it was first isolated. The first two species, *Zaire ebolavirus* and *Sudan ebolavirus*, were discovered in near simultaneous outbreaks that occurred in 1976 in Yambuku and Sudan respectively. While the Sudan out-break was traced to a worker in a cotton factory, in Yambuku the index case was a male instructor at a Belgian Catholic mission school who had brought fresh antelope and monkey meat on his way to the village, suggesting the outbreak had a zoonotic origin. The following year, a nine-year-old girl died of Ebola at Tandala Mission Hospital, in Zaire, but no one else in her family was infected and the virus spread no further. This was followed, in 1989, by the isolation of a third species, *Reston ebolavirus*, during an outbreak that occurred at a primate quarantine facility in Reston, Virginia. That outbreak was blamed on a shipment of wild monkeys—long-tailed macaques—that had been imported to the United States from the Philippines for use in animal research. However, although the outbreak resulted in four subclinical infec-tions in laboratory workers, no humans died, suggesting that the Reston strain did not present a disease risk to humans. The fourth species, *Côte d'Ivoire ebolavirus*, was the one isolated from the Swiss zoologist in the Tai Forest in 1994. The fifth and final subtype, *Bundibugyo ebolavirus*, was named after a small outbreak in the Bundibugyo district of western Uganda in 2007, in which just thirty people were killed (by contrast, seven years earlier, an out-break of *Zaire ebolavirus* in Gulu, Uganda, resulted in 425 cases and 224 deaths). In addition, in 1995 there was an outbreak of *Zaire ebolavirus* in Kikwit, a city in the DRC with a population of 400,000.[16]

The sporadic appearance of Ebola coupled with the genetic variation between the different subtypes is both a puzzle and a challenge to viral ecolo-gists. On average the genomes of each species show a 30–40 per cent diver-gence, suggesting that each subtype has evolved in a different animal reservoir or occupies a different ecological niche. Moreover, as no one knows where the virus goes between outbreaks or the evolutionary history of the different strains, it is impossible to say why some, such as *Zaire ebolavirus*, are especially lethal to humans, while others, such as *Bundibugyo ebolavirus*, are associated with far lower rates of mortality. The fact that so much about Ebola remains shrouded in mystery underlines the importance of paying attention to factors that are known to increase the risk of infection and that lie within human control. One of these is the consumption of bushmeat. The other is social behaviours and cultural practices. In the context of West Africa, perhaps none are more significant than the rituals surrounding death, mourning and burial. These rituals are informed by Christian and Muslim religious beliefs as well as people's subscription to sodalities or secret societies. Although few outsid-ers have gained access to these societies, it is known that their members worship ancient bush spirits that are thought to reside in the forest and are usually represented by a masked figure that is part crocodile, part human. For instance, during the initiation into *Poro*, as the traditional men's society is known, young boys are led into the forest to be "eaten" by the masked bush spirit, after which they undergo circumcision and ritual scarification. Female initiates into the women's society, *Sande*, undergo similar ritual scarification, as well as, on occasion, genital mutilation.[17]

Peoples' subscription to such societies, however, is probably far less important than syncretistic beliefs and practices, including mortuary practices, designed to ensure that the deceased are reunited with their ancestors in the afterlife. For the Kissi and other ethnic groups indigenous to the region, including the Mende and Kono, this so-called "village of the ancestors" is not like the Christian idea of heaven or hell—how people have conducted themselves on Earth has no bearing on their destiny in the afterlife. Rather, it is determined by the accomplishment by the living of certain mortuary practices that are owed to the dead. These include washing and dressing the corpse, a practice that is repeated twice, first when the corpse is initially clothed or wrapped in a fine cloth, and second when it is re-clothed for burial (usually in a cheaper material). These rituals may also include treatments and sacrifices to dispel angry spirits or to address imagined acts of "sorcery" and "witchcraft." Such rituals assume even more significance when an Ebola patient collapses in a remote rural area and is removed to an Ebola Treatment Unit (ETU) many miles from their home village. If these rituals are not performed in the prescribed manner, or crucial steps are missed, it is thought that the deceased will be condemned to wander eternally, in which state they will visit curses upon their family and community—something survivors fear more than Ebola itself.[18]

Finally, in times of sickness, it is common for local people to turn to *zoes* or traditional female healers for help. Sometimes these healers will treat the sick with herbal remedies. On other occasions they may touch them and offer magical incantations in an effort to dispel the "evil spirits" that are thought to be the source of the affliction. In the case of Ebola, of course, such practices represent a considerable infection risk. Washing and touching the bodies of Ebola cadavers is similarly dangerous, as studies have shown that Ebola can persist in blood and organs for up to seven days after death.[19]

* * *

Perhaps no one knows more about the significance of these traditions and the challenges they present for the management of Ebola in rural areas of Africa than Jean-Jacques Muyembe-Tamfum. A short, vital man who always seems to be on the point of breaking into a grin, Muyembe is the director of the National Institute for Biomedical Research (INRB) in Kinshasa, and has attended more Ebola outbreaks than any other scientist alive. Known in his home country as "Dr Ebola," Muyembe points out that bushmeat is a traditional part of Africans' diet, which is why, rather than seeking to ban the practice, he supports efforts in the DRC to train hunters to butcher and prepare carcasses safely. He is also critical of Ebola control measures such as mandatory cremations and bans on burial rituals. "By seizing their cadavers we hurt peoples' spirit," he explained.[20]

Muyembe's first encounter with Ebola came during the 1976 outbreak at Yambuku, although, like other people involved in the response to the mysterious illness at the Belgian mission hospital, he had no idea at the time that he was dealing with a new filovirus. "We heard that a lot of people were dying, even the Catholic sisters," he said. "The minister of health ordered me to go there and assess the situation." At the time, Zaire was ruled by the dictator Joseph Mobutu, and when Muyembe, then a young professor of microbiology at Kinshasa Medical School, was told Mobutu had offered the use of his private jet, he realized he had no choice in the matter. He arrived at the mission late in the evening after a gruelling four-hour journey by jeep from the nearest landing strip to find that all the staff had fled and the wards were deserted save for a single sick child. "The mother said it was malaria but I think it was probably Ebola because the child died in the night." The next day, he awoke to find the hospital full of anxious villagers, many of whom were also feverish.

> Word had got out that we had come from Kinshasa with medicine. I thought it was typhoid fever so I lined them up and collected blood. I was immediately struck by the fact that when I removed the syringe from the site of the puncture wound it bled profusely. My fingers and hands were soiled with blood. I just used water and soap to wash it off.

The next outbreak Muyembe attended was in 1995 when, after a nearly twenty-year hiatus, *Zaire ebolavirus* re-emerged in the Congolese city of Kikwit. The outbreak had almost certainly begun in January in a forested area close to the city but had initially been mistaken for typhoid. It was only when a surgical team at Kikwit General Hospital fell ill in March after carrying out a risky operation on a laboratory technician, and Muyembe was sent to investigate, that he realized it was probably Ebola.[21] He forwarded blood samples to the CDC in Atlanta for testing. In all, the Kikwit outbreak resulted in 315

with either confirmed or probable Ebola reached a new low in mid-April, leading many experts to believe that the world had dodged a bullet. However, at the same time as a dip in cases was observed in Conakry, MSF physicians saw a dramatic spike in the mortality rate in Guéckédou. "All of a sudden we're having patients who have to come in, they cannot hide their illness, they're so obviously deathly ill that in their communities they cannot hide from us any-more," said Sprecher. "That's not what the end of an outbreak looks like." Sprecher would subsequently label the dip in cases observed in Conakry in April and May "the dog that didn't bark."[25]

Guinea was not the only country that had an invisible and growing problem. In early March 2014, a young woman named Luisey Kamano had approached a fisherman on the Guinean border with Sierra Leone and asked to be ferried across the river. Kamano had just seen her mother, grandmother, and two of her aunts die of Ebola and was terrified that she was about to be forcibly removed to an ETU. "I was told white people were looking for me, that they wanted to take me to Guéckédou," she said. "I was told they'd kill me with an injection. So I ran away."[26]

Once in Sierra Leone, Luisey easily evaded the authorities who had been alerted by WHO officials that she might be harbouring the virus. She was not the only one. By late March other people who had cared for sick relatives had also fled across the border. Many of them made for Koindu, a village set deep in the rolling hills and diamond mines of Kailahun. There they visited a tradi-tional healer, Finda Mendinor, drawn by the belief that she had the powers to expel the evil spirits that were the source of their affliction. It is not known how many people Mendinor treated or how—most likely she gave them herbal medicines and uttered incantations as she touched their foreheads and other parts of their body. One thing is certain, however: her ministrations were no protection against Ebola, and soon she had also contracted the dis-ease. Her death at the end of April sparked a week-long mourning period that brought scores more people to Koindu to attend her funeral. There, local women prepared her for burial by washing and dressing her corpse, while others crowded around the cadaver and showered it with kisses. The result was that within a month of Mendinor's death, authorities were reporting thirty-five laboratory-confirmed cases of Ebola across Sierra Leone and at least five active chains of transmission. Nowhere was the impact of this new phase of the outbreak more dramatically felt than at Kenema General Hospital—the same hospital where researchers had detected Ebola antibodies in stored serum samples from Lassa patients a year earlier.

* * *

Kenema is located in the heart of diamond-mining country, and feels like a frontier town. Approached via a new Chinese highway that abruptly turns into a red dirt road just beyond the city limits, the town is a magnet for prospectors en route to the rich alluvial diamond beds that dot the surrounding hills and valleys. In boom times the main square teems with dealers ready to pay hard cash for the right stone, but the city has also seen its fair share of terror. In the early 1990s, Kenema was overrun by the Revolutionary United Front (RUF), a rebel militia led by a former Sierra Leone Army corporal, Foday Sankoh, who specialized in amputations and the abduction of child soldiers. Trading diamonds for arms, Sankoh advanced as far as Freetown, occupying and reoccupying the Sierra Leone capital for several years before finally being repulsed in 2002 by a British-backed force of UN peacekeepers. With the cessation of the civil war, diamond production increased tenfold and good times returned to Kenema. But the conflict had taken its toll on Sierra Leone's health system, and many doctors fled the country. One of the few to return was Dr Sheik Humarr Khan.

Born in 1975 in Lungi, a small town just across the bay from Freetown which also happens to be the site of the country's international airport, Khan had grown up dirt-poor, the youngest of ten children. Despite these unpromising beginnings, Khan graduated at the top of his class in 1993 and won a place at a prestigious medical school in the capital. He hoped to become a Lassa Fever specialist, but in 1997, as the RUF closed in on Freetown, he was forced to flee to Conakry. His family urged him to apply for a visa to the United States, where several of his siblings had already settled. But in 2004 Khan learned that the director of Kenema's Lassa program, Dr Aniru Conteh, had died after accidentally pricking himself with a needle; Khan decided to apply for the position. His application was accepted.

In those days, there was no Chinese highway and it took eight hours to reach Kenema from Freetown, a gruelling drive along untarred dirt roads. On arrival, Khan was pleased to find that the public hospital was no longer a scientific backwater but had a state-of-the-art laboratory courtesy of a partnership with Tulane University. Researchers could now screen patients for Lassa and treat them on the spot. Dividing his time between the laboratory and the maternity ward, Khan quickly won the respect of nursing staff and was soon also a well-known figure about town, particularly on the nights when his favourite football team, AC Milan, was playing in the European Champions League and he could be heard cheering them loudly from his regular spot in a local bar.

When Khan learned about the outbreak in Guinea, he warned nurses they should be prepared in case Ebola came to Kenema. At the very least there was a good possibility that suspected Ebola bloods would be sent to the hospital for testing since the Tulane laboratory was the only one in the country with PCR equipment. Unfortunately, by the time he verified the first positive blood sample on 24 May from a nurse who had attended Mendinor's funeral, it was too late: staff had already admitted a pregnant woman to the maternity ward unaware that she was infected with Ebola. A few days later the woman miscarried, spreading the virus to other patients.

In response, Khan set up a triage zone in front of the hospital and tried to impress upon the staff the importance of avoiding contact with blood, vomit and other fluids whenever they entered the red zone—the area of the hospital reserved for Ebola patients. When a Tulane research colleague arrived with surgical gloves and personal protection kits, Khan demonstrated the correct procedures for disrobing and disinfecting the suits and gloves with chlorine. Unfortunately, within weeks the hospital was overrun with new Ebola cases—many of them people who had attended Mendinor's funeral—and nurses were under so much pressure that many disregarded the protocols. In the hope of stemming the outbreak, Khan travelled to Kailahun, where he met with village headmen and tried to convey the dangers Ebola presented to the local population. However, many community leaders were in denial and resisted Khan's entreaties to evacuate suspect cases to Kenema for testing. On one occasion, a local chief seized Khan's government-issued Toyota and held it overnight, warning him to stay out of Kailahun. Opposition was fiercest of all in Koindu, where the population erected roadblocks and threw stones, shattering the windshield of Khan's car. "There were rumours that we were coming to give them the disease," recalled Robert Garry, the Tulane researcher who had travelled to Kenema to assist Khan. "They said we would take people away and never come back. The attitude was, 'Leave us alone.'"[27]

The news that Ebola had crossed the border sent government officials in Freetown into a spin. Over the next few days Khan fielded increasingly frantic calls from the president's office and the Ministry of Health. By now, a Seattle-based nonprofit, Metabiota, one of whose members shared the Kenema laboratory, had also confirmed the presence of Ebola in Sierra Leone and was being asked to send a representative to Monrovia where there were reports of suspected Ebola cases in New Kru Town. However, WHO officials on the ground were in denial, telling members of local NGOs, "Ebola doesn't cause urban outbreaks" and that there was no danger of the virus reaching Freetown.[28] Judging by a series of memos and emails between senior WHO officials in Geneva that were obtained by Associated Press, this denial went all the way to the top of the UN organization. Treating Ebola as an international emergency "could be seen as a hostile act … and may hamper collaboration between WHO and affected countries," warned Keiji Fukuda, the WHO's Assistant Director-General for Health, Security and Environment, in an internal briefing note to WHO Director-General Margaret Chan on 2 June. "This outbreak must be considered as a sub-regional public health issue."[29] Sylvie Briand, the director of WHO's Pandemic and Epidemic Diseases Department, concurred. "I don't think declaring a PHEIC [Public Health Emergency of International Concern] will help fight the epidemic at this stage," she emailed a colleague on 4 June. "The problem with declaring a PHEIC is that one has to make recommendations and these risk hurting the country without helping public health. … I see [it] as a last resort." As a result, it was not until late July that Chan upgraded the emergency to Grade 3 and it was not until 8 August that, bowing to international pressure and concerns that, in the words of MSF, the outbreak was "totally out of … control,"[30] Chan finally declared Ebola a PHEIC.*

Unfortunately, that declaration came too late for Khan. In the hope of containing the outbreak, the Ministry of Health had decided to refer all suspected cases from Freetown to Kenema—a gruelling four-hour journey by road in overheated ambulances. On one level, the policy made sense: Kenema was one of the few hospitals in the country whose staff had previous experience treating haemorrhagic fever, albeit Lassa. However, Kenema was also a stronghold of the opposition Sierra Leone People's Party. The result was that when ambulances carrying Ebola patients began arriving at the hospital, rumours spread that the epidemic was a plot by the ruling All People's Congress Party and that nurses on the wards were deliberately infecting patients with Ebola in order to attract foreign aid for the benefit of the political elite in Freetown. In early July these tensions reached a boiling point when a woman set up a makeshift pulpit in Kenema's market area. Claiming that she was a former nurse and had seen Khan poisoning patients with her own eyes, she incited an angry mob to march on the hospital. In response Khan barred the gates and ordered his staff to evacuate while police fired tear gas to disperse the crowd.

The claims were nonsense, of course. The people who were in most danger of getting Ebola were not other patients but Khan and his staff. As Will Pooley, a newly qualified British nurse who volunteered to work on the Ebola ward in June, recalled, conditions inside the hospital were "chaotic." Arriving for

---

* The term is commonly pronounced "pike" or "fake."

duty in the morning, it was common to find five or more corpses lying sprawled in the toilets surrounded by pools of vomit and bloody diarrhoea. There were maggots and flies everywhere, and the heat inside the PPE suits was oppressive. To Pooley's horror, many nurses were unable to bear it and removed their suits when they got too hot. Others would perform cursory decontaminations, then splash water on their faces. Most alarming of all, he frequently saw staff eating from shared bowls of rice, oblivious to the fact that someone who had just emerged from the Ebola unit may have dipped their hands into the same bowl. "For that reason I always left the hospital to eat," said Pooley.[31]

The first member of the medical team to fall ill was Khan's colleague, Alex Moigboi. In a rare breach of protocol for the usually meticulous doctor, Khan reached for Moigboi's face to examine his pupils. In doing so, he inadvertently touched Moigboi's skin. Moigboi was diagnosed with Ebola soon after, and died on 19 July. By now Mbalu J. Fonnie, the hospital's much-loved matron, was also feverish. Refusing to believe she had Ebola, Khan allowed her to stay in the annex reserved for "suspect" cases long after her blood samples tested positive. Fonnie was given antimalarials and IV fluids but there was little Khan could do, and on 22 July she died. By now, Khan was also feeling unwell and kept his distance from colleagues as a precaution. When his blood tested positive for Ebola it was decided that rather than remaining in Kenema, where his sickness might panic patients and staff, he should be moved to an MSF facility in Kailahun. It would prove a fateful decision. In Kenema, the treatment protocol was to give patients fluids intravenously, but MSF took the view that the risk of death from bleeding was greater than the potential benefits so placed Khan on the standard regimen of oral treatments—paracetamol for pain relief, antibiotics for diarrhoea, and rehydration salts. In addition, MSF considered giving Khan an experimental drug called ZMapp that had shown great promise in monkeys but had never been tested in humans. In June a researcher from Canada's public health agency had brought three treatment courses to Kailahun to test the drug's viability in a tropical environment, depositing the vials in a freezer adjacent to Khan's ward. MSF agonized over whether it should give Khan the drug. On the one hand the ZMapp might save his life; on the other, if he died, people might accuse MSF of hastening his death, or worse, poisoning him, thereby further eroding trust in its medical staff. In the event, MSF decided not to give Khan the drug. Critically ill, Khan was apparently never told about the ZMapp. As his white blood cell count dropped, there was talk of evacuating him in an air ambulance, but there were no protocols in place for managing such a risky procedure, and many doubted that in his fragile condition Khan would survive the arduous journey to Lungi airport where, in the shadow of the town where he grew up, a plane was waiting to fly him to Europe. The debate proved moot; Khan died on 29 July before a final decision could be made. However, his case focused attention on the need for procedures for airlifting other health workers to safety, particularly foreign nationals working for NGOs or under contract to the WHO. The result was that when Will Pooley fell ill in August after handling a baby whose parents had died of Ebola but who had initially tested negative for the virus, he was airlifted to London in a Royal Air Force ambulance. Removed to a high-level isolation unit at the Royal Free Hospital, London, Pooley was sealed in a pressurized tent and treated with ZMapp. He survived. Around the same time, two American missionaries who had been caring for patients at Samaritan's Purse's Eternal Love Winning Africa (ELWA) treatment centre in Monrovia also fell ill. After a debate about what to do, the decision was taken to airlift Kent Brantly and Nancy Writebol to Georgia for emergency treatment at Emory Hospital, Atlanta; they were first given ZMapp to stabilize their condition. They also survived.

The contrast in the treatment accorded the American missionaries was not lost on Khan's elder brother, C-Ray, who argued "if it was good enough for Americans, it should have been good enough for my brother."[32] Many experts had sympathy for his point of view. Worrying that the better outcomes enjoyed by foreign health workers might further undermine trust in ETUs, they opined that it was important to replace the "stick" of confinement with the "carrot" of treatment.[33] Just as importantly, Khan's death sent shock waves through Sierra Leone's medical community that were also felt in Freetown. In a country with one doctor for every 45,000 inhabitants (in the United Kingdom, the ratio is one per eighty-eight), the government could ill afford to lose the figurehead of its fight against Ebola and a man whom Sierra Leone's president Dr Ernest Bai Koroma had described as a "national hero." The result was that the day after Khan's death, Koroma declared a state of emergency and established a presidential task force to oversee the country's response to Ebola.

* * *

It was not only in Sierra Leone that the free passage of people across the porous borders of the Mano River region ceded an advantage to the virus. In Liberia too, health facilities were completely unprepared for the arrival of Ebola from Guinea, and medics had to learn the lessons of previous outbreaks all over again. A good example came at Foya Borma hospital in Lofa district, the site of what is widely believed to have been Liberia's index case. CDC epidemiologists traced the introduction of Ebola there to a woman who had arrived in Foya from Guéckédou in the first days of April. At the time, Liberia had no laboratory capable of conducting an ELISA test for Ebola, much less PCR, and because the woman presented with severe diarrhoea, the attending physician assumed she had cholera. Even when on the second day she began to display haemorrhagic symptoms, the physician did not consider Ebola, assuming she was coinfected with Lassa. The absence of diagnostic facilities was not the only reason Ebola was able to take hold in Foya. Nursing staff also had limited training in infection control, no rubber gloves or masks, and very limited access to running water— all basic requirements that had been identified by Ebola experts decades earlier but which, due to chronic underinvestment in health care in Liberia, were notably absent. The result was that in a matter of days several health workers and patients had also been infected with the virus. Once it was in Foya, there was little the authorities could do to prevent Ebola from travelling to Liberia's capital. It is thought the virus was introduced to Monrovia by a patient who travelled by motorcycle taxi to the Firestone treatment centre on the outskirts of the city. En route, he infected the taxi driver and others. The result was that by 7 April, Liberia was reporting twenty-one cases and ten deaths from Ebola. However, by the end of May, no new cases had been recorded since 9 April, and by June the WHO was confident that Liberia was free of Ebola, having gone through two full incubation periods (twenty-one days times two) without any new cases being registered.

As in Guinea, the official case counts would prove misleading. Far from disappearing, Ebola had gone underground. Indeed, retrospective phylogenetic analysis suggests there were now at least three related strains of the virus circulating concurrently in the tri-border region.[34] The first hint of a resurgence in infections in Liberia came in early June when six people in New Kru Town fell ill. Before long other cases were turning up at the John F. Kennedy Medical Center, the country's only referral hospital. The hospital had been badly damaged during Liberia's protracted civil war and lacked an isolation ward or personal protection equipment. The result was that, as in Kenema, the virus quickly spread to doctors and nursing staff, prompting the authorities to close the hospital in mid-July. The only other facility in Monrovia equipped to treat Ebola was the Eternal Love Winning Africa Hospital, known as ELWA, operated by the missionary group Samaritan's Purse. ELWA was rapidly overwhelmed. Then, on 22 July, Kent Brantly collapsed, prompting the discussions that would lead to his evacuation to Atlanta at the end of the month together with his Samaritan's Purse colleague Nancy Writebol. By contrast, Liberians enjoyed no such privileges. So incensed was one Liberian by this disparity in medical treatment that in late July he stormed the government's Emergency Operations Center and set off a fire-bomb, destroying computers that were being used to track Ebola cases. By now, Samaritan's Purse had closed ELWA and had opened a new facility—ELWA 2—next door, but there were still too few beds, prompting patients to camp outside the unit. The pictures of desperately ill people collapsed in the road for want of spaces inside ELWA 2 should have been a game changer, driving home MSF's earlier warnings that the epidemic in West Africa was out of control. However, it would seem that officials in Geneva were still reluctant to treat the outbreak as anything more than a regional health crisis, albeit a severe one.

The event that arguably changed this was the arrival of a Liberian-American lawyer in Lagos, one of the most populous cities in Africa. Patrick Sawyer had boarded a flight to the Nigerian capital on 20 July. An employee of the mining company ArcelorMittal, he was en route to a conference in Calabar, in southern Nigeria, as a representative of the Liberian ministry of finance. At least, that was the story Sawyer gave officials on arrival at Murtala Mohammed International Airport in Lagos. In fact, Sawyer, who had been caring for his sick sister in Monrovia a few days earlier, was already infected with Ebola. One theory is that he was desperate to get to Nigeria, calculating he would have a better chance of receiving high quality care there. Unfortunately, on the flight to Lagos, Sawyer started vomiting and passing bloody stools, endangering other passengers. Taken on landing to the First Consultant Hospital in Lagos, Sawyer at first denied having had any infectious contacts and insisted on being discharged so he could continue his journey to Calabar. Initially, the nursing staff thought he might have malaria, but as his symptoms worsened, one of the consultants grew suspicious and decided to test him for Ebola. When his blood test came back positive, she quickly insti-tuted barrier nursing controls and alerted the authorities to trace other pas-sengers on the flight. In all, Sawyer infected nineteen people and it was only thanks to the consultant's quick thinking that the outbreak spread no further. However, she could do nothing to stop the infection running its course, and five days later Sawyer died. Then in August she also fell ill and died, adding another health worker to Ebola's tragic toll.

The Sawyer case was a wake-up call. In response, Liberia's president Ellen Johnson Sirleaf ordered the country's borders sealed and banned diplomats from traveling abroad. The United States followed suit, issuing a travel warning advising its citizens to stay away from the former American-freed slave colony. Meanwhile, prompted by the news that the Samaritan's Purse missionaries had arrived in Atlanta, Donald Trump, then a New York property developer, tweeted, "Stop the EBOLA patients from entering the U.S." and "The U.S. cannot allow EBOLA infected people back. People that go to far away places to help out are great—but must suffer the consequences!"[35] As panic spread, several major carriers, including British Airways and Air France, cancelled their services to Liberia, Guinea and Sierra Leone, leaving just two operators, Brussels Air and Air Maroc, to continue flying health workers and vital aid in and out of West Africa. "Let's face it," lamented Peter Piot, "there is an epidemic of Ebola in West Africa, then there is a second epidemic, an epidemic of mass hysteria."[36]

Through all of this, Margaret Chan held steadfast to her belief that the outbreak did not warrant an escalation in the WHO's response. However, by now it was clear to everyone that Ebola was spreading faster and further than the WHO had anticipated, and when on 6 August Sirleaf announced a national state of emergency, the pressure on Chan became irresistible. The result was that on 8 August she finally bowed to international pressure and declared Ebola a PHEIC. Joanne Liu, the international president of MSF, would later comment acidly that Chan's decision had less to do with the growing humanitarian crisis in Africa than the fear that Ebola was just a plane ride away from a major American or European metropolis. "The lack of international political will was no longer an option when the realisation dawned that Ebola could cross the ocean," she says. "When Ebola became an international security threat ... finally the world began to wake up."[37]

Unfortunately, by now the epidemic was also testing the limits of MSF's medical and humanitarian capacity. At the onset of the epidemic in March, MSF had a handful of Ebola veterans it could call on. Since then, it had called up all its haemorrhagic fever experts, plus experienced medical and logistical staff, and put an additional 1,000 volunteers on crash courses in Ebola management. At the same time, the agency had begun construction of the ELWA 3 centre in Monrovia, which would become, when it was fully operational in late September, the largest Ebola treatment centre in the world. However, the immediate impact of the evacuation of the American missionaries was paralysis. Samaritan's Purse quickly suspended operations at its two Ebola management centres in Monrovia and Foya—the only centres in the country at that time—leaving MSF to absorb the full brunt of the crisis. Nor did WHO's declaration of a public health emergency trigger a direct intervention from other humanitarian aid organizations on the scale witnessed during natural disasters such as the 2010 Haiti earthquake or Typhoon Haiyan in the Philippines in 2013. On the contrary, in the short term, it worsened matters. "We didn't want to say it but everybody was dragging their feet to come and play a role," said Liu.[38]

One reason for this paralysis was fear. Ever since the publication of *The Hot Zone*, the best-selling 1994 book by *New Yorker* journalist Richard Preston, Ebola had occupied a terrifying place in the public imagination. Drawing on the outbreak at the Reston primate facility in Virginia in 1989 and interviews with survivors of the Yambuku outbreak, Preston's account focused on the most lurid and visually shocking symptoms of Ebola, such as the way that in the last stage of illness patients sometimes "bled out," leaking blood and haemorrhagic fluids from their eyes, noses, and intestines. Even though such symptoms are mercifully rare, they helped fix in the public's mind the idea that Ebola was, as Preston put it, a "molecular shark."[39] Through the imaginative use of flypapers marked with biosafety hazard warnings and extensive passages devoted to the Reston incident, Preston also reinforced the impression of Ebola as a potential biowarfare agent, one that could emerge from the jungles of Africa, or the laboratory of a deranged terrorist, at any time, spreading panic and threatening the future of humankind. "A tiny change in its genetic code," he warned, "and it might turn into a cough and zoom through the human race."[40] Experts subsequently concluded that concerns of Ebola becoming a viable aerosol were overblown. Nevertheless, the proximity of the Reston outbreak to the US capital underlined Ebola's potential as a biosecurity threat, resulting in its selection for a war game exercise* at a meeting of the American Society of Tropical Medicine and Hygiene in Honolulu.[41] More significantly, the Reston incident contributed to Ebola appearing alongside AIDS in the Institute of Medicine's iconic 1992 list of EIDs.

* * *

By the middle of August, as dead bodies piled up in the streets of Monrovia, Sirleaf was becoming desperate. In a moment of panic she ordered for Ebola patients to be moved to a temporary holding centre in a converted school in

---

* The war game exercise uncannily presaged the 2013–16 Ebola epidemic, imagining an outbreak at the border of three fictitious equatorial countries where civil war had led to a dangerous concentration of refugees living in unsanitary border encampments.

West Point, a slum area of Monrovia that is home to some 50,000 people, most of them desperately poor. In response, West Pointers ransacked the centre, and seventeen Ebola patients fled into the slum. Four days later, on 20 August, Sirleaf ordered police and soldiers to block all the exit roads and placed the entire community under quarantine.

West Point is an opposition stronghold, and soon rumours were rife that Ebola was a hoax and that Sirleaf's real motivation was to quash an armed rebellion. As food prices soared, the imprisoned slum dwellers took to the streets in protest. Then, when a government-appointed commissioner tried to escort her family out of West Point under armed guard, an angry mob stormed the barricades. Police and armed soldiers drove them back with their batons and shields, but when the rioters began throwing stones they opened fire, wounding two young men. Tragically, one of them, a 15-year-old called Shakie Kamara, died. Incredibly, Kamara's death brought Sirleaf to her senses, and ten days later she lifted the quarantine, but the damage had been done and public distrust of the health measures deepened.

In late August, shocked by the scenes of police brutality, CDC director Tom Frieden travelled to West Africa to assess the situation, meeting with Sirleaf and other West African leaders. Although he was no stranger to explosive outbreaks of infectious disease, Frieden found the conditions in Liberia "beyond belief." Stopping at a hastily constructed MSF treatment unit in Monrovia, he was appalled to find just one doctor for 120 patients.

> There were people ... struggling for their lives, right next to people that had died ... but to remove someone who's died you have to have six people come in in full body suits and they didn't have enough staff to do it. ... I particularly remember one tent I went into, there were eight beds, or eight mattresses on the ground, and there was one woman lying face down with beautiful cornrow braided hair, and as I looked more closely I realized that she was dead. There were flies on her legs and she was one of the ones that couldn't be removed. So to have so many deaths that you can't even keep up with burying the dead is just a horrific situation.[42]

Frieden warned Sirleaf that bad as the situation was it was "going to get worse very quickly" and that if she wanted to get to grips with the epidemic she needed to put Ebola management on a professional footing. He also advised her to engage with communities, as there was no possibility that extra bed capacity could be provided quickly enough. On his return to the United States, Frieden briefed President Barack Obama, telling him that the epidemic was even worse than he had feared. He then issued a statement to reporters in which he compared the WHO's lacklustre response to Ebola to the foot-dragging he'd witnessed during the early years of AIDS. By now, Liu had also decided to up the ante. In an emotional address to the UN in New York on 2 September, she decried the "coalition of inaction" and warned that severing links with the affected countries in the hope that the epidemic would burn itself out was not a solution.

> To curb the epidemic, it is imperative that states immediately deploy civilian and military assets with expertise in biohazard containment. . . . To put out this fire, we must run into the burning building.[43]

At this point, there had been nearly 1,400 probable and confirmed cases of Ebola in Liberia and nearly seven hundred deaths. However, with new infections doubling in Liberia every fifteen to twenty days, and Sierra Leone not far behind, CDC disease modellers were predicting the two countries could see as many as 16,000 cases by the end of September. In the absence of additional interventions, and extrapolating from existing behavioural patterns, by the new year the situation could be catastrophic, according to the CDC, with as many as 550,000 cases across Liberia and Sierra Leone, or 1.4 million when corrected for underreporting.[44] "Something is different in Monrovia," MSF's Armand Sprecher told a reporter from the *New York Times* in August. "We've never seen this kind of explosion in an urban environment before."[45]

Just at the point when it seemed the situation in Liberia could not get any worse, it did. August is monsoon season, and as the rains fell on the graves of hastily buried Ebola victims, the dead began floating to the surface. The sight of the decomposed corpses sparked outrage, prompting Sirleaf to institute mandatory cremations. Although cremations are deeply offensive in Liberian culture, this time Liberians acquiesced. "People accepted it and it didn't cause any riots," said Kevin De Cock, the head of the CDC's mission to Liberia. "There was some resistance, but basically it was done."

Then came another surprise: people stopped touching one another. At first this sudden behavioural change astonished De Cock and other Western observers, but when they thought about it later it made sense. As Bruce Aylward, assistant director-general for polio and emergencies, argued, it was precisely because in Monrovia the crisis had been so extreme and the WHO's failure so marked that the behaviour change happened there earliest:

> Suddenly the entire Monrovia knew Ebola was real—Ebola kills. Ebola's going to kill me unless I do one or two things differently. There was a huge fear and people didn't know what this was. They wouldn't know a virus from a bacteria from whatever, but they knew we had to do something differently. . . . the first

thing you do in that kind of overwhelming fear is you retreat, and they changed their behaviours in ways which suddenly slowed down and took the heat out of this thing.[46]

Similar behavioural shifts also occurred spontaneously in Sierra Leone around the same time, particularly in Kailahun and Kenema, the two districts that had been hit earliest and hardest by Ebola. Elsewhere, however, resistance to the Ebola control measures persisted. Noncompliance was a particular problem in the Western District, the area that includes Freetown and its extra urban sprawl, and Port Loko, a 2,000-square-mile district to the north of the capital scored with swamps and rivers. For instance, in March 2015, shortly before Liberia released its last Ebola patient from the hospital, a fisherman infected with Ebola evaded government contact tracers and persuaded three colleagues to ferry him to a remote island in the Rhombe swamps within sight of Lungi airport. There, he consulted a traditional healer before continuing by sea to Aberdeen, a township on the outskirts of Freetown, where he alighted at Tamba Kula wharf, a stone's throw from the Radisson Blu Yammy, the city's premier luxury hotel. By now the fisherman was a walking virus bomb, and on disembarking he made straight for an Oxfam-built toilet block where he vomited haemorrhagic fluids. As a result, twenty villagers in Tamba Kula were infected with Ebola, prompting the authorities to quarantine the Aberdeen community for twenty-one days. In theory that should have been the end of the transmission chain, but despite the best efforts of contact tracers, one of the men who had accompanied the fisherman by boat got away, hitching a ride on a motorcycle to Makeni, three hours' drive from Freetown, where he infected three more people, including a local healer. All four were eventually traced and taken to a nearby Ebola treatment centre. However, once there, they refused medical care, fearing that staff were trying to murder them with what the healer called their "Ebola guns"—a reference to the hand-held electronic thermometers used to measure patients' temperatures.

In an attempt to eliminate the last hot spots of infection, the government launched a public health campaign under the Krio slogan, "*Leh we tap Ebola* (Let us stop Ebola)." At the same time, officials met with local paramount chiefs and asked them to use their authority with village headmen to pass on information about suspicious behaviour. However, while in many parts of the country this reporting system was successful, in Port Loko there were several cases of village headmen concealing Ebola patients and turning a blind eye to secret burials. The result was that in Sierra Leone, unlike in Liberia, there was no spontaneous behaviour change and sudden decline in cases: instead, the outbreak persisted into the summer of 2015.

In the end, what made the difference was the mobilization of additional resources by the international community. On 19 September 2014, in recognition of the security threat posed by the ongoing outbreak, the UN secretary general established the United Nations Mission for Ebola Emergency Response (UNMEER) to scale up the response and coordinate the delivery of logistical and technical support to the Ebola zone. It was only the second time in history that an infectious disease outbreak had been debated on the floor of the UN—the first time had been AIDS in 1987—and it had a similarly galvanizing effect. President Obama pledged to send 3,000 troops to Liberia, and by the end of the year the US Congress had agreed to emergency funding of $5.4 billion for Ebola, more than had previously been allocated for any EID. The result was that by March 2015, Britain, France and the United States had mobilized significant military assets, and thousands of health workers and contact tracers from more than twenty countries were on their way to West Africa to assist in the "getting to zero" drive.[47] Nevertheless, it would take a further year for the WHO to certify the end of the epidemic. In all, Ebola had sparked nearly 29,000 infections, 11,300 of them fatal. It was the worst outbreak of the disease in history, but while five countries in West Africa had been affected, the Armageddon scenario of a pandemic had been averted.

* * *

Like SARS, the Ebola epidemic drove home the risks that the emergence of novel pathogens in previously remote regions posed in an increasingly interconnected world. The West African outbreak was exactly the sort of scenario that had been envisaged by the Institute of Medicine in the early 1990s when it warned of the dangers that the growth in international air travel and commerce posed for the spread of EIDs. These risks had been brought home to Americans first by the arrival of Patrick Sawyer in Lagos, and secondly, by the presentation in September 2014 of another Liberian national infected with Ebola at a hospital in Texas. Thomas Duncan had walked into the Emergency Department at Dallas Presbyterian Hospital on 25 September complaining of abdominal pain and nausea, but despite his telling staff that he had recently visited Liberia, no one thought to screen him for Ebola and he was sent home with Tylenol and a course of antibiotics. For three days, the 42-year-old lay feverishly ill at a friend's apartment in Dallas, before being picked up by paramedics and returned to the hospital on 28 September. It was only then that Duncan was tested for Ebola. Unfortunately, by now he was vomiting copious fluids and was highly contagious. He died ten days later, having infected two nurses.[48]

Like the 9/11 attacks, the Duncan case exposed the porosity of American airspace and the United States' vulnerability to exotic pathogens which, thanks to commercial air travel, could be in any city on the globe within seventy-two hours.[49] Little surprise then that even before Donald Trump began calling for bans on Ebola patients and health workers returning from abroad, the inquests had started. Most people blamed the WHO. There was a clear lack of direction and "vacuum of leadership" at the highest levels of the UN organization, concluded Christopher Stokes, the general director of the Brussels branch of MSF, a year into the epidemic. "Instead of limiting its role to providing advisory support … the WHO should have recognized much earlier that this outbreak required more hands-on deployment."[50] Dame Barbara Stocking, the chair of the Ebola Interim Assessment Panel, the independent panel of experts tasked by the WHO with examining its response to the crisis, was similarly scathing. Finding that the Ebola epidemic exposed shortcomings in both the WHO's functioning and the operation of the International Health Regulations, she argued that what had been needed was "independent and courageous decision-making" by the director-general and the WHO Secretariat—qualities that had been notably "absent" in the early months of the crisis.[51]

But if the WHO was at fault, then so were other organizations. For instance, in March 2014 the CDC had dispatched one of its top Ebola experts, Pierre Rollin, to Guinea. The deputy head of the CDC's Special Pathogens branch, Rollin is a veteran of several Ebola outbreaks and an affable Frenchman with a talent for putting the science of filoviruses in layman's terms. Frieden hoped that, as a French speaker, Rollin would establish a rapport with Guinea's president Alpha Condé and convince him to extend an invitation to the CDC to assist with surveillance and control efforts. Rollin did not disappoint, quickly persuading Condé he needed the CDC's help and that it would be counterproductive to close Guinea's borders. Next, he set up an information management system to log cases and trace contacts who may have been exposed to the virus. For most of the five-and-a-half weeks he was in Guinea, Rollin stayed in Conakry, the better to monitor cases at Donka Hospital, but he also found time to tour prefectures close to the capital and dispatch staff to Guéckédou to report from the epicentre of the outbreak. By the end of April Conakry had not seen a new patient in over a week, and Rollin noted that cases had also slowed to a trickle in Guinée Forestière. Sierra Leone, meanwhile, had yet to report any cases, while Liberia had not seen a case in four weeks. As far as Rollin was concerned, the job was done. Returning to CDC headquarters in Atlanta on 7 May, he recalls thinking to himself, "It looks like, smells like, tastes like regular outbreaks in previous areas."[52]

However, by the fall of 2014 as Ebola spread to Liberia and Sierra Leone, prompting border closings and the suspension of international flights by panicked airlines, Rollin was desperately backpedalling. "It was an unprecedented outbreak; it never happened before," he told the *New York Times* in December. "There were a lot of things we didn't know at that time. No one could have imagined that it would be what we have now."[53] Peter Piot, director and professor of global health at the London School of Hygiene and Tropical Medicine and a veteran of the original 1976 Yambuku outbreak, was similarly humbled by the experience. "Together with the Swiss Franc this was probably the Black Swan event of the last 12 months," Piot informed global health policy makers gathered at the World Economic Forum in Davos on 21 January 2015, two weeks after Switzerland's surprise announcement that it was abandoning the cap on the franc to allow the Swiss currency to float against the Euro. "It was totally unanticipated and we could not have predicted what would happen based on the experience of the previous thirty-seven years."[54]

What was it that had so blinded these experts to the risks posed by the outbreak in Guinée Forestière? And why, even as Ebola spread across the border to Sierra Leone and Liberia, threatening urban outbreaks, were health agencies so slow to respond?

There are several answers to those questions. One is that while Ebola previously been amplified in hospital settings and, on occasion, had sparked urban outbreaks, those outbreaks had been rapidly contained by the institution of strict barrier nursing controls and the isolation of infectious contacts. Another is that while books like *The Hot Zone* had reinforced the impression of Ebola as a highly unstable and virulent virus, by the turn of the millennium the concerns that Ebola might mutate into an "Andromeda strain" were diminishing. This was because for all that the reservoir of the virus was unknown, each of the five identified subtypes showed a high degree of genomic stability. Moreover, while the Yambuku outbreak had seen case mortality rates as high as 90 per cent, in Kikwit the mortality rate had been 78 per cent, while in an outbreak in Gabon the following year the mortality rate had been 57 per cent.[55] Clearly, for all the concerns about Ebola's virulence, infection was not an automatic death sentence. Indeed, in the two dozen outbreaks of Ebola in Africa prior to 2013, the virus had been responsible for a total of just 2,200 infections and no single outbreak had caused more than four hundred deaths.[56] Compared to AIDS or more widely prevalent tropical diseases such as malaria, this made Ebola more of a security risk than an urgent public health threat.

Unfortunately, the experts had forgotten the importance of social behaviours and deeply entrenched cultural practices, such as the consumption of bushmeat and people's adherence to traditional funerary rituals. Nor had they factored in the mobility of local populations living at the border of three countries or the fact that new highways had greatly reduced travel times to urban areas. Nor had they considered the impact that the widespread distrust of foreigners and government elites might have on the willingness of affected communities to accept that Ebola was real, and not a hoax. No doubt there were other reasons too: in the early days of the epidemic, the absence of laboratories in West Africa capable of testing for Ebola had been critical, as had the Guinean government's insistence on only counting laboratory-confirmed cases. Nor had medical research agencies and pharmaceutical companies shown much interest in conducting safety studies of Ebola vaccines and drugs that had shown promise in animal models, much less in advancing the medications to license. Instead, ZMapp and other experimental medical products had languished on the shelves of biotech companies.[57]

The absence of doctors and nurses trained and equipped to handle Ebola, plus the fragmentation of health systems due to chronic underinvestment and civil war, also played a role. But perhaps the biggest lesson of the West African Ebola epidemic was that *Zaire ebolavirus* had most likely been circulating undetected in the tri-border zone for years. Indeed, the strain that sparked the outbreak—known as the Makona variant—was all but identical to strains isolated in previous outbreaks in Central Africa (in the language of viral genomics, the subtypes were 97 per cent homogenous). Moreover, phylogenetic analysis suggested that the outbreak had been triggered by a single spillover event, a finding consistent with the epidemiological evidence and reports that the index case had originated in Meliandou in December 2013. There was one other intriguing finding: the Makona variant had diverged from other *Zaire ebolavirus* variants only about a decade earlier. This suggested that it was a relatively recent introduction to West Africa.[58] Little wonder then that when medical researchers discovered that some local people presenting for Lassa also carried antibodies to Ebola, no one gave the report much attention.

The question is, how did *Zaire ebolavirus* get all the way to Guinea and why Guéckédou? Introduction from a human traveller seems unlikely: there is little regular travel or trade between Central Africa and Guéckédou, and the town is a twelve-hour drive from the nearest international airport at either

Conakry, Freetown or Monrovia. The more likely culprit is a fruit bat. Besides the hammer-headed fruit bat, *Hypsignathus monstrosus*, the leading candidates are Franquet's epauletted fruit bat, *Epomops franqueti*, and the little collared fruit bat, *Myonycteris torquata*. These bats are common across sub-Saharan Africa, including Guinea, and some are thought to be capable of migrating long distances. Perhaps a wayward fruit bat introduced the virus to Guinée Forestière, from where it spread to local bat populations, including the colony of *Mops condylurus* sheltering in the tree stump in Meliandou. As for why Guéckédou, one need look no further than the clearance of formerly forested areas by loggers and farmers. Clear-cutting in particular has had a devastating impact, driving bats from their roosts and forcing them ever closer to human habitations.

Finally, why did the outbreak occur in 2014 and not earlier? Without further ecological investigations and a better understanding of Ebola transmission patterns and where the virus goes between outbreaks, it is difficult to say. However, several observers noted that the outbreak coincided with the beginning of the dry season in Guinée Forestière, prompting speculation that the drier conditions may somehow have influenced the number or the proportion of infected bats in the region—presuming, of course, that bats are in fact the reservoir of Ebola—and the frequency of their contact with humans. Or perhaps Emile and his friends had a knack for extracting the *lolibelo* and were simply unlucky.

9

Z IS FOR ZIKA

"The ideal is to think globally and to act locally."
René Dubos, "Despairing Optimist"

Recife in north-eastern Brazil is a city of contrasts. Take a stroll along the grand Haussmann-style boulevards that radiate from Recife's renovated harbour area and you could be in Paris. The sense of dislocation increases as you board a catamaran on the Rio Beberibe and sail past the brightly painted baroque buildings that line the waterfront of Santo Antonio, the city's historic centre. With its network of canals and ornate churches and monasteries dating back to the colonial period, Recife rightly calls itself the "Venice of the South." Built with the profits of the seventeenth-century sugar trade, it is a monument to the ingenuity and vision of the original Portuguese and Dutch settlers. However, first impressions can be misleading, and as you turn your back on the lavishly gilded *Capela Dorada* and head west toward Boa Vista, you enter a world of modern apartment buildings and outsized shopping malls, and, in the gaps and crevices between, the places the poor call home.

Like other cities in Brazil, Recife (pronounced "he-see-fey") is infamous for its favelas and urban slums. They hug the highways running parallel to the coast and encroach on the canals that feed into the Beberibe and other tributaries that drain from what used to be a massive mangrove swamp. One of the largest, Jaboatão dos Guararapes, lies south of the seaside resort of Boa Viagem, a five-mile stretch of prime beachfront lined with international hotels and luxury condominiums.

It was here that in 2015 Brazilians awoke to a disturbing new reality. In August of that year several women from Jaboatão dos Guararapes and adjacent communities gave birth to babies with an unusual congenital syndrome. The infants had normal faces up to the eyebrows, but virtually no foreheads,

227

and when paediatricians ran a tape measure around their heads they found they were far smaller than normal, less than 32 centimetres, and in some case as small as 26 cm (a typical newborn's head measures 35 cm). Many of the babies cried continually, as if they were in constant pain, and could only be comforted by being bathed in warm water or by resting their stomachs on pilate balls. Others had trouble focusing on their mother's faces, while the worst affected were racked by seizures and spasms and had grotesquely twisted limbs and clubfeet.

One of the first physicians to recognize the new syndrome was Vanessa van der Linden, a neuro-paediatrician of Dutch descent who practices at Hospital Barão de Lucena, a public hospital in the northeast of the city. In early August, van der Linden examined a pair of twins. One of the boys had a severe case of congenital microcephaly, and when van der Linden ordered a CT scan she was alarmed to see that instead of having the usual walnut formation, the child's brain was smooth and white, with calcified patches marring the cortex. "I'd never seen anything like it," she said.[1] The boy's mother recalled that in the first month of pregnancy she had developed a rash, but nothing that was overly concerning. Puzzled, van der Linden ordered tests for rubella, syphilis and toxoplasmosis, a parasite harboured by cats that is extremely common in Brazil and which, like rubella and syphilis, is known to be associated with congenital birth defects, but all the tests were negative. Next, she looked for genetic mutations, such as Down's syndrome, but again the tests were negative.

However, for all that van der Linden was concerned, the twin was just one of hundreds of children delivered in Recife hospitals every month. Then, two weeks later, while doing her usual maternity rounds, she came across three more babies with microcephaly, and the following week two more. At a loss to explain the pattern of neurological damage, she shared her concern with her mother, Ana van der Linden, also a paediatrician. "Hà algo errado," she told her. "There is something very wrong."[2] Her mother agreed, informing her that she had seen seven similar cases. Soon, the van der Lindens had identified fifteen cases in hospitals in Recife. In a normal year, physicians in Pernambuco might see five cases across the whole state. It could not be a coincidence.[3]

The van der Lindens immediately informed the Pernambuco Health Department and asked them to check for reports of other cases of neurological malformations in newborns. In all, fifty-eight had been registered in hospitals across the state, most of them within the space of four weeks. In addition to rubella, syphilis and toxoplasmosis, tests had been run for cytomegalovirus, HIV and parvovirus, but they had all been negative. At a loss to explain the pattern, the Pernambuco Health Department did the only thing it could: it called a disease detective, Carlos Brito.

A slim man with wiry hair, Brito is constantly in motion. Trained as an infectious disease clinician, he seems never happier than when parsing epidemiological data or tapping furiously at his laptop. Brito's first experience of outbreak control came in 1991 when Brazil's Ministry of Health invited him to draw up diagnostic guidelines for physicians during a cholera epidemic. Since then he has consulted on several outbreaks in Brazil including, most notably, those caused by the arboviruses dengue and chikungunya, and he works closely with the Osvaldo Cruz Foundation (Fiocruz), Brazil's premier public health and medical research organization. In August 2014, shortly after the FIFA World Cup final, Brito was summoned to Bahia, a state adjacent to Pernambuco famed for its coconut-fringed beaches and agreeable climate. A few weeks earlier an epidemic of chikungunya had broken out in Feira de Santana, a city sixty miles north of Salvador, Bahia's populous capital. The Ministry of Health was concerned that physicians needed better guidelines to help them diagnose and recognize the mosquito-borne disease. As it turned out, this experience would make Brito the ideal person to investigate the mysterious cases of microcephaly in Pernambuco two years later.

* * *

Arboviruses (short for arthropod-borne viruses) are endemic to South America. The deadliest arbovirus, yellow fever, was most likely introduced to Brazil in the late seventeenth century when slave ships from West Africa began arriving at Recife and other coastal ports with slave labourers for the sugar plantations. Those ships also brought the *Aedes aegypti* mosquito, the main vector of yellow fever, dengue and chikungunya. A small, dark mosquito with white lyre-shaped markings and banded legs, *A. aegypti* is extremely common in areas lacking regular public water services and adequate sanitation systems. Virtually eradicated from Brazil in the 1950s with DDT and other pesticides, in the 1970s the mosquito launched a comeback, gradually colonizing Brazil's fast-growing cities and, in particular, urban slums and favelas. The result is that today *A. aegypti* is ubiquitous in Recife and other Brazilian cities, and in far greater densities than in the past.

The mosquito prefers to lay its eggs in fresh water (during the slave trade, the *Aedes* larvae would have bred in the casks of drinking water kept below decks, next to the slaves whose chains made them sitting targets for the mature mosquitoes). Ideally, *Aedes* looks for a shady uncovered container with a wide opening, but it is not fussy and its larvae have been found in everything from flowerpots to water bowls, to car tires and discarded plastic bottles.

While the male mosquitoes feed exclusively on nectar, the females need blood to produce their eggs and are extremely active in the two hours after sunrise and at dusk. Their preferred mode of attack is to sneak up from behind and insert their sharply pointed proboscises into ankles or elbows, though knees will also do. The bad news is that one bite is usually sufficient to transmit whatever virus the mosquito happens to be harbouring. Unlike other types of mosquitoes, such as *Culex*, *Aedes* is also a "sip" feeder, meaning it likes to bite again and again. But perhaps *Aedes*'s most important characteristic is that it is a house-haunting mosquito that seldom leaves any dwelling where it has once fed.

Yellow fever is the most feared virus transmitted by *A. aegypti*. Though most people will experience little more than a mild headache, fever, and nausea, in something like one-fifth of cases patients enter a highly toxic phase with ghastly symptoms characterized by high fever, severe jaundice (hence its name "yellow fever"), bleeding from the mouth and gums, and the retching of black vomit (*vomito negro* in Spanish) due to the haemorrhaging of the stomach lining. In such cases, the disease is nearly always fatal. The good news is that there is a vaccine against yellow fever and one shot offers protection for life. This is not the case with dengue, a painful and debilitating disease caused by one of four closely related serotypes, or chikungunya. For both diseases there are, as yet, no vaccines approved for general use, nor are there any cures.

In the case of dengue, symptoms usually appear three to seven days after infection. Most patients experience a high fever, intense headaches, and severe joint and muscle pains. It can feel as if someone has taken a sledgehammer to your arms, legs and neck; hence the common name for the disease, "breakbone fever." Sometimes, patients will also develop a rash on the face and limbs two to five days after the onset of fever. After a period of four to seven weeks of illness, most patients will recover. However, some may go on to develop dengue haemorrhagic fever, a rare complication characterized by high fever, bleeding from the nose and gums, and failure of the circulatory system. In the worst cases of all, these symptoms may terminate in massive internal haemorrhaging, shock, and death.

The symptoms of chikungunya are almost identical, the main difference being that the virus is very rarely fatal and has a longer incubation period (one to twelve days). In addition, the characteristic rash of the disease usually appears within forty-eight hours of the onset of symptoms, and can be found practically anywhere on the body (the trunk, limbs, face, palms or feet). Whereas with dengue the pains tend to be muscular, with chikungunya the pain is located in the joints and there may be noticeable swelling or oedema in the morning. These joint pains may become chronic, particularly in the case of the elderly or those with underlying medical conditions.[4]

Dengue has been a recurrent problem in Brazil since 1981, when an epidemic broke out unexpectedly in the state of Roraima. In 1986, and again in 1990, there were significant outbreaks in Rio de Janeiro, and by 2002 dengue was being reported in sixteen states, including in Sao Paolo, the most populous city in the Americas. Since 2008, when Brazil recorded 734,000 suspected cases and 225 deaths, and 2010, when cases exceeded one million for the first time, these epidemics have been growing in severity.[5] Most worrying of all, there is now active circulation of all four serotypes with outbreaks of one or sometimes two or more dengue serotypes simultaneously every two to three years (while patients infected with one serotype enjoy lifelong immunity, cross-immunity to other serotypes is partial and temporary, and subsequent infections with other serotypes increase the risk of the haemorrhagic form of the disease). Little wonder then that the Pan American Health Organization (PAHO) has made the control of dengue a regional priority and that the WHO has been urging the uptake of an experimental vaccine developed by Sanofi Pasteur in areas of endemic transmission.[6]

It was against this background of growing concern about dengue and the spread of arboviruses generally that Brito was dispatched to Bahia to take stock of the chikungunya outbreak in Feira de Santana. There he was introduced to another physician, Kleber Luz, who specialized in arbovirus infections. Based in Natal, the state capital of Rio Grande de Norte, two hundred miles north of Recife, Luz had recently returned from Martinique, the site of a recent large chikungunya outbreak, so was well versed in differential diagnosis of the disease—the process of distinguishing a disease or condition from one with which it shares similar signs or symptoms. By the end of September, Feira de Santana had seen more than 4,000 cases, and Luz feared that chikungunya was primed to spread to neighbouring states and cities, including Natal (chikungunya would eventually spark 20,000 infections across Brazil in 2015). However, when patients began turning up at clinics in Natal complaining of fever, rashes and itchy red eyes the following January, Luz decided their symptoms did not fit either chikungunya or dengue, and shared his concerns with Brito. "These patients had mild fevers, but with dengue the fever is usually very high," Brito explained. "About 40 per cent of the patients complained of joint pains, but unlike with chikungunya the pains were not severe. By contrast, there was a very high frequency of rashes, something you see infrequently in dengue and which is not all that important in chikungunya." It was at this point that Brito and Luz made a crucial decision. Rather than writing a report and waiting for it to be circulated to interested parties, they decided to make use of the social messaging service WhatsApp, so that they could share their thoughts instantly with other like-minded physicians. Inspired by the example of the early Jesuit missionaries to Brazil, they named their WhatsApp group, "Chikungunya: The Mission."[7]

By now similar cases were appearing in Recife. Then in March came reports of further outbreaks in Salvador and Fortaleza, another city in the northeast, prompting journalists to begin talking about the "*doenca exantematica misteriosa*"—the "mysterious disease with a rash." Frantically, Luz and Brito began searching the medical literature for clues. Eventually, in the medical textbook *Fields Virology*, under the section on arboviruses, Luz found a brief report of a virus whose symptoms seemed to fit the pattern of illness he had observed in patients in Natal. The virus was called Zika and had last been associated with an outbreak in 2013 in French Polynesia in the South Pacific, five thousand miles from the coast of Chile. As in Natal, patients presented with a mild fever, an itchy pink rash, bloodshot eyes, headaches, and joint pains. In all, 18 per cent of the population of French Polynesia had been affected, but no one had died and the outbreak had been rapidly forgotten. Could this be the mysterious disease?

With growing conviction, Luz sent Brito a message on WhatsApp. It read: "*Isso deve sere Zika virus. Veja. Aqui esta todo munde doente … vai ter que dar Zika virus.*" ("This must be Zika virus. Look. Here everyone is sick … it can only be Zika virus"). The date stamp read 21:19 on 28 March 2015. Brito, who admits he had never heard of Zika, recalls the moment clearly as he was in a restaurant having dinner with his family at the time and immediately typed "Zika" into a search engine, coming up with several references to the outbreak in French Polynesia, as well as another smaller outbreak that had occurred in Micronesia in 2007. Although Micronesia is in the western Pacific and even further from South America than French Polynesia, Brito was intrigued. "I will begin working on it first thing tomorrow," he replied, toasting Luz with a glass of wine.[8]

Brito was not the only person who had never heard of Zika. Except for a handful of arbovirus experts, no one had. Rarely diagnosed, most Zika infections are mild and even fewer require hospitalization. Certainly, in the seventy years since the first description of the virus, no one had recorded a fatality from the disease. Worse, Zika lacked a reliable animal model. The only way to study the virus's properties was to passage it repeatedly through mice specially adapted for the purpose, but in so doing the risk was that the virus would cease to bear much resemblance to the pathogen seen in nature. In short, as the *New York Times*'s science correspondent Donald McNeil put it: "In the hunt for research funding, a virologist specializing in Zika would struggle to get grants."[9]

Indeed, as he delved into Zika's history, it became apparent to Brito that knowledge of Zika was largely a by-product of historical research into yellow fever and laboratory studies that focused on the Aedés mosquito. In 1942 Alexander Haddow, a Scottish-educated zoologist with an interest in mosquito-borne diseases, had moved to Africa to work as an entomologist at the Rockefeller Foundation's Yellow Fever Research Institute in Entebbe, Uganda (now the Uganda Virus Research Institute). There, he teamed up with another Rockefeller researcher, Stuart F. Kitchen, and George W. A. Dick from the UK's National Institute for Medical Research, and began looking for a suitable site to trap mosquitoes. They found it in the Zika forest, a swampy inlet of Lake Victoria adjacent to the Entebbe-Kampala highway which was home to several species of *Aedes*, including *A. africanus*, the vector of yellow fever in Uganda. Placing traps on steel towers that rose forty metres above the forest floor, they began by measuring the density of mosquitoes at different levels of the tree canopy and the times they were most active. Next, they placed monkeys in cages at the elevations where they knew there were a lot of *Aedes* and allowed them to be bitten repeatedly. Afterwards, they checked the monkeys' temperatures and, if they were sick, took a blood sample to see whether they were infected with yellow fever or some other virus. It was from one of these monkeys that, in April 1947, Haddow and his colleagues succeeded in isolating the Zika virus for the first time. Nine months later, they also isolated the virus from an *A. africanus* mosquito, though it would take five more years for them to prove that mosquito and monkey were infected with one and the same virus and that it had an affinity for nerve tissue.

Today Zika is classified as a flavivirus, from *flavus*, the Latin word for yellow (in the case of Zika the name is somewhat misleading as, unlike yellow fever, the virus rarely causes jaundice). Under an electron microscope both viruses look like twenty-sided polygons called icosahedrons, each containing a single strand of RNA. It is these strands that invade and hijack the machinery of animal cells, including human cells, and cause the characteristic symptoms of Zika: a raised red rash, headache, conjunctivitis and myalgia.[10]

In the 1950s, following reports of the first human infections, several researchers tried to show that *A. africanus* was not the only vector, but that *A. aegypti*, which thrives in urban environments, could also transmit the virus (they did this by infecting themselves with Zika and allowing *A. aegypti* to bite them on the arm repeatedly, something that would not be permitted by university ethics committees today). However, the experiments proved unsuccessful, and it was not until 1966 that the virus was isolated from *A. aegypti* for the first time. That this occurred in Malaysia, not Africa, should have rung alarm bells, indicating that the virus was on the move and might be capable of infecting people in urban areas. Indeed, by the early 1980s Zika had spread to India and other parts of equatorial Asia and was being reported as far west as Indonesia. However, since cases requiring medical attention were rare and seroprevalence studies showed there was wide population exposure, there was little concern. In retrospect, researchers suspect that the fact that just sixteen human Zika infections were recorded between 1947 and 2007 probably resulted from underreporting due to the disease's similarity to dengue and chikungunya,[11] and because 80 per cent of people infected with Zika never develop symptoms and so do not seek medical attention.*

The first outbreak to make an impression on doctors and public health professionals came in 2007 when five hundred Yap islanders suddenly fell ill. At first the outbreak was mistaken for mild dengue, but when the CDC sent samples to the United States for testing, they turned out to be positive for Zika. This was a shock, as Yap is a long way from Africa and there were no monkeys present on the island. In theory, the virus could have been introduced by windblown mosquitoes from Indonesia. However, it is far more likely the virus was carried to Yap in the blood of an infected patient or by an *Aedes* mosquito that hitched a ride on a ship. Whatever the source, within five months more than two-thirds of the island's 7,000 residents were infected.**

The next significant outbreak occurred in 2013 when physicians on Tahiti and other islands in French Polynesia reported an "eruption" of fevers, rashes, and bloodshot eyes.[12] At first the French suspected dengue, but by the end of October half of the samples had tested positive for Zika, and by December cases were being reported on all seventy-six islands that comprise the archipelago. In addition, patients began arriving at emergency rooms in varying degrees of paralysis, something that had not been noted or reported in previous

---

* It is also likely that due to repeated exposure to the virus, most Asian populations were immune to Zika.

** There have been no further outbreaks on Yap since 2007. This is most likely because the majority of islanders now possess immunity to Zika. It is only when herd immunity wanes and there are sufficient numbers of susceptibles again that a new epidemic may erupt.

Zika outbreaks. The cause of the paralysis was Guillain-Barré syndrome, a rare autoimmune condition that in the most extreme cases can result in permanent nerve and muscle damage and even death if the paralysis extends to the diaphragm. As fears of Guillain-Barré spread and the government stepped up mosquito spraying, rumours began to circulate that the insecticide, deltamethrin, was responsible. By the time the outbreak concluded the following April, 8,750 people had fallen sick and forty-two had been diagnosed with Guillain-Barré.[13] Fortunately, most of these cases resolved with time, but if the world needed another wake-up call that Zika deserved to be taken seriously, this was it. That is not what happened, however. Instead, as Zika continued its westerly spread across the Pacific, reaching New Caledonia in March 2014 and Rapa Nui (Easter Island), a territory of Chile, soon after, the world's attention was seized by a far more visible emerging disease threat: the Ebola outbreak in West Africa. The result was that when at some point in 2014 Zika arrived in Brazil, no one noticed.

* * *

By April 2015 Brito and Luz were becoming increasingly convinced that Zika was responsible for the spate of rashes and fevers in the northeast, but in order to convince the Pernambuco health authorities and Brazil's Ministry of Health that these were not "dengue light" cases, they needed hard laboratory evidence. Unfortunately, antibodies to Zika cross-react with those of dengue and other flaviviruses, so conventional serological testing using ELISA or immunofluorescence would not be sufficient. To be certain that Zika was the cause, positive results would have to be obtained by the detection of viral nucleic acids using RT-PCR. Accordingly, in April, Luz sent serum samples from twenty-one suspected cases to Claudia Nunes Duarte dos Santos, a virologist at the Carlos Chagas Institute in Curitiba in Paraná. Eight of the patients, seven of whom were women, tested positive for Zika by RT-PCR. All lived in Natal and all had relatives with the same symptoms. At around the same time, another group of virologists based at the Federal University of Bahia in Salvador also detected the presence of Zika RNA in seven cases from Camacari, 650 miles to the south. There could now be no doubt, and on 14 May the Ministry of Health released a statement confirming that Zika was circulating in Brazil. However, while the statement prompted PAHO to issue an epidemiological alert, no further action was forthcoming, and the announcements prompted little alarm among Brazilian physicians or the wider global health community. By now, however, Brito had read up on the

Guillain-Barré cases in French Polynesia and had issued an alert to members of the WhatsApp group warning them to look out for neurological symptoms. That's how he came to learn about a group of patients being treated by Lucia Brito (no relation), the head of neurology at the Hospital da Restauracao in Recife. Some had inflammation of the optic nerve, others of the brain and spinal cord, and several had Guillain-Barré syndrome.[14]

As yet, the link between Zika and Guillain-Barré was unproven—it was merely a temporal association and could have been a coincidence. To show the two were causally connected, a virologist would need to test the cerebrospinal fluid (CSF) of patients with Guillain-Barré for Zika virus—something that had not happened during the outbreak in French Polynesia. In short, Brito needed a microbiologist to help him connect the dots. Fortunately, Brito knew the perfect person: Ernesto Marques, the head of virology at Fiocruz in Recife and an expert on dengue.

The grandson of a pharmacist from Recife, Marques was raised in Recife and has long felt a duty to use his knowledge to serve the people of his home town. That sense of purpose took Marques to medical school in Recife and, after graduation, to Johns Hopkins to study for a PhD in pharmacology. Drawn to research with practical applications for health problems, he decided to specialize in dengue, developing a tool to help doctors predict the health outcomes of patients infected with the virus. On obtaining his doctorate in 1999, Marques was offered a prestigious faculty research position, but he knew that in order to study dengue and other mosquito-borne diseases he needed to be close to the people most affected, so in 2006 he left Baltimore and returned to Recife to head up Fiocruz's virology department at the Instituto Aggeu Magalhães (IAM). Among his first cohort of research students was Brito. While Brito was interested in the clinical symptoms of dengue, Marques was interested in mapping the T cells involved in clearing the virus with a view to identifying segments on the surface of the virus known as epitopes to which antibodies bind and which might be relevant to vaccine design. The two men soon became close friends, discovering in the process that they shared an enthusiasm for medical detection.

In 2009, Marques was offered an associate professorship at the University of Pittsburgh's Graduate School of Public Health, and began dividing his time between Pittsburgh and Recife. However, he and Brito stayed in touch, swapping notes and helping to recruit patients for Fiocruz's ongoing research into dengue. The result was that when Marques first heard about the outbreak in Recife, he assumed the mysterious disease was mild dengue. Even when, in late April, Brito visited Fiocruz with a list of candidate viruses, including

Zika, and raised the possibility of a connection with Guillain-Barré, Marques, who watched the meeting on a video link from his office in Pittsburgh, saw little reason to alter his opinion. Nevertheless, he agreed to order reagents to conduct tests for Zika and instructed his laboratory to concentrate on patients recently diagnosed with Guillain-Barré. Not long after, the laboratory took delivery of samples from thirty of Lucia Brito's patients. By May Brito and Marques had their answer. Zika was present in the blood of seven of the patients. Not only that, but CSF from some of the same patients also tested positive—strong evidence of a causal link with Guillain-Barré.

When other laboratories in Brazil had first reported the presence of Zika in dengue light patients, Marques had shared the news with his Pittsburgh colleagues, including Donald Burke, the dean of the Graduate School of Public Health and an expert on arboviruses (it was Burke who had written the chapter on arboviruses in the textbook that Luz had consulted in March). Although at this stage it was assumed that such infections were largely benign, with Marques's input Burke agreed to draft an email to a former colleague in the Biological Threats Department of the White House. The email read:

> If Zika is in fact spreading in Brazil, it is of concern for several reasons. 1. It will cause confusion about what is dengue and what is Zika, and what will be vaccine preventable. 2. It could spread more widely in the Americas. 3. There may be surprising interactions of Zika and dengue.

The email concluded by urging the implementation of surveillance for Zika "as soon as possible."[15] Now, with hard evidence of a causal link between Zika and Guillain-Barré, and possibly other neurological conditions as well, the case for surveillance was even more urgent. At the very least, Marques expected Fiocruz to issue an announcement about their findings. Instead, as Brito briefed the press, officials at Fiocruz urged caution, then issued a statement denying the reports. Marques was furious, but in the meantime he had filed a report to the Ministry of Health, so he knew it was only a matter of time before the truth came out.

Events now moved quickly. When van der Linden began noticing the cases of microcephaly, one of the first persons she shared her concern with was Marques, her old medical school classmate. Soon Brito was also on the case. His first move was to gather together sixteen women who had recently given birth to babies with microcephaly at the Instituto Materno Infantil de Pernambuco (IMIP) and distribute detailed questionnaires asking whether they had recently experienced a rash, conjunctivitis, or oedema. "Because of the discovery of Zika virus in cerebrospinal fluid and the neurological conditions seen in previous outbreaks, he was already thinking Zika," said Marques when I met him at his office at IAM.[16]

As Brito expanded his inquiries, circulating questionnaires to women at other maternity wards, his conviction grew that he was on the right track. All the women had tested negative for the common causes of microcephaly, and all had experienced a rash and a fever during the first trimester of pregnancy. Besides, the dispersal was too extensive. "It could not be an outbreak transmitted by saliva, such as rubella, or a sudden decline in immunity that would allow the spread of cytomegalovirus," says Brito. "It needed a vector."[17] However, although Brito was enthused by the thought that he might be on the brink of solving the mystery, his excitement was tempered by sadness. Many of the women he spoke to were as young as fourteen and barely out of childhood. "It was their first child and when they burst into tears it was hard for me not to cry too."[18]

By now Luz had also identified several women in Natal who had given birth to microcephalic babies and had experienced symptoms characteristic of Zika early in their pregnancies. Increasingly convinced that Zika was responsible for the increase in microcephaly cases, in October Brito presented his findings to the Ministry of Health and the Pernambuco health authorities. At this juncture, 141 cases of microcephaly had been detected in Pernambuco (by comparison, in 2014 Pernambuco had registered 12 cases). Similar increases in microcephaly and other peculiar neurological malformations were being reported in Rio Grande do Norte and other nearby states, and although the authorities were reluctant to accept that Zika was to blame, it was obvious there was a problem. Accordingly, on 11 November the Ministry of Health declared a national public health emergency and the Pernambuco Health Department issued an order requiring the compulsory notification of all microcephalic births.

Still, rumours abounded. Some people speculated that the supposed increase in microcephaly cases could be an artefact of Brazil's live-birth reporting system and better surveillance. Others clung to the theory that it was a bad batch of rubella vaccine or the fault of insecticides and larvicides. What scientists needed was live virus from a pregnant woman. But the Zika virus is typically detectable only in the first two to five days after the onset of symptoms, after which it usually disappears from the blood.* Because no one

---

* By contrast, Zika virus has been isolated from semen up to 188 days after the onset of symptoms.

in Brazil was aware of the threat posed by Zika in the early part of the year, presumably the most common time when pregnant women had contracted the disease, no one had thought to test their blood for the virus during this critical period. Nor could they have—even as late as December 2015, when epidemiologists began to study the microcephaly births intensively, there was no routine diagnostic test available for Zika, and PCR was only available in specialist labs such as Marques's. Of course, antibodies to Zika might still be detectable, but such antibodies could have been produced during prior exposures and were not evidence that the women had been infected with Zika during their pregnancies. The only possibility was to look for the virus in the amniotic fluid of a pregnant woman. The question was, where could such a candidate be found?

Unbeknownst to Brito and Marques, while they were puzzling over these questions, Adrian Melo, a researcher in foetal medicine in Paraíba specializing in high-risk pregnancies, was treating two women whose sonograms showed unusual foetal brain development. The first woman had developed a rash, followed by fever and myalgia at eighteen weeks of gestation, and had been prescribed intravenous cortisone. She recovered, and at sixteen weeks her ultrasound was normal, but further ultrasounds at twenty-one and twenty-seven weeks indicated foetal microcephaly (the woman would eventually give birth to a baby with a head circumference of 30 cm).[19] The second woman had similarly suffered Zika-like symptoms during pregnancy—in this case, at the tenth gestational week—with an ultrasound at twenty-five weeks also indicating foetal microcephaly. What particularly concerned Melo was that both foetuses had marked deformations of their cerebellum, the part of the brain that controls muscular movement, hearing, and eyesight, something that was not usual in microcephaly.* A few days later, Melo received a text about the suspected link between neurological malformations in newborns and Zika. That's when it hit home. "It was the only possible explanation," she said.[20]

In early November Melo succeeded in making contact with a researcher at Fiocruz in Rio de Janeiro and arranged for amniotic fluid to be drawn from the women at twenty-eight weeks. Both samples tested positive for Zika virus. It was exactly the proof Brito needed, but still the Ministry of Health hesitated. Only when on 28 November another research group in the state of Pará announced it had also isolated the virus, this time from the brain of a

---

* These malformations and nervous system deficits would later be labelled Congenital Zika Syndrome (CZS).

stillborn baby with microcephaly and other congenital abnormalities, did the ministry agree to issue a statement confirming the findings. It was official: something as innocuous as a mosquito bite might be causing severe neurological damage in newborns across Brazil, the most populous country in South America; and pregnant women exposed to Zika, especially during their first trimester, should be presumed to be at risk of microcephaly. On 1 December, with nine other countries in South America, including Venezuela, Colombia, and Mexico, reporting transmission of Zika, PAHO also fell into line, issuing an alert warning member states about the virus and advising them to prepare health centres and antenatal centres for a "possible increase in demand ... for neurological syndromes." At this point, Brazil was investigating 1,248 cases of microcephaly, including seven deaths, in fourteen states. That gave a prevalence of 99.7 microcephaly cases per 100,000 live births—a twentyfold increase over the 2010 rate.[21] The question was how much of this increase was down to Zika, as opposed to heightened awareness of microcephaly and the efficiency of Brazil's live births information system. Were other countries in Latin America experiencing similar increases? As 2015 drew to a close, no one knew the answers to those questions, least of all the WHO's then-director general Margaret Chan, to whom it now fell to assess the level of the threat and whether it constituted a public health emergency of international concern (PHEIC).

* * *

In a filing cabinet somewhere at WHO headquarters in Geneva is a document listing the world's leading infectious disease threats. Only to be referred to in the event of an emergency, the document, known as a "decision instrument," provides a step-by-step guide for assessing outbreaks that may pose a "serious" threat to public health. At the top of that list are smallpox, polio, pandemic influenza and SARS. Outbreaks of any of these pathogens automatically trigger a PHEIC. In second place come cholera, pneumonic plague and viral haemorrhagic fevers such as Ebola and Marburg. Yellow fever, dengue and West Nile, another arbovirus, also make the list, but in 2015 there was no mention of Zika. This is not because the virus was unknown to public health experts—it had first been identified in 1947—but because until the outbreak in Brazil no one had imagined it might pose a threat to expectant mothers and their babies, let alone require a coordinated international response.

By any measure Zika's rise through the microbial threat rankings had been astonishing. In the corridors of the WHO some officials were suggesting it might even constitute a bigger health risk than Ebola. The timing was particularly unwelcome for Chan. After she had weathered months of criticism over her handling of the Ebola epidemic and stinging reports questioning her leadership abilities, the epidemic was finally over and officials were returning from West Africa to enjoy Christmas with their families. In the closing months of the outbreak, the WHO had even scored a significant victory, supervising the trial of an experimental vaccine that, according to preliminary data, conferred complete protection against Ebola. Now, with just eighteen months of her term as director-general left to serve, Chan was faced with another critical decision, one that could forever define her stewardship of the WHO as a success or failure. She could not afford to make another wrong call. But in the case of Zika, it was by no means clear what was the right thing to do. As yet, there was no proof the virus caused birth defects—it was simply an association in time and space. Moreover, any suggestion that there might be a causal relationship risked needlessly panicking expectant mothers. There was another consideration, too: the Olympic torch was on its way to Rio ready for the official launch of the Summer Games on 5 August. The Olympics would bring thousands of spectators and tourists flocking to Brazil. As few of them would have been exposed to Zika before, few would possess immunity, risking further outbreaks and the introduction of the virus to their home countries once the games were over. Finally, there were the athletes and the Brazilian economy to consider. The Olympics was a mega-event, one in which the Brazilian government and corporate sponsors had invested millions. Stadium construction was already behind schedule, and with the government facing growing criticism over its clearance of urban slums and other favela "beautification" measures, there was a risk athletes might withdraw rather than risk exposing themselves and their families to Zika.

When faced with a tricky decision there is nothing like safety in numbers. In weighing whether or not to announce a PHEIC for Ebola, Chan had taken advice from thirteen experts. In the case of the Zika emergency committee Chan recruited eighteen experts and invited David Heymann to chair their deliberations. It was a shrewd choice. Heymann had been a key architect of the 2005 revisions to the International Health Regulations and one of those who, behind the scenes, had criticized Chan's handling of Ebola, believing she had been too slow to challenge claims by WHO's Africa office and member states that they had the outbreak under control. After leaving WHO's Communicable Disease Division, Heymann had taken up a position as professor of infectious disease epidemiology at the London School of Hygiene and Tropical Medicine and accepted the chairmanship of Public Health England, an executive agency of Britain's Department of Health and Social Care tasked with the surveillance and control of contagious disease outbreaks. A regular contributor to *The Lancet* and the *New England Journal of Medicine*, he also headed Chatham House's Centre on Global Health Security, giving him a powerful platform to expound on global health issues and network with other key opinion makers.

From Heymann's point of view, chairmanship of the emergency committee would give him a chance to push for the sort of systems that had proved so successful during the SARS outbreak when the WHO had put its faith in virtual networks of experts and allowed them the space and security to collaborate and share confidential research data. Still, it must have come as a shock when four days before the committee was due to meet, Heymann got the call to say he had been selected as chair.

In the case of Ebola, once an emergency committee had been convened, the determination of a PHEIC had been relatively easy. After all, by August 2015 Ebola had killed thousands of people in West Africa and was known to be highly virulent. But in the case of Zika there was so much that was not known about the virus and its pathology, and although it was clear that transmission was widespread and likely to affect other countries in the Americas, it was unclear to what extent Zika posed an ongoing health threat, let alone a "serious" one, which is the first test of a PHEIC. Another problem was that although the relationship between Zika and microcephaly was unknown, the virus was not: on the contrary, it had first been described in 1947 only to be dismissed by experts as a virological curiosity (in epistemological terms this made it an "unknown known"). Nor was it possible to say whether Zika's emergence in Brazil was truly "unexpected" or "unusual"—the other tests of a PHEIC—or simply an artefact of better surveillance. Adding to the pressure on Heymann and other committee members were the heartbreaking pictures of babies with tiny heads that were beginning to fill the morning news shows and Twitter feeds and a recent travel advisory from the CDC recommending that pregnant women consider postponing travel to Brazil and twelve other countries with Zika transmission.

If Heymann had been hesitating about recommending a PHEIC before, as soon as the committee began reviewing the evidence his doubts evaporated. The first shock was the presentation of new evidence from French Polynesia indicating that there had been an increase in neurological disorders, including Guillain-Barré, coincident with the 2014 Zika epidemic, something that had not been reported at the time.[22] In addition, it was discovered that the authorities had overlooked several cases of neurological damage in foetuses.

None of the affected mothers had recalled being ill during pregnancy, but four had subsequently tested positive for flavivirus antibodies, suggesting they could have been carrying silent Zika infections. These discoveries were game changers. As Chan was to put it: "Now it wasn't 'only Brazil' any more."[23]

Another critical determinant was Heymann's realization that the clusters of microcephaly and neurological disorders required "intensified research." Without this research, and the deployment of rapid diagnostic tests to enhance the surveillance and diagnosis of Zika infections, it would be very difficult to establish a causative link or, conversely, to rule one out. Declaring a PHEIC would have a galvanizing effect, Heymann calculated, making a coordinated international response and the development of a vaccine that much easier. On precautionary grounds, then, and to avert a potentially bigger crisis, the committee was justified in ruling that the clusters represented an "extraordinary event" and a public health threat to other parts of the world. "That is the PHEIC," Heymann explained, sitting alongside Chan as she announced the decision to the world's press on 1 February 2016. "The PHEIC has to do with proving whether the clusters are or are not linked to the Zika virus."[24]

* * *

Even before the WHO's announcement, speculation about Zika and its effects on women's gestation cycles was sparking hysterical headlines around the world. Now that hysteria had ramped up several notches, the Rio Olympics committee decided it had no choice but to issue its own travel advisory. Standing in front of a poster showing a mosquito with a red line through it and the caption "*Mensagem sobre Zika*" ("Message about Zika"), João Granjeiro, the director of medical services for Rio 2016, advised athletes and visitors attending the games to smother themselves in mosquito repellent, shut their windows, and use air conditioners to minimize the risks of being bitten. He could offer little reassurance to pregnant women, however. Instead, he echoed previous government advice that expectant mothers should think twice about travel to Brazil.[25] By now, imported Zika cases in travellers who had recently visited South America were being reported from Ireland to Australia, and the United States had confirmed a rare case of sexual transmission of the virus in Texas, further ratcheting up the hysteria. "No one is safe from Zika," screamed the *Daily Mail* in an article revealing that more than 21,000 Colombian women had contracted the virus.[26] "Living with Zika," declared another story illustrated with pictures of women cradling microcephalic babies at a rehabilitation centre in Recife—victims of what the *Daily Mail* referred to as the "head-shrinking bug."[27]

By June, with reports that the virus had spread to Mexico and the Caribbean and that the CDC was monitoring 279 pregnant women with confirmed or suspected Zika infections in the United States, the outbreak took on panic proportions. Newlyweds who had been looking forward to honeymoons in Puerto Rico and Costa Rica cancelled their trips, while retirees, whose chil-drearing days were long behind them, reconsidered plans for leisurely Caribbean cruises. Soon athletes were also exhibiting signs of Zika hysteria. One of the first to fall victim was the world's number one golfer, Jason Day, whose wife had recently given birth to their second child. When Day announced he would not be competing at the Olympics because of his con-cerns about Zika, several other famous golfers followed suit. Meanwhile, Greg Rutherford, the British Olympic long jump champion who was a hot favourite to repeat his gold medal-winning performance at Rio, revealed he had taken the precaution of freezing his sperm (even so, his partner, Susie, and their son Milo would not be attending). Even normally level-headed commentators such as Amir Attaran, professor of law and medicine at the University of Ottawa, got publicly involved, signing an open letter with one hundred other public health experts calling on the International Olympic Committee to move or postpone the games. "The fire is already burning but that is not a rationale not to do anything about the Olympics," Attaran explained. "It is not time now to throw more gasoline on the fire."[28]

By now fumigation brigades, their numbers swelled by 55,000 Brazilian military personnel, were going door-to-door in Rio and other Brazilian cities, spraying insecticides and handing out educational leaflets aimed at persuading people to remove sources of standing water. The *Aedes* had not seen an assault of this magnitude since the 1930s when the Brazilian dictator Getúlio Vargas, with financial support from the Rockefeller Foundation, authorized a mili-tary-style program of larval reduction in an effort to eradicate yellow fever. Then, city and town dwellers had been compelled to destroy mosquito breed-ing sites or risk fines for noncompliance, but by 2016 Brazil was no longer a dictatorship and the authorities could not force disadvantaged communities living in the shadow of the Olympic village to cooperate. Instead, the last-minute blitz fuelled conspiracy theories that insecticides and larvicides were to blame and that medical technology, not the mosquito, was the culprit.[29] However, it was in Miami, another subtropical city 4,000 miles to the north, that the buzz and clamour around Zika reached fever pitch when in August the CDC issued a travel warning advising pregnant women to avoid a one-square-mile area of the city. Fourteen people had been diagnosed with Zika after being bitten by mosquitoes in and around the trendy Wynwood arts district, and although Florida's governor, Rick Scott, insisted that Miami was still open for business, the CDC begged to differ. As planes loaded with an insecticide called Naled stepped up their aerial bombing missions, Wynwood became a ghost town, prompting protests about "chemical warfare."[30] The protestors' voices were soon joined by those of hotel and casino operators in and around South Beach, nervous about the impact the Zika scare was having on summer tourist bookings. The only silver lining was that the panic persuaded politicians in Washington to pass a $1.1 billion funding package for Zika that had been deadlocked in Congress for months. Though by the time Congress approved the bill in late September the summer mosquito season was drawing to a close, those funds were desperately needed for future Zika control measures and, just as important, research into vaccines.

Today, the panic over Zika is a fading memory. The Olympic Games went ahead as scheduled, and while a few athletes tested positive for the virus none developed serious illnesses or neurological complications. Nor did their wives return home to be confronted, nine months later, with the news that their children had microcephaly. And while the epidemic eventually spread to eighty-four countries, and the virus is now firmly entrenched throughout the Americas, at the time of writing Zika is no longer considered an international health emergency. The WHO lifted the PHEIC in November 2016 after a systematic review of the scientific evidence left experts in no doubt that Zika *was* a cause of congenital brain abnormalities, including microcephaly seen in newborns (six months later, in May 2017, Brazil's Ministry of Health followed suit). There are even several candidate vaccines in the pipeline, but given the ethical problems of conducting trials with pregnant women—the main target for such vaccines—and the fact that vaccines themselves can sometimes trigger Guillain-Barré, making it difficult to distinguish the effects of vaccination from those associated with infection, such vaccines are unlikely to be available for several years. Meanwhile, the social and environmental conditions that turn Brazil's favelas into fertile breeding grounds for *Aedes* and other Zika-bearing mosquitoes that transmit the virus have not gone away, nor have mosquitoes stopped taking blood meals.

* * *

In July 2017 I travelled to Recife to speak to the Brazilian doctors, epidemiologists, and virologists who had been at the forefront of the outbreak.

At that point Zika was no longer front-page news; in the first six months of 2017 the CDC had registered just one case of local transmission in the United States. Moreover, with a huge cholera outbreak raging in Yemen, the WHO's attention was firmly back on Africa. Arriving at my hotel in Boa Viagem within sight of Recife's famous reefs, I found that the news shows were preoccupied with a yellow fever outbreak that had begun in Minas Gerais state and was now encroaching on the environs of Sao Paolo and Rio. But though Zika was no longer a pressing public health issue, there were still many unanswered questions.

For instance, though it had been established that the virus that triggered the outbreak in Brazil in 2015 was the same as the one that had caused the outbreak in French Polynesia two years earlier, and that both were descended from an Asian strain of Zika, it was still not known how the virus had reached Brazil. It used to be thought that Zika arrived during the FIFA World Cup that had kicked off in Rio in June 2014. This seemed plausible, particularly as one of the host cities had been Natal, until it was pointed out that no Pacific countries had sent teams to the competition. The next suggestion was that the virus may have been introduced during the Va'a World Sprint Championship held in Rio de Janeiro in August of the same year. This was more likely, as four Pacific countries (French Polynesia, New Caledonia, Cook Islands and Easter Island) had sent canoe squads to the competition. However, this theory was undermined by a letter published in *Nature* in May 2017 in which an international team of scientists announced they had collected fifty-eight Zika virus isolates from Brazil and other countries in the Americas and sequenced their genomes. Using phylogenetic analysis to run the molecular clocks of the isolates backwards in time, the scientists showed that all the strains descended from an ancestral virus that had arrived in northeast Brazil around February 2014. If the analysis was accurate, that suggested Zika had been in Brazil six months before the sprint championship and fifteen months before the confirmation of the first Zika cases by Brazil's Ministry of Health.[31] Zika's precise relationship to microcephaly presented a similar puzzle because it was still not known how and why the Zika virus triggered birth defects in some women but not others, or whether apparently normal newborns might present with developmental problems in later childhood. Nor could anyone say what the long-term prognosis was for Brazil's Zika babies and what the risks were of sexual transmission of the virus.

I was keen to find out what Brito and Marques made of these questions and to hear their thoughts as to why the outbreak had proved so explosive in Pernambuco (by now, a paper in *The Lancet* had shown that the northeast had accounted for 70 per cent of microcephaly cases during the first wave of the epidemic). I also wanted to visit Jaboatão dos Guararapes and other impoverished communities in the greater Recife metropolitan area and speak to entomologists investigating mosquito breeding patterns and Zika's transmission dynamics. But most of all I wanted to meet the women who had given birth to the first cohort of microcephalic babies, and find out what provisions had been made for them and how they were coping now that the world's interest had moved on. In short, I wanted to see what the epidemic looked like since Zika had once again become an object of neglect.

I was hoping to find some of the answers at the IAM, the research centre where Marques has his laboratory. Located on a sprawling campus in northeastern Recife, it was here that Brito first presented his theory of a link between Zika and Guillain-Barré, and that Marques's colleague, the Fiocruz epidemiologist Celina Turchi, coordinated the initial investigation into microcephaly. Realizing the scale of the threat, Turchi was instrumental in reaching out to other researchers around the world and lobbying the authorities to issue a public health alert. Such were the consequent offers of support, the director of IAM offered to lend her his office. It was here that, two years later, I caught up with Turchi sitting at a large glass desk surrounded by her assistants still busily sorting papers and responding to queries from the public. "Even today there are people who still believe the rumours that the epidemic was due to insecticides or the rubella vaccine," she said. "The latest conspiracy theory is that the virus is being spread by transgenic [genetically modified] mosquitoes," she added, rolling her eyes. "We have no choice but to respond to each and every one."[32]

A soft-spoken woman, Turchi's voice becomes louder, her speech more urgent, as she recalled the shock of the first wave of microcephaly cases and the challenges facing Brazilian mothers of Zika babies as they struggle to raise severely disabled children in a climate of mounting austerity and cuts to public health programs. Visiting the maternity wards in the early days of the epidemic was "frightening," she said. "I remember seeing four or five babies with no forehead and a very strange skull structure. They looked very different from babies with congenital microcephaly. My grandmother could have diagnosed it."

One of Turchi's first moves, once she had been briefed by Brito ("he had the whole thing worked out"), was to call other epidemiologists both in Recife and abroad and ask whether they had noticed similar increases in microcephaly, including during the epidemic in French Polynesia. A retrospective investigation of birth records there subsequently turned up seventeen cases of neurological malformations and showed that the peak had been missed because most women had terminated their pregnancies rather than give birth to microcephalic children. By contrast, in Brazil, where abortion is illegal, it is very difficult to get a termination unless you are wealthy and can afford to travel abroad for the procedure.

At this point, Turchi began to worry that the cases in maternity wards in Recife might be the tip of an iceberg. "We didn't know how it was going to turn out, but we could see that it was going to be something really big." It was around this time that some paediatricians began urging the Pernambuco health authorities to revise the reporting criteria for microcephaly. Contrary to the suggestion that it was Brazil's live birth system that had led to the increase in reported microcephaly cases, prior to December 2015 the Ministry of Health had lowered the head circumference limit from 33 cm to 32 cm,[33] reducing the number of newborns likely to be categorized as microcephalic.[34]

Now the figures are in, it is clear that the upsurge was not a reporting artefact. In all, Brazil recorded 4,783 suspected cases of microcephaly and 476 deaths in 2015, as opposed to 147 cases in 2014. The highest rates were in the northeast, with 56.7 cases per 10,000 live births at the peak of the epidemic in November 2015. That rate was twenty-four times higher than the historical mean in Brazil. By contrast, in the southeast, where Zika appeared later and was generally less severe, the rates were far lower—5.5 cases per 10,000 live births, which is similar to the rates observed in the United States (the overall rate for Brazil was 18 per 10,000). The question is, how much of this increase was due to Zika, as opposed to another cofactor, and why was the peak observed in the northeast so much higher than in other areas of Brazil?[35]

In an attempt to answer that question, in 2016 Turchi initiated a case control study with colleagues from the London School of Hygiene and Tropical Medicine in which women attending antenatal clinics in Recife were screened for Zika. The laboratory-confirmed cases were then followed to term, together with those of two controls who had tested negative for the virus. The babies were examined for microcephaly and other manifestations of congenital Zika syndrome with clearly defined denominators.

At the time of the epidemic, rumours abounded that the higher prevalence of microcephaly in the northeast might be due to exposure to insecticides used to control mosquitoes. Another widespread conspiracy theory was that the fault lay with vaccines administered during pregnancy. Now that the results of the study are in, both theories can be ruled out. Researchers found no statistically significant correlation between the incidence of microcephaly and exposure to insecticides or vaccines. By contrast the odds of association with prior Zika infection was 95 per cent.[36]

Unfortunately the study was unable to investigate the association—long suspected by researchers—between the incidence of microcephaly and a mother's socioeconomic background. That would require better Zika sero-prevalence data in order to ascertain whether women included in the study are representative of the wider population. More importantly, because Zika was not a reportable condition at the time of the epidemic, researchers have no way of gauging the total number of babies born to pregnant women infected with Zika in 2015–16 and thus whether the high rates of microcephaly observed in the northeast were really as high as they seem. Laura Rodrigues, a professor of infectious disease epidemiology at the London School of Hygiene and Tropical Medicine who works closely with Turchi, suspects that northeast-ern Brazil may have had a fast-moving outbreak of a particularly severe strain of Zika. However, Rodrigues also acknowledges that this is "a gut feeling" and without better data she cannot be sure.[37]

Another open question is the extent to which the higher microcephaly prevalence rates may have been due to higher mosquito densities and women's greater risk of exposure to Zika because of social behaviours and environ-mental conditions. Climate scientists point out that 2015 was an El Niño year in South America, with higher than normal amounts of rainfall in northeast Brazil, increasing the risk of flooding. Coupled with rising temperatures due to climate change, this could have accelerated the reproductive cycle and density of *Aedes* and the mosquito's transmission of the virus. "I do feel it's got to do with the environment and social conditions," said Turchi. "Recife is a highly urbanized area, and it's a city crossed by rivers with a lot of swamp areas, so there are a lot of mosquitoes. And because it's hot, people do not cover up: they are very exposed." Indeed, in Jaboatão dos Guararapes and other poor communities it is not unusual to find upwards of a thousand people crammed into an area measuring one hundred square metres, and since many accommodations lack screened windows and even fewer have air conditioning, occupants are frequently bitten many times in the same night by the same mosquitoes. Then there is the fact that piped water supplies are erratic, meaning that many residents have no choice but to store water in bottles and buckets in their backyards, or that when it rains channels behind people's homes fill with sewage and rubbish, providing perfect breeding sites for mosquitoes.

In addition, there is the ongoing question of whether prior exposure to another arbovirus infection or vaccination against yellow fever confers cross-immunity to Zika or, conversely, makes an individual more susceptible. Turchi points out that prior to the 2015 Zika outbreak, Pernambuco had not suffered a major dengue epidemic for several years, whereas in central Brazil and the southeast, dengue had been a more recent visitor. Moreover, the highest rates of CZS were seen in younger women—precisely the group who had less time to be exposed to dengue or to get the yellow fever vaccine. On the other hand, in vitro studies by Marques and his colleagues using serum from pregnant women suggest that the presence of dengue antibodies can make Zika infections more severe.[38] The technical term is antibody-dependent enhancement (ADE). In layman's language the Zika virus latches onto the dengue antibodies and uses them as camouflage to evade the immune system and ease its entry to a human cell. "Think of it as the viral equivalent of a Trojan horse," said Marques. When the epidemic broke, such was the demand for testing that his laboratory became a public reference laboratory. Later, Marques and his colleagues developed a rapid diagnostic test for dengue, making it easier to diagnose and differentiate it from Zika. His principal focus now is whether or not ADE might explain the high microcephaly prevalence rates in the northeast and whether high anti-dengue titers confer protection against Zika. However, he does not discount the possibility that the high rates might be due to an unknown environmental cofactor. "There is still so much we do not know about Zika," Marques acknowledged. "We have decades of work ahead of us."

Like Turchi, Marques was full of praise for Brito, and I was looking forward to meeting him face-to-face. Although we had previously spoken by Skype, his English was halting and as my Portuguese was non-existent I feared much may have been lost in translation. Fortunately, when we did eventually meet at a restaurant near my hotel, he brought his daughter, Celina, a second-year medical student, to translate. The restaurant specialized in tapioca, the traditional accompaniment to any meal in Pernambuco, and after ordering some tapioca flour pancakes we got down to business. Why, during previous Zika outbreaks, had the association with microcephaly and neurological disorders been missed? Why did he think that no one had made the connection before?

"My father says that when the first microcephaly cases appeared it was easy for him to make the connection because he had been following the Zika epidemic from the beginning," said Celina. "So naturally one of the first questions he asked the women was whether they remembered having a rash during pregnancy."

Yes, but what was it about Pernambuco that made the microcephaly cases so obvious? In other words, why did it become visible here and not somewhere else?

Brito furrowed his brow as Celina translated my question. Then, nodding intensely, he explained that it was all a matter of numbers. French Polynesia has a population of just under 300,000, whereas the population of Pernambuco is nine million, of which four million live in Recife and the greater urban area. Pernambuco also has a very high birth rate, with some 170,000 babies being delivered at maternity wards across the state every year. In addition, in French Polynesia the microcephaly cases were scattered across the archipelago, whereas in Pernambuco they were concentrated in a handful of hospitals in and around Recife. The result was that it did not require much of an increase in the prevalence rate of microcephaly for these cases to come to paediatricians' attention. "If you have twenty cases in one room in one week you can't miss it. That's why it was easier to recognize here."

It was a good answer, the answer you would expect an epidemiologist to give, and as I mulled it over afterwards I was reminded of Turchi's comment that "her grandmother" could have spotted the microcephaly cases. However, it did not address the deeper questions of causation, of why the risk of microcephaly seemed to be so much higher for women from poor neighbourhoods, what the role of social conditions was, and how the provision of adequate water services and sanitation systems affected the transmission dynamics of Zika in Recife and other cities in Brazil. Nor did it address the issue of what measures were needed to interrupt the transmission of the virus by mosquitoes and reduce the risk of Zika infections in the future. Those were questions that were best answered by an entomologist and perhaps by a sociologist.

Ever since Haddow and Dick isolated Zika from an *A. africanus* mosquito in Uganda in 1948, it has been assumed that *Aedes* is the principal vector of the virus in the wild. In Brazil and other parts of South America, most studies have focused on *A. aegypti*. In addition, Zika can be transmitted by the "Asian tiger mosquito," *Aedes albopictus*, which ranges as far north as Chicago and New York during the northern summer.* However, Zika has also been isolated from several species of *Culex*, including *C. quinquefasciatus*, which is abundant in Brazil, as well as in Asia. Moreover, unlike *Aedes*, which prefers clean water, *C. quinquefasciatus* favours dirty water and is happy to breed in sewer runoffs and canals clogged with refuse and other debris.

In an office a few doors from Turchi's, another Fiocruz researcher, Constância Ayres, had been taking a closer look at the *Culex* mosquito and the evidence that it might play a role in transmission. A slim energetic woman

---

* *A. albopictus* is also the principal vector of West Nile virus.

with the posture of a ballet dancer, Ayres began by collecting *Culex* and *Aedes* mosquitoes from different neighbourhoods around Recife and raising them in an insectary. Next, she allowed both sets of mosquitoes to feed on infected blood in her laboratory. Then, a week later, she collected saliva from the mosquitoes and assayed them for Zika. Positive results were obtained for both sets of mosquito. In addition, Ayres was able to recover Zika virus from the salivary glands of the *Culex*, a necessary condition for a "competent" vector. However, despite these results, many experts refused to accept that *Culex* might be responsible for spreading Zika in the wild, so in 2016 Ayres returned to the field and, using an aspirator, collected more mosquitoes, this time vacuuming them up from residences occupied by individuals with symptoms of Zika. When she returned to the lab and examined her catch, she found she had nearly four times as many *Culex* as *Aedes*. Next, she separated out the female mosquitoes of each species, divided them into pools, and assayed them for Zika. Three of the *C. quinquefasciatus* and two of the *A. aegypti* pools were positive for Zika.

Unlike *Aedes*, *Culex* is not a sip feeder—the mosquito typically takes just one blood meal per night. However, they are about twenty times as abundant as *Aedes* in urban areas of Recife with the highest concentrations of microcephaly. The mosquito is similarly ubiquitous in Micronesia and French Polynesia. Interestingly, in these areas researchers were unable to detect Zika in wild-caught Aedes. Unfortunately, no one thought to test *C. quinquefasciatus* in these places, so it is not known if it could have been a vector for the Zika epidemics there, but the possibility cannot be ruled out.

If Ayres is right, her findings have important implications for ongoing vector control strategies aimed at reducing the threat of Zika and other arboviruses. At present, mosquito fumigation measures are directed at the *Aedes*. This is not surprising given its role in transmitting dengue, but Ayres is furious at suggestions by local health chiefs that this is why Recife has not witnessed another outbreak. "The reason we have not seen another Zika epidemic is because the majority of the population now has antibodies. It is not because the mosquitoes that transmit the virus have been eliminated. Unless something is done about *Culex*, I predict that once immunity wanes, Zika will return."

Unfortunately, that is a message no one appeared interested in hearing. Instead, the week I visited Recife, a German biotech company was gearing up to release male *A. aegypti* mosquitoes artificially infected with *Wolbachia* bacteria in Corrego do Jenipapo, a sprawling favela in the northeast of the city. The bacteria, which is harboured by 60 per cent of the world's insect species but not *Aedes*, renders the offspring of the mosquitoes infertile, thereby reducing the size of *Aedes* populations and their ability to transmit Zika and other arboviruses. Similar trial releases of *Wolbachia*-modified mosquitoes have taken place in Rio and Medellin, in Colombia, and similar genetic modification techniques are being used on the *Anopheles* mosquitoes that transmit malaria.[39] The trials have the backing of major charitable funders, including the Bill and Melinda Gates Foundation in Seattle, Washington, and the London-based Wellcome Trust, not least because they can be conducted in distinct geographic areas and the effects are relatively easy to quantify using scientific measures—one of the key requisites for global health interventions "from above." Meanwhile, low-tech ground-up control measures, such as providing bednets and screens for windows, are neglected, as are urban renewal programs that might improve waste management and the provision of water services to the poorest, mosquito-blighted communities.

One day I accompanied Ayres's mosquito collectors on one of their regular sweeps through Jaboatão dos Guararapes. The aim was to visit ten addresses in the favela and vacuum up mosquitoes from people's bedrooms and living rooms, but in the event one of the portable aspirators failed, so it was only possible to visit five addresses. The residents were for the most part elderly and crammed into narrow two-or-three-room cinderblock dwellings, one on top of the other. Only two had indoor toilets, and all the cooking and washing took place in the same room, or, if they were lucky, a backyard. Ayres's top mosquito collector, Miguel Longman, led the way, running his battery-powered Horst Armadilhas aspirator along the walls and countertops, before concentrating on the ceilings and hard-to-reach corners. A typical haul, he told me, was fifty to sixty mosquitoes. While he unhooked the net on his aspirator to inspect his catch, I asked the couple whose home we were in how often they got piped water. Twice a week, came the reply. And the other days? They pointed to two plastic tubs filled with dirty dishwater in their kitchen and a series of water containers lined up on their windowsill. As with the other homes we visited, the windows had no screens, although in this case I noticed their bedroom had a mosquito net. Had she or her husband had Zika? No, came the reply, but several of their neighbours had.

Later that day, back at IAM, Ayres introduced me to Andre Monteiro, a Fiocruz public health engineer. Monteiro is an expert on the hydrology of the greater Recife area and has made a close study of the city's sanitation system. Only 6 per cent of households in Jaboatão dos Guararapes have access to sewage services, he told me. By contrast, for Recife as a whole the figure is 30 per cent. Most of the waste is sluiced into rivulets that flow through people's backyards and empty into the canals and storm sewers designed to prevent flooding. Up until the 1800s most of the city comprised mangrove swamp, so excess rain water was easily absorbed or was able to flow out to sea with the falling tide. But in the nineteenth century, as Recife expanded, the mangrove swamp was gradually covered to make way for new buildings and roads. To compensate for the loss of natural drainage, Recife's engineers, inspired by the example of the Dutch, built 200 kilometres of canals, threading them through Recife's backstreets and alongside the city's rivers. However, by the 1970s many of the canals had fallen into disrepair and were not being properly maintained, leading to frequent floods (the largest, in 1975, saw 80 per cent of the city under water). At the same time, favelas in hills to the north of Recife begun suffering catastrophic mudslides, culminating in one in 2002 in which fifty people lost their lives. But perhaps the city's most embarrassing moment came in 2013 when a Reuters photographer captured the image of a nine-year-old boy bobbing about in a refuse-filled canal near his home in Canal do Arruda, a favela in northeast Recife. It later transpired that Paulinho da Silveiro was combing the canal for bottles and other recyclable material he could sell and, together with his brothers, was a regular visitor to the polluted waterway. The shocking images prompted the municipal authorities to launch a clean-up campaign, and, although Recife's canals and rivers are flowing freely again, at low tide it is common to see the river banks choked with plastic bottles and other litter. "The rubbish is a big problem," says Monteiro, "not only because it affects drainage but because of the mosquitoes that breed in the trapped water."

At the end of our interview, Monteiro showed me a heat map of Recife with the areas with the highest numbers of microcephaly cases marked in oranges and reds. Although there were orange dots sprinkled throughout the city, including in middle-class districts such as Boa Vista, the deepest reds coincided with the favelas to the north and south.

The following day, in search of the mothers of some of these microcephalic babies, I visited a specialist rehabilitation centre for sight-impaired children in Iputinga. Nearly half of children with CZS have severe vision problems due to lesions in their retinas or optic nerves, as well as, in some cases, neurological and cortical-based impairments. To address their vision deficits, Altino Ventura, a medical charity specializing in the treatment of ophthalmic conditions, had already provided several children with corrective magnifying goggles and intensive rehabilitation. Now it had also designed a multisensory kit to help mothers train their children to focus on objects and interact with them better, and had invited several women to test the devices at its Menina dos Olhos rehabilitation centre.

I arrived to find mats with cushions for the children already spread out on the floor and volunteers removing items from the kit—ping pong paddles with bright, painted faces, shakers with long glittery tassels. The session began with a prayer from Altino Ventura's president, Liana Ventura. "Today is the Sabbath so let us take a moment to recognize all our hard work and the challenges we face in our lives. Lord, show us the light and make us instruments of inspiration and, above all, hope." Ventura, a professor of ophthalmology, and her husband Marcelo Ventura have won numerous awards for their work. Their foundation, which is open around the clock seven days a week, processes up to five hundred patients a day at its emergency ophthalmic clinic in downtown Recife. Patients come from all over Pernambuco, drawn by the promise of free eye care and corrections for cataracts and other common vision problems. Altino Ventura conducts research into ophthalmological conditions associated with diseases like toxoplasmosis, syphilis, rubella and cytomegalovirus, which are common in Brazil, and also runs an outreach program on Recife maternity wards. So when babies began presenting with microcephaly and unusual optical lesions in the fall of 2015, it was not long before Liana Ventura was showing an interest. Many of the babies had eyes that were crossed or swivelled aimlessly from side to side. In some cases, the vision loss was profound. "We realized the babies could see only 30 per cent of the normal visual field and in a few cases they couldn't see anything," she told me. "It was heart-breaking. They could not see their mothers' faces, they had no interest in anything around them. They cried the whole time."[40]

90 per cent of vision develops in the first year of a child's life. Without the ability to see, a child's ability to interact with their primary caregiver and to develop normally is greatly impaired. With corrective goggles, however, the transformation was dramatic. "Their faces lit up immediately and for the first time they smiled," said Ventura.

Ventura removed a ping pong paddle from one of the bags and handed it to Joane and Marcilio da Silva, a young couple from Olinda. Their son, Hector, was born with a severe astigmatism but with goggles can now see 60 per cent of his visual field. Nevertheless, at twenty months he still could not sit up on his own unaided and had to be propped up with pillows in order to interact with the trainers. Sitting beside them, observing their progress, was another young woman, Mylene Helena dos Santos. Aged twenty-three, dos Santos is the mother of three sons, including her youngest, David Henrique. Born in August 2015, David was one of the first cohort of Zika babies and is profoundly disabled. Strapped to a baby seat, with braces supporting his legs, he is unable to swallow properly and has a severe astigmatism. He developed a lung infection when some food got caught in his trachea and had to be rushed to the hospital. The doctors inserted a tube in his stomach so that he could be fed antibiotics, but, according to dos Santos, the tube caused him considerable discomfort. "It is too big so he wriggles the whole time," she explained. "The doctors have warned me to keep it clean, otherwise it could become infected. I would like to get him goggles but as long as he has stomach problems it is impossible. Hopefully, when he is better."

Dos Santos was five months into her pregnancy when an ultrasound revealed David might have a congenital malformation, but no one mentioned microcephaly and she had never heard of Zika. "I only knew about dengue," she said. She does not recall a rash, but as her pregnancy progressed there was a series of complications, including a leak of amniotic fluid, and she very nearly miscarried. In the event, David was born seven weeks premature. A year later, both mother and son tested positive for Zika.

Dos Santos is currently living with her parents in Jaboatão dos Guararapes, having separated from David's father shortly after his birth, and relies on her extended family to care for her other children while she and David travel to medical appointments. "In the beginning everybody wanted to help," said dos Santos. "But after a year it slowed down and I was removed from a government program. That's when I turned to Altino Ventura for help."

It is an all too common story. In the wake of the epidemic, the Brazilian government approved cash-transfer programs for poorer families and promised to invest $35 million a year in specialized rehabilitation centres. At the same time, the Pernambuco state authorities pledged $5 million for the construction of regional centres for infants with CZS. But at the close of 2016, the National Congress approved a constitutional amendment freezing public spending for twenty years, and at the time of writing most of the centres have yet to be built. Instead, as austerity measures bite, women like dos Santos struggle to find the money for essential medicines and care. Nor is there any indication that the authorities are prepared to make the investments necessary to rectify the systemic water and sanitation problems. Instead, the government has been shifting the responsibility for mosquito control back onto households through awareness campaigns targeting housewives.

This is not the only way that the underlying social and environmental conditions that gave rise to the outbreak continue to be neglected. As Human Rights Watch discovered when it visited Brazil to interview women in Pernambuco and Paraiba on the first anniversary of the epidemic, roughly a quarter of the women and girls who gave birth to babies with microcephaly were below the age of twenty. Yet this is precisely the group least likely to have access to contraception and sexual and reproductive health information. Nor was Human Rights Watch impressed by the state of the favelas they visited, reporting that it was common to find channels running with raw sewage and mosquitoes breeding in refuse-clogged canals and marshes behind people's homes.

"Brazilians may see the health ministry's declaration of the end of the Zika emergency as a victory," commented Amanda Klasing, senior women's rights researcher at Human Rights Watch. "But ... Brazilians' basic rights are at risk if the government doesn't reduce mosquito infestation over the long term, secure access to reproductive rights, and support families raising children affected by Zika."[41]

That is a verdict with which Liana Ventura concurs. Of the 325 children being treated by her foundation, just two were private referrals—everyone else came through the public health system. Yet two years on from the epidemic, nearly half are still awaiting the results of Zika serology tests. "There is still so much that we don't know about the pathology of Zika and microcephaly, but at the moment, frankly, it's a struggle," she told me. "Let's hope it doesn't take another epidemic to make the world sit up and take notice."

* * *

Before checking out of my hotel I decided to go for a stroll on the promenade at Boa Viagem. When I had left for Ipitunga in the morning the waves were covering the rocks that form a barrier with the roadside and there was no beach to be seen, but by 4pm the tide had receded to reveal Recife's famous reefs, and the sand was now studded with beach umbrellas and children splashing happily in the channels and puddles left by the ebbing waters. With a light offshore breeze, the conditions were perfect for surfing, but to my surprise there were no surfers to be seen beyond the breakers, nor did anyone appear to be venturing into the sea to swim. The reason soon became apparent when within a few yards of the beach I was confronted by a fierce red and white sign that read "Perigo" (danger) and below it, in English, "Danger—Shark Zone." This was followed by the outline of a shark in yellow and advice on when to avoid bathing. Some of the advice was commonsensical. Swimmers should not venture into the sea "with bleeding or wearing bright objects" or when they were "drunk" or "alone." However, bathing was also not advised "in open waters," "at high tide," or at "dawn and dusk." In other words, pretty much anytime except the daylight hours when the tide was out.

A little further along the beach, I spotted a lookout station and approached the lifeguard for an explanation. Until the early 1990s, he explained, Boa Viagem had been a popular surfing destination. Then, in 1992, came the first in a series of shark attacks. By 2013 Boa Viagem had suffered fifty-eight such attacks, twenty-one of them fatal, forcing the authorities to ban surfing and post shark warning signs. No one was sure of the reason for the sudden change in the sharks' behaviour, but most experts blamed it on the construction in the 1980s of a new container port at Suape, twelve miles south of Recife. During construction, workers had dredged the estuaries and built docks that protruded far out into the ocean. The dredging of the estuaries was thought to have been particularly disruptive to the breeding and feeding patterns of bull sharks, who generally stay close to shore and are able to tolerate fresh water. However, the more serious shark infestation coincided with the completion of the container port and the subsequent explosion in ship traffic in the 1990s. The larger ocean-going vessels brought with them migratory tiger sharks, attracted by the waste and rubbish thrown overboard. Drawn into Port Suapes, it is thought that these tiger sharks, which are expert scavengers, rapidly developed a taste for the coastal waters and began feeding on the untreated sewage that spills into the sea every day from Recife's canals and rivers. The result is that today even lifeguards avoid swimming at Boa Viagem, preferring to train in chlorinated pools, and if they are forced to intervene in a life-or-death situation at sea their preferred mode of transport is a jet ski.[42]

It was transatlantic shipping and the international search for profits that had first brought *Aedes* to this coast, too. No one can be sure when *Aedes* first made landfall in Brazil. Perhaps it was as early as the 1530s when the first Portuguese colonists arrived at Olinda, a colonial town just north of Recife, and discovered the natural harbour formed by the confluence of the Capibaribe and Beberibe Rivers and the long sea wall guarding the estuary. But most likely the mosquito arrived later in the sixteenth century when Portuguese ships loaded with slaves destined for Pernambuco's sugarcane plantations began crossing from the west coast of Africa.[43] By 1637, when the Dutch took possession of the plantations and moved the colonial capital to Recife, the sugarcane business was booming. However, by now British and Dutch slavers making the middle passage to the Caribbean had introduced the virus of yellow fever to Barbados. In 1685 the first outbreak was recorded in Recife, inaugurating a cycle of arbovirus epidemics, the threat of which—except for a brief period in the 1940s and 1950s—has never gone away.

Today, mosquitoes are once again making the crossing,[44] this time breeding in car tires filled with rain water as they once bred in the casks of fresh drinking water beside slaves chained below decks.* And as they do so it is unlikely that Zika will be the last arbovirus to accompany them. Nor, when you factor in the growth of international jet travel, would you wish to bet against other viruses and microbial pathogens, to which local people may have little or no immunity, hitching a ride to Brazil in airplanes.

Predicting what that pathogen might be and when it will make landfall is a fool's errand. Like the lifeguards at Boa Viagem, all we can do is scan the horizon for dorsal fins and other lurking threats, and while we may not be able to alter the facts of global travel and commerce, we can address the local sanitary and environmental conditions that have made Recife and other Brazilian cities so hospitable to the *Aedes* and other disease-carrying mosquitoes. That is not a matter of knowledge but of political will.

---

* This is almost certainly how *Aedes albopictus*, the principal vector of chikungunya, and a mosquito previously restricted to Southeast Asia, reached the Americas, reproducing in ornamental bamboo and disused car tires on ships destined for Texas, from whence it spread via interstate trucking routes to Mexico and Latin America.

DISEASE X

"It came and went, a hurricane across the green fields of life"

The Times, 1921

On the evening of 30 December 2019, Dr Marjorie Pollack was relaxing at her home in Cobble Hill, Brooklyn, when she received an email about a peculiar cluster of pneumonias in Wuhan, the capital of Central China's Hubei Province. A graduate of the CDC's Epidemic Intelligence Service, Pollack is a medical epidemiologist with more than thirty years' experience in the field. She is also the deputy editor of ProMED, a program that trawls the internet looking for chatter about unusual disease outbreaks. That made her the perfect person to evaluate whether the reports, which a colleague had spotted on the Chinese chatroom, Weibo, merited further investigation or could safely be placed on hold until after the new year.

What Pollack saw when she opened the email immediately raised her hackles. "The alert gave me some tweets about stuff that was going on in Wuhan – a cluster of four cases, then 27 cases - along with a picture theoretically of a document sent out by the Wuhan public health commission stating something about pneumonia cases that seemed to be associated with a seafood and wildlife market," she recalled. "Having lived through and worked through the SARS outbreak, it just rang a bell. This was a déjà vu."[1]

Pollack immediately issued her own appeal on the ProMED network and within hours had located a Chinese media report confirming that the Wuhan health commission document was real. Four hours later, an artificial intelligence system based at Boston Children's Hospital also issued an alert about the unidentified pneumonia cases in Wuhan, rating the seriousness as three on a scale of five. That was all the prompting Pollack needed and shortly before midnight she issued a more detailed warning to ProMED's 80,000-strong international community of doctors, epidemiologists, and public health officials.

Pollack did not realise it at the time, but she had just picked up the first signal of a major new coronavirus outbreak. Within a matter of months Covid-19 would become a true global pandemic, one with uncanny echoes of the 1918-19 Spanish influenza. The difference was that in 1918 the world had been at war and, although the flu sparked a wave of deaths, factories and schools for the most part had stayed open and, except for troop transports, there was far less movement of people between countries and continents. By contrast, Covid-19 struck a world that had never been more interconnected, setting off a chain of infections that crashed world stock markets, grounded international aviation, and silenced the most advanced cities on the globe.

* * *

We now know that the pandemic of Covid-19 began in December 2019 in or around the Huanan Seafood Wholesale Market in Wuhan, a city of 11 million inhabitants. Despite its name, the market also sold the meat of a huge range of wild animals, including wolf cubs, crocodiles, and snakes. "Patient zero" was a 70-year-old man who fell ill on 1 December. Given that SARS-CoV-2, to use the official name of the virus, has an average incubation period of fourteen days, that suggests he must have been infected in mid-November—or possibly earlier. A week later, there were seven more cases, two of them with direct links to the seafood market. This was followed on 12 December by the illness of a 49-year-old market vendor, followed, seven days later, by his father-in-law. Ominously, the father-in-law had not visited the market, suggesting that he had caught the infection directly from his son-in-law.

By the end of the week, at least three hospitals in Wuhan were reporting similar cases. However, the patients were told they had flu or bronchitis and were sent home. Even doctors who had begun to suspect a connection with the market were relatively unconcerned by the presentations, rationalising there was no evidence of community spread. As the head of one of Wuhan's hospital's emergency departments told the *Wall Street Journal*: "The early stages made us drop our guard."[2]

The event that would change that—and which would result in the signal that Pollack picked up in New York—was a chatroom post by a young Chinese whistle-blower, Dr Li Wenliang. After graduating from Wuhan University School of Medicine in 2011, Li had specialized in ophthalmology, eventually landing a position at Wuhan Central Hospital. Despite having joined the Chinese Communist Party in his sophomore year, Li was not afraid to criticize the authorities. When, in 2011, a journalist was suspended for raising questions about a train crash in Wenzhou that had left 40 dead and 170 injured, Li demanded the journalist be reinstated.[3] Two years later, following a spate of unprovoked attacks on Chinese doctors, Li posted a screenshot on Weibo of a paper in the British medical journal, *The Lancet*, calling for the authorities to do more to protect medical staff.[4] It was only natural, then, when he heard from a colleague in the hospital's emergency department that seven patients had presented with atypical pneumonias and their tests had come back positive for "SARS coronavirus", that he would want to share the news. "7 SARS cases confirmed at Hua'nan Seafood Market," read his Weibo post on 30 December. "Quarantined in the Emergency Department of our hospital."[5] Li also shared a CT scan of one of the patient's lungs. Instead of the air tubes and arteries silhouetted against a dark background, as in a healthy lung, the respiratory tree was obscured by hazy white patches punctuated by peculiar dark opacities. It looked as if the air sacs were full of pus and other fluids, but the lung consolidation was uneven, with some lobes and areas more severely affected than others.

In China, communicating outside of official channels is a serious offence and the post earned Li a stern rebuke from Wuhan's Public Security Bureau, which accused him of "illegal rumor mongering" and of disturbing public order.[6] A few days later, Li was summoned to Zhongnan Police Station and was made to sign a statement declaring that his Weibo messages were incorrect and promising not to repeat the offence.

In fact, the Wuhan branch office of China's Center for Disease Control (CCDC) had already dispatched a team to the seafood market to conduct an investigation. There, they identified 27 cases of "unexplained pneumonias", prompting the Wuhan Municipal Health Committee to issue its own Weibo post on 30 December in which it acknowledged that seven patients were in a critical condition. The following day China's CDC dispatched another team to the seafood market to disinfect it, and on 31 December they notified WHO's China office of the pneumonia cases—though whether this was to pre-empt any more rumours on social media, or in response to Pollack's ProMED post, is impossible to say. Two days later, the Wuhan Institute of Technology isolated the virus from one of the patients and ran it through an RT-PCR machine.*

---

* Reverse Transcription Polymerase Chain Reaction, RT-PCR for short, is a sensitive and highly specific test that looks for tiny fragments of virus and amplifies them so they can be typed and studied more closely. It can be likened to a magnifying glass.

Like SARS and Middle East Respiratory Syndrome (MERS), which had been the cause of sporadic outbreaks in the Middle East since 2012, the virus belonged to the coronavirus family. However, it wasn't SARS or MERS. It was a completely new virus.

This was China's Chernobyl moment. By January 2020, the novel coronavirus, later named Covid-19, was almost certainly already transmitting freely in Wuhan. As it was a new virus, which no one anywhere in the world had immunity from, it was imperative to act quickly before it escaped the city's boundaries. But rather than sounding the sirens and alerting citizens to the possible fallout, the Wuhan authorities hesitated. The Chinese Lunar New Year was approaching and Wuhan, the cradle of the Chinese Revolution, was about to host a big banquet. The last thing Wuhan's mayor needed was adverse publicity ahead of the country's most important family holiday.

Another factor may have been fear: since Xi's election as General Secretary of the Chinese Communist Party, power had become even more concentrated in Beijing and dissent from the party line could spell the end of a bureaucrat's career. The result was that officials lower down the party hierarchy were reluctant to take decisions without the say-so of the politburo and its "paramount leader". Nor did anyone want to be the harbinger of news that might undermine Xi's "China dream", a project of national rejuvenation fuelled by a dynamic globalized economy and respect for China's unique political and cultural traditions. So instead of sounding the alarm, Wuhan officials covered up the news of the signal in the hope that it would go away. It was not until the third week in January that Xi, who, it was later revealed, had been apprised of the true situation in Wuhan on 7 January, took the decision to quarantine Wuhan.[7] Within days, the quarantine had extended to ten other Chinese cities, placing 50 million people under lockdown. By then, an estimated five million people had already left Wuhan, many of them for overseas destinations. It was too late.*

Tragically, one of the first casualties of this new plague was Li Wenliang. After being reprimanded by police, the whistleblowing doctor had continued seeing patients, including an elderly man who presented with symptoms of Covid-19 on 7 January. Five days later, Li developed similar symptoms and was admitted to the respiratory ward of Wuhan Central Hospital. There, a tube was inserted into his trachea to support his breathing, but his condition deterior-

---

* Located at the centre of China's airline network, Wuhan is both a domestic and international hub, with more than one hundred non-stop flights to twenty-two countries worldwide.

ated. Despite being hooked up to a blood oxygenation machine to relieve the pressure on his lungs, on 7 February he died.[8] Li was just 34.

News of his death sparked a howl of rage on Chinese social media. People hailed him as a martyr and used his death to call for an apology from the Wuhan authorities and for greater freedom of speech.[9] That evening, in tribute to their fallen hero, the citizens of Wuhan threw open their windows and stood on balconies to chant the lyrics to "Do You Hear the People Sing?" from the musical *Les Misérables*. "Singing the songs of angry men," the people would "not be slaves again."

The most scathing attack of all came from the Chinese military surgeon and Tsinghua University professor Xu Zhangrun. In a philippic comparing the censorship of Li's posts to China's cover-up of the SARS outbreak in 2002, Zhangrun wrote: "The cause of all of this lies, ultimately, with The Axle [that is, Xi Jinping] and the cabal that surrounds him . . . They stood by blithely as the crucial window of opportunity that was available to deal with the outbreak snapped shut in their faces."[10]

* * *

Coronaviruses take their name from the array of menacing proteins that protrude from their surface, giving the coat the appearance of a crown. That coat is comprised of fatty lipid molecules that are easily degraded by soap; outside of an animal cell, SARS-CoV-2 can survive for no more than 24 hours on cardboard, and about two to three days on steel and plastic. To prosper it needs an animal cell.

Like influenza viruses, coronaviruses are composed of single strands of RNA that are highly prone to copying errors. RNA is the molecule that carries instructions from DNA to the body's cells, but because it is much less stable than DNA, RNA viruses tend to be smaller than DNA viruses. They are measured in kilobases (kb) of information. For instance, polio is relatively lightweight, measuring just 7kb. By contrast, influenza and Ebola are middleweights, measuring 14kb and 19kb respectively. Sars-CoV-2 is a heavyweight coming in at 30kb. That is about as long as a strand of RNA can be without accumulating so many errors during replication that it self-destructs (a problem known as "error catastrophe"). What makes coronavirus a particularly cunning adversary is that, because of the length and complexity of its RNA genome, it has evolved to carry its own proofreading enzyme to correct the errors it makes as it goes along. That gives us grounds for hope that the virus is less likely to mutate in response to our immune response or to vaccines or drugs we might develop against it.

The virus most commonly enters the nose through minuscule droplets expelled in coughs or sneezes, but it can also enter via the eyes or mouth. Once the virus's particles are inside the body, they attach to a particular receptor on the surface of cells, using the crown-like spike protein, or S-protein. This S-protein is designed to fit a receptor protein called ACE-2 (short for angiotensin-converting enzyme 2) found on the surface of cells that line the mucous membranes of the respiratory tract.[11] In the case of SARS-Cov-2, the exact contours of these S-spikes allow it to stick far more strongly to ACE-2 than in the case of SARS-CoV-1 (classic SARS), which is why the new version of the coronavirus may be able to transmit more efficiently.[12] These spikes also latch on to ACE-2 sites deep in the lungs, which may be why SARS-CoV-2 causes more persistent and stubborn lung infections.

Having latched onto the cell membrane, the virus enters and disassembles, releasing its RNA and begins to reproduce it. This is what triggers the initial symptoms of a sore throat and, sometimes, a runny nose. As the virus continues to replicate, it produces millions of viral particles that carry the infection deeper into the respiratory tree. In response, the immune system sends signalling molecules called cytokines to the site of the infection, triggering the inflammation response. It is these proinflammatory cytokines that cause a fever and possibly the other characteristic symptoms of Covid-19, such as a persistent dry cough, sore throat, head and body aches, plus other pains. On average, these symptoms present themselves five days after exposure but they can also arrive sooner or up to fourteen days later.

For the vast majority of people that is the end of the matter and, after a few days, their symptoms dissipate and they begin to feel better. But in some people, such as the elderly (70 and over) and those with underlying medical conditions, the virus keeps traveling down the respiratory tract and invading cells deep within the lungs. For these patients, the critical moment comes when the virus reaches the five-sided satchels that hang from the terminal bronchioles. These satchels, which measure about 2.5cm in diameter, are full of tiny air sacs known as alveoli, whose function is to regulate respiration by exchanging oxygen and carbon dioxide molecules to and from the bloodstream. As these sacs become inflamed, more and more cytokines flood to the seat of the infection, followed by antibodies, and other proteins and enzymes. The process can be likened to a snowstorm. Eventually, the sacs become so full of fluids and damaged cells that they become blocked and oxygenation is no longer possible. This is the point where patients struggle to breath and report feeling as if their chests are being crushed. On a CT scan, this partial filling of the satchels shows up as a patchwork described as "ground glass opacities".[13]

This patchwork is composed of polygonal shapes corresponding to the satchels and can, in combination with the thickening of adjoining walls, create an appearance similar to crazy paving, or drifting snow glimpsed through a shower door. As the satchels continue to fill, further consolidation ensues and on the CT scan the lung takes on an increasingly white appearance. The patients may now be heading toward Acute Respiratory Distress Syndrome (ARDS) and, unless supported with a ventilator, death may follow within a matter of hours.

* * *

How did it come to this? How is it that despite a century punctuated by repeated outbreaks and pandemics, we failed to heed the warnings about Covid-19 and act when our actions could have prevented the outbreak from spinning out of control? After all, this was not the first time that a coronavirus had emerged from a hidden animal reservoir to encircle the globe. In November 2002, something very similar happened when SARS emerged in Guangdong in southern China. From there, the virus was carried by bus to Hong Kong and by commercial airliners to Vietnam, Singapore, Thailand, and Canada. By July 2003, when the WHO officially declared the epidemic over, the world had recorded more than 8,000 cases and 774 deaths. Within three months of the start of the Covid-19 pandemic, we have already seen twice as many cases, and with experts predicting a second wave of illness in the fall of 2020 that could continue into the winter of 2021, there is no telling when the misery might end. Little wonder that many experts have compared Covid-19 to the first great pandemic of the 20th century, the 1918-19 Spanish influenza.[14] That it should coincide with the centenary of that cataclysmic event is a coincidence no historian could have imagined or a novelist would have dared to invent.

One of the tragedies of the Covid-19 pandemic is that, unlike earlier missed alarms canvassed in this book, veterinary ecologists—whose job it is to monitor remote animal habitats for emerging infectious disease threats—had seen it, or something like it, coming. There had also been no lack of warnings from organizations and institutions who monitor global health security and advise governments on how to prepare for pandemics.

In the last one hundred years we have witnessed a succession of pandemics, some of which, like parrot fever, have been mild; others, like AIDS, extremely severe. However, the first wake-up call of the twenty-first century was the SARS outbreak. Originating in civet cats sold at "wet markets" in

Guangdong,* SARS brought to light the risks that the consumption of exotic sources of protein, urban overcrowding, international jet travel, and the growing interconnectivity of global markets presented in the modern world.[15] Those risks were underlined by the 2009 swine flu pandemic, which despite being less severe than initially feared nonetheless resulted in 120,000 to 200,000 deaths globally, and the Ebola outbreak that began in southeast Guinea in 2014.[16] Much to the surprise of viral haemorrhagic fever experts at both the CDC and WHO, the haemorrhagic virus had spread very rapidly to nearby countries, sparking a major regional emergency in West Africa, and lockdowns in Monrovia and Freetown. To contain the epidemic and prevent Ebola from spreading more widely, the United Nations, at the prompting of Médecins Sans Frontières and the Obama administration, launched the biggest humanitarian response in peacetime backed by the combined military might of the US, France, and Britain. The response averted a bigger disaster, and perhaps a pandemic, but at a huge economic cost that reduced the gross domestic product of Guinea, Sierra Leone, and Liberia by $2.8 billion, an average of $125 per person.[17]

The Zika outbreak that began in Brazil in 2015, while the world was still focused on Ebola in West Africa, was the twenty-first century's fourth wake-up call. The difference was that Zika was not a new pathogen but one that virologists had known about for decades. But like other neglected diseases that are usually confined to the tropics, few scientists had thought that Zika, which had first been identified in 1947 in a remote forested region of Uganda, could pose a threat to the most populous cities in South America, let alone spread to the Caribbean and the southern United States.

Ever since the Institute of Medicine issued a report on "emerging infections" in 1992, biologists and other experts have been warning that globalization, coupled with climate change and the increasing demand for animal protein, had made the world "intrinsically more vulnerable" to infectious diseases, both known and unknown, than in the past. But it was SARS that brought home just how interconnected the world had become and how many of these potentially pandemic viruses were harboured by bats. The first breakthrough came in 2005 when researchers isolated a virus very similar to SARS in horse-

---

* "Wet market" is a term that originated in Hong Kong and Singapore English to distinguish markets selling fresh meat and produce from "dry" markets selling packaged and durable goods such as textiles. Chinese wet markets typically sell fresh meat, fish, and seafood.

shoe bats in China. However, the virus was missing a crucial protein spike needed to infect human cells. That changed in 2013 when a group of scientists working for the EcoHealth Alliance, a global non-profit organization based in New York, ventured into a limestone cave in Kunming, southern China, occupied by similar horseshoe bats. Dressed in hazmat suits for protection, they drew blood from the bats and collected faecal samples from the cave floor. Nearly a quarter of the 117 animals sampled contained coronavirus, including two new strains almost identical to SARS, especially in the part of the genome that codes for the spike protein. As the president of EcoHealth Alliance, Peter Daszak, and one of the authors of the report told *Science*: "This shows, that right now in China, there are bats carrying a virus that can directly infect people, and cause another SARS pandemic."[18]

Bats, which constitute about a fifth of all mammals on the planet, are not only a natural reservoir of coronaviruses.* They also harbour the Marburg, Nipah, and Hendra viruses, which have caused human disease and outbreaks in Africa, Malaysia, Bangladesh, and Australia. Bats also transmit rabies and are thought to be the natural reservoir of Ebola. Why bats are able to tolerate such a wide range of viruses is the subject of ongoing research, but one theory is that, as part of their adaptation to flight (they are the only mammals with wings), bats have evolved dampened immune systems. This dampened response could be an adaptation to the stress of flight which causes cells within bats' bodies to break down and release bits of DNA. Ordinarily, these cell fragments would cause inflammation, but thanks to the bat's weakened immune system they don't. The hypothesis is that the same response that protects bats from inflammation from cell debris also stops them from becoming sick when infected with foreign viruses.[19]

Daszak, who holds degrees in zoology and parasitology from the University of London and has devoted most of his career to wildlife conversation, was initially sceptical about the extent to which bats posed a threat to human health. However, in 2017, together with the ecologist Kevin J. Olival and other members of the EcoHealth Alliance, he created a database of 754 mammal species and 586 viral species, and analyzed which viruses were harboured by which mammals and how they affected their hosts. Their analysis, published in a letter in *Nature*, showed that bats hosted a significantly greater proportion of zoonoses than all other mammals combined. Indeed, for every species of bat, Olival and Daszak estimated there were about 17 zoonoses yet to be discovered,

---

* Bats are found on every continent except Antarctica.

versus about ten for rodents and primates.[20] This was not the end of their revelations. Following the publication of their letter in *Nature*, Daszak and his intrepid band of virus hunters continued probing caves and other remote bat habitats in China and other parts of Southeast Asia. To date, they have discovered about 500 coronaviruses in Chinese bats alone. In 2018, they also reported that an outbreak of a disease on four pig farms in Guangdong province that had been identified as a type of porcine diarrhea was due to a novel coronavirus almost identical to a bat coronavirus isolated from horseshoe bats in Guangdong and Hong Kong in 2007. Intriguingly, the outbreak had occurred only 62 miles from the home of the index patient of SARS.[21]

In all, during fifteen years of probing caves and taking swabs from bats, Daszak and his colleagues have identified five hundred new coronaviruses. Even more alarmingly, based on the current rate of discovery, Daszak estimates there may be as many as 13,000 unknown coronaviruses still out there waiting to be discovered. Daszak and his colleagues have also identified 335 emerging infectious disease events between 1940 and 2004, with a peak incidence in the 1980s at around the time of the AIDS pandemic.[22] Their survey leaves little doubt that these events have been increasing in incidence since the mid-point of the last century.

* * *

Daszak was not the only person to caution that a coronavirus – or some other unknown pathogen emerging suddenly from bats or another wild animal— might be the trigger for the next pandemic. In a 2015 TED talk that quickly "went viral", Bill Gates warned that "if anything kills over 10 million people in the next few decades, it's most likely to be a highly infectious virus." The West African Ebola outbreak had given the world a preview of the dangers lurking in nature. It was only thanks to the heroic efforts of health workers who had chased down the Ebola transmission chains—and the fact that infected individuals rapidly developed severe symptoms and tended to be bedridden rather than moving around—that Ebola hadn't infected more urban centres. But what if the next emerging pathogen was an airborne virus, like the 1918 Spanish flu, and what if people didn't exhibit symptoms right away, but boarded planes without realising they were infectious? "Next time," Gates concluded, "we may not be so lucky."[23]

One organization had not forgotten about the threat posed by emerging and re-emerging viruses. Since the 2003 SARS epidemic, the WHO had declared public health emergencies on four occasions: during the 2009 swine flu pandemic; the 2014 polio and Ebola outbreaks; and the 2016 Zika epidemic. Determined not to be caught out by another unexpected emergence event, in 2018 the WHO decided to update its Research and Development Blueprint. This was a priority list of pathogens which the world lacked adequate vaccines and/or therapeutics for, and which the WHO had determined required additional research funding. In 2015, the list included Crimean-Congo haemorrhagic fever, Ebola and Marburg, MERS-CoV and SARS, Lassa Fever, Nipah, and Rift Valley Fever. In seventh place the WHO also pencilled in "R&D preparedness for a new disease", but the category was little more than a placeholder and, at the time, few people paid it much attention.[24] However, in 2018 the WHO decided not only to add Zika to the priority list but also that it needed to apprise the world of the danger posed by a different order of threat triggered by a completely unknown pathogen. The name they proposed for the new category was "Disease X".[25]

Daszak recalls the moment vividly. "It was at the end of the meeting and we were getting ready to finalise the list. Then, the guy who does the [mathematical risk] analysis, gets up and says, 'I know you'll support the idea of including this unknown pathogen. We're going to call it Disease X'. I thought, wow, for the WHO that's pretty cool phraseology."[26]

A few weeks later, on his return to New York, Daszak recalls seeing a reference to Disease X in a newspaper and thinking, "that's really good, finally we've got a simple way for the public to understand what we're trying to do."

For Daszak and his colleagues in the EcoHealth Alliance, the buzz generated by Disease X presented an opportunity to leverage additional funding for research, for not only known coronaviruses, such as MERS-CoV and SARS, but also unknown ones and other potentially pandemic viruses lurking in the animal kingdom. Two years earlier, at a summit of disease ecologists at the Rockefeller Foundation's Bellagio Conference Center on the shores of Lake Como, Italy, Daszak and other infectious disease experts had noted the world's growing vulnerability to emerging viral threats. Pointing out that only 0.1 per cent of the estimated 1.6 million viruses with "epidemic/pandemic potential" had been identified, they called for the establishment of a Global Virome Project (GVP).[27] Modelled on the Human Genome Project, which had ushered in the era of personal genomics, the GVP would leverage funds for vaccines, drugs and other medical countermeasures "in advance" of future emergence events. Building on the success of USAID's PREDICT program, which since 2010 had discovered more than 900 new viruses in thirty countries, the aim of the GVP, according to a briefing document, was to "fill the knowledge gap" by creating a comprehensive database of "all naturally-occurring viruses". The document continued, "Despite the potential impact of viral threats, the world remains unable to predict when, where, or from what species the next emerging virus will break out. To be fully prepared, we need to know the enemy before it emerges."[28]

While Daszak was seeking funds for the GVP, the Coalition for Epidemic Preparedness Innovations (CEPI) was trying to raise money for new vaccine platforms. An Oslo-based non-profit, CEPI had been established at the 2017 World Economic Forum in the Swiss ski resort at Davos as an initiative of the Norwegian and Indian governments. Its self-stated goal was to "outsmart epidemics" by investing in novel vaccine platforms ahead of outbreaks, thereby breaking the boom-and-bust cycle that had characterized research into emerging infectious diseases for the past thirty years.[29] With backing from the Bill & Melinda Gates Foundation and the Wellcome Trust, and additional support from the European Union and several governments, by 2018 CEPI had raised $760 million towards its $1 billion five-year funding goal. Most of those funds went to support vaccine development for three priority pathogens: Lassa, Nipah and MERS.* However, in late 2019 CEPI also issued a new call for innovative vaccine platforms that could be employed against any suddenly emerging infectious disease, whether known or unknown. Earlier that year, the World Bank and WHO had issued an annual review of the world's preparedness for a pandemic. The report made for stark reading. Between 2011 and 2018, the WHO had tracked 1,483 outbreaks in 172 countries. Based on the current rate of emergence, the board was growing increasingly concerned. "There is a very real threat of a rapidly moving, highly lethal pandemic of a respiratory pathogen killing 50 to 80 million people and wiping out nearly 5 per cent of the world's economy," the board warned. "For too long, we have allowed a cycle of panic and neglect when it comes to pandemics . . . It is well past time to act."[30]

The degree to which time was running out was underlined by a prescient exercise held in New York on 19 October 2019. Organized by the Johns Hopkins Center for Health Security in partnership with the Bill and Melinda Gates Foundation and World Economic Forum, the exercise sought to model a pandemic with a simulated virus, called CAPS, short for Coronavirus Associated

---

* Like SARS, MERS-CoV originates in bats but the intermediate host is dromedary camels rather than civet cats. Although MERS does not transmit as efficiently between humans as either SARS or SARS-Cov-2, its mortality rate is far higher, killing about 30 per cent of people it infects (by contrast SARS has an average mortality rate of 10 per cent, while SARS-Cov-2 is fatal between 2-4 per cent of cases).

Pulmonary Syndrome. In the exercise, the pandemic begins with the transmission of the novel coronavirus from bats to pigs on a farm in Brazil. Next, pigs pass the virus to Brazilian farmers, igniting a chain of human-to-human transmission that rapidly spreads to low-income neighbourhoods in Sao Paulo and other megacities in South America. From South America the virus is exported by air to Portugal, the US and China, setting off a chain of global infections in which cases are seen to double every week. As no one has immunity from the virus, the model predicts the pandemic will only end when 80 per cent of the world's population has been infected. In the exercise, this takes 18 months and results in 65 million global deaths.[31]

One thing that would have made a difference to those projections – and to Covid-19 casualties in the real world – is a vaccine. But, despite the 2003 SARS epidemic and the 2012 outbreaks of MERS-CoV, coronavirus research has been a victim of boom-and-bust funding. Prior to SARS, coronavirus research was considered a dead end. The first coronaviruses were identified in pigs, chickens and other animals in 1937. Since that time only four had been found to infect humans, but while the viruses were responsible for a third of common colds, they rarely caused fatal outcomes. Indeed, the only truly nasty coronavirus was the avian infectious bronchitis, which killed chickens but was incapable of infecting people. The result was that coronaviruses had a reputation of being the "Cinderellas" of the virus world and ambitious young microbiologists hoping to build a research career were advised to steer clear of them.

This changed after SARS, but not for long. In the US, the NIAID, which had previously allocated $3 million to $5 million a year for coronavirus research, raised funding to $51 million annually. But within a few years the average annual research spend dropped to $20 million. The 2012 MERS outbreak saw another flurry of funding, but by 2019 it had levelled off at $27 million.[32] The picture was not much better in Europe. Yes, CEPI managed to make up some of the shortfall, but the funds raised were less than it had targeted and had to be split between several different priority diseases. As a virologist at the Francis Crick Institute in London put it, "virologists need more than clever tricks: we also need cash."[33] And cash for coronavirus research was precisely what was missing in the run-up to the Covid-19 pandemic.

* * *

I am writing these words from my sickbed in London. It is 26 March and I am nursing a temperature and an intermittent cough. Because of the lack of

National Health Service testing kits, I have no way of knowing whether I have Covid-19 or a cold, much less when it will be safe to hug my 88-year-old mother again (several friends have reported worse symptoms, including an unsettling loss of sense of smell, and a diminished sense of taste).

Just as China was too slow to respond to the warning signs in early January, the British government has also been too slow to follow China's example and impose the sort of draconian measures that might have halted the spreading infection chains. Instead, the great British public, like the Americans, has been asked to practise "social distancing" in order to "flatten the curve"—terms that until last week, few people had heard of and even fewer could define.

Certainly, the virus has spread with uncommon speed since it emerged in Wuhan. China informed the WHO of the outbreak on 9 January and published the complete genetic sequence of the virus on 12 January; but on 13 January, Thailand became the first country outside of China to be infected and on 20 January, cases were also being reported in Japan and the Republic of Korea. That same day, the US saw its first case when a traveller returning from Wuhan introduced the virus to Washington State. Within a month, thirteen people had been infected at a nursing home in Seattle and Washington State had recorded sixteen deaths, though now it is New York that seems destined to bear the brunt of the contagion in the US.

Around the world, health systems have begun to buckle under the onslaught of Covid-19 patients. This is nowhere more true than in Italy, which has recorded 8,215 deaths, nearly three times as many as in Hubei. Shockingly, the casualties include not only the elderly and those with underlying health conditions, but scores of doctors and nurses, some of whom are in their 30s. "It's as if a storm hit us," said an infectious disease doctor from Brescia, in northern Lombardy, currently the worst affected region of Italy.[34]

For some, these deaths have recalled the sacrifice of other health workers in other outbreaks, such as the Italian physician Carlo Urbani, who perished of SARS in 2003. At the same time, we have also been treated to anxious episodes such as the quarantining of the *Diamond Princess* cruise ship in Yokohoma harbour. The passengers, the majority of whom were retirees, thought it was simply a matter of sitting out the quarantine, after which they'd be free to resume the cruise. Instead, the delay by Japanese officials to lock down the vessel—seventy-two hours after they received notification of the first case—turned the ship into a floating petri dish.[35] Unlike maritime quarantines at other periods in history, viewers were able to follow this one in real-time, as tech-savvy passengers like the elderly British couple, David and Sally Abel, posted regular updates on social media that were immediately rebroadcast on

TV. The Abels' plight, imprisoned in their cabins as the virus mysteriously spread below decks, deeply recalled the experience of the residents of the Amoy Gardens apartment complex in Hong Kong during SARS. By the time the quarantine of the *Diamond Princess* was lifted on 19 February, two passengers were dead and 621 had been infected with the virus.[36] However, it has not been all doom and gloom. Amidst the grief there has also been cheering; from Rome to Madrid, Lisbon to London, people stood on their balconies to pay tribute to their brave health workers or, as the hashtag for Britain's National Health Service puts it, "clap for carers".[37]

There has been little sign of clapping in Iran, however. The official death count is 1,812, but pictures posted on social media show bodies stacked in hospital corridors, and mass graves filled with lime near the holy city of Qom. These are images reminiscent of the fourteenth-century Black Death. By rights, they should have no place in the twenty-first century.

That is the bad news. The good news is that on 23 March, for the first time since the outbreak began, China recorded no new cases of Covid-19, and if the trend continues, Xi intends to lift the quarantine in Wuhan and other Chinese cities on 8 April. Despite its initial cover-up of the outbreak, China has since won wide praise for the scale of its response, which is now seen by the WHO as a model for other countries. Suspicion that China had been under-reporting cases, and that official figures could not be trusted, has been replaced by a newfound respect for the speed with which Xi was able to construct new hospitals and roll out tests for Covid-19—a key factor in China's ability to suppress the transmission chains and restrict its death toll to 3,270.

It is now 1 April and I am feeling much better. Unfortunately, the same cannot be said for Italy, the European epicentre of the pandemic where testing has been lax and other preparations have also been poor. There, the death toll has risen to 12,428. The US is on a similarly catastrophic path, with disease modelers estimating that between 100,000 and 240,000 Americans might be dead by the time the pandemic has run its course. These projections are due, in no small part, to the CDC's failure in February to supply working test kits to state, city, and county public health laboratories, and may be wildly optimistic—based on the current ratio of infections to fatalities the death toll could be in the order of half a million.[38] Critics are also condemning Trump for his 2018 decision to disband the pandemic unit in the national security council, whose job it was to prepare for health emergencies like the present one, as well as for his refusal to use a Korean war-era law to force American companies to manufacture ventilators.[39] The result is that the US currently has over 190,000 cases – more than any other country, including China, Italy, and Spain Over a third of these cases are in New York State. In response, New York's governor, Andrew Cuomo, has closed all non-essential services, and with the help of the Federal Emergency Management Center, transformed Manhattan's Javits Center into an emergency medical station (the Excel Centre in London Docklands has undergone a similarly impressive refit that has seen the exhibition space transformed into a 4,000-bed hospital). For the moment the cots and cubicles are empty, but if the disease modelers' projections are accurate, New York could soon be facing a tsunami of patients, overwhelming the capacity of the city's public hospitals (at the beginning of the outbreak, New York State had 4,000 ventilators; Cuomo estimates that at least 30,000 will be needed over the next six weeks). Already, nurses at hospitals in Queens and Brooklyn are likening hospital wards to "war zones" as the death toll in the city surpasses the 1,000 mark. In response, on 30 March, the hospital ship USNS *Comfort*, with its 1000-bed capacity, arrived in New York City, but it was not outfitted for coronavirus patients, and it remains to be seen whether it can be isolated from Covid-19.

The speed with which the virus has spread to the US and Europe has shattered the complacency of scientific "experts", and punctured the hubris of populist politicians such as US President Donald Trump who insisted, contrary to the evidence, that Covid-19 was going to "disappear . . . like a miracle" and was no worse than a "common flu".[40] In fact, SARS-CoV-2 spreads more rapidly than seasonal flu and is ten to twenty times more lethal, killing about two per cent of confirmed cases - a mortality rate similar to that of the Spanish flu.* Little wonder that Bruce Aylward, who headed up a WHO mission to China in February, has dubbed it the "Wayne Gretzy of viruses", after the Canadian ice hockey Hall-of-Famer whose white gloves and dazzling speed earned him the soubriquet, "The White Tornado".[41] Contrary to hopes that there were many more mild or asymptomatic cases in China than had been reported, Aylward insisted there was no evidence that the confirmed cases in China were the "tip of a grand iceberg". "What we're seeing is a pyramid: most of it is above ground."[42] Aylward's insight was crucial as it suggested that the percentage of the population at risk of developing severe Covid-19 disease, as opposed to mild or asymptomatic infections, was much higher than had been supposed and that it was imperative to prepare hospitals for floods of patients. But in Britain the government's scientific advisors were not listening. Instead, on 3 March, Boris Johnson, who would subsequently be hospitalised with Covid-19, cheer-

---

* By contrast, seasonal flu has an average mortality of 0.1 per cent.

fully informed the British public that the country had "fantastic testing systems" and was "extremely well prepared".[43]

In the US, "experts" were guilty of a similar complacency. As I write, New York City has recorded more than 43,000 cases, exceeding China's Hubei province and making it ground zero of America's outbreak. The scale of threat has shuttered public buildings and theatres on Broadway, and prompted Governor Cuomo to issue a stay-at-home order to protect the elderly and most vulnerable members of the community (the measure is called "Matilda's Law" after his 88-year-old mother). "This is an invisible beast, it is an insidious beast," he said in a clear-eyed address from the Javits Center that has resulted in calls for him to run for the Democratic presidential ticket.[44] Meanwhile, all Trump thought he needed to do to keep America safe from the "China virus", as he insists on calling Covid-19, was to bar Chinese citizens and other foreign nationals from entering the US. Nor does he accept Cuomo's projections that as many as 140,000 New Yorkers could be infected and that up to 40,000 might require ventilation. "[I have] a feeling that a lot of the numbers are just bigger than they're going to be," he told Fox News.[45] It is also a cruel beast that, because of the risk of infection, Covid-19 condemns patients to die alone, isolated from their families.

No sooner were those words out of his mouth, however, than a Manhattan hospital announced the death of its first health worker, Kious Kelly. A 48-year-old assistant nursing manager at Mount Sinai West, Kelly had tested positive for Covid-19 on 17 March, seven days after helping another nurse, who had been working with an infected patient, remove a flimsy plastic gown she had been given by hospital managers in lieu of personal protective equipment. Pictures subsequently posted on social media by other nurses at Mount Sinai showed them dressed in black trash bags above the caption "No more gowns in the whole hospital".[46] It is three months since Li Wenliang's chatroom post, warning the world of the outbreak in Wuhan, was picked up by Pollack and her colleagues at ProMED. Unfortunately, much of that time has been squandered by politicians, and now the virus has caught up with the signal.

* * *

One hundred years ago, when the planet was swept by a similarly devastating plague, the world was at war and the Spanish influenza made curiously little impact on the collective consciousness of society. "Americans took little notice of the pandemic," remarked the environmental historian, Alfred Crosby, "then quickly forgot whatever they did notice."[47]

The Times of London was similarly puzzled by the pandemic's failure to leave more of an emotional residue. "So vast was the catastrophe and so ubiquitous its prevalence that our minds, surfeited with the horrors of war, refused to realize," opined its leader column in February 1921. "It came and went, a hurricane across the green fields of life, sweeping away our youth in hundreds of thousands and leaving behind it a toll of sickness and infirmity which will not be reckoned in this generation."[48]

Even now, just three months into the pandemic of Covid-19, there seems little danger of the coronavirus being similarly forgotten. Indeed, newspaper columnists are already referring to the pandemic as "our new historical divide", and looking forward to the first year AC - "After Corona".[49] When that will be, however, no one can say.

The latest disease model from Imperial College London suggests that, even with effective suppression measures, the pandemic could continue for another year, and possibly as long as eighteen months. Based on all available data on deaths in and outside of China, the Imperial modelers have pegged the average case fatality ratio at 1.4 per cent.[50] Assuming eighty per cent of the world's population is infected, that could mean 13 million deaths globally, a number that, after adjusting for population growth, is a far cry from the toll wrought by the Spanish flu, but devastating nonetheless.[51] The big unknown is India, a nation of 1.4 billion people. Although Kerala boasts 38,000 government hospitals, the same is not true of other Indian states where the public health system has been starved of funds and few tests are being conducted. The result, according to the novelist Arundhati Roy, is that "we may never know the real contours of the crisis" in India.[52]

One thing that would make a difference is a vaccine – currently, there are 43 candidates in the pipeline, but given the complexities of clinical trials and licensing procedures, it is unlikely any will be deployed before 2021.[53] The other thing that could shorten the duration of the pandemic and reduce global mortality is if infection with SARS-CoV-2 were to provide protection against reinfection with the virus. But at present, no one knows whether people who fall ill and recover enjoy *any* immunity, let alone how long immunity might last.

What is abundantly clear, however, is this: thousands of lives have already been lost, not due to our lack of knowledge—we have had plenty of warnings—but because of our collective failure, abetted by complacent politicians, to take those warnings sufficiently seriously and to prepare for the pandemic that virologists and other experts told us was coming our way. It is to be hoped that, after Covid-19, no one will be foolish enough to make the same mistake again.

EPILOGUE

THE PANDEMIC CENTURY

"Gentlemen, it's the microbes that will have the last word."

Louis Pasteur

Sharks never attack swimmers in the North Atlantic. Flu is a bacterial disease and a threat to infants and the elderly, not young adults in the prime of life. Ebola is a virus endemic to forested regions of equatorial Africa—it can't reach a major city in West Africa, let alone one in North America or Europe. Coronaviruses are uninteresting—the "Cinderellas" of the viral world; they might present a threat in hospitals and other closed environments, such as cruise ships, but they are unlikely to cause a global pandemic.

As the pandemic century that began in 1918 ends, we know better than to trust the pronouncements of experts. Battered by their repeated failure to predict deadly outbreaks of infectious disease, even the experts have come to recognize the limits of medical prognostication. This is not only because microbes are highly mutable—that has been *known* since Pasteur's time—but because we are continually lending them a helping hand. Time and again, we assist microbes to occupy new ecological niches and spread to new places in ways that usually only become apparent after the event. To judge by the recent run of pandemics and epidemics, the process seems to be speeding up. If HIV and SARS were wake-up calls, then Ebola, Zika, and Covid-19 confirmed it. "Despite extraordinary advances in medical science, we cannot be complacent about the threat of infectious diseases," acknowledged the National Academy of Medicine in an influential report published in 2016. "The underlying rate of emergence of infectious diseases appears to be increasing."[1]

Why this should be the case—if it *is* the case—is a matter of ongoing research and conjecture. Certainly urbanization and globalization would appear to be key factors. By concentrating large numbers of people in cramped and often unsanitary spaces, the mega-cities of Asia, Africa, and South America, like

Athens in the time of Thucydides, provide ideal conditions for the amplification and spread of novel pathogens. Sometimes technology and alterations of the built environment can mitigate the risks that such overcrowding presents for the transfer of pathogens to people. The plague abatement measures in the Mexican quarter of Los Angeles in 1924 may have been brutal and morally questionable (certainly, it is hard to imagine environmentalists and community activists in California tolerating the wholesale demolition of minority neighbourhoods and the mass slaughter of squirrels today), but at the time they were effective in removing the threat of plague from downtown LA and its harbour. Likewise, air conditioners and modern cooling systems are very effective ways of insulating people from the mosquitoes that breed in and around urban high rises and favelas, but as the Legionnaires' disease outbreak demonstrated, and SARS confirmed, water towers and fanned air can also present new disease risks, particularly in closed environments such as hotels and hospitals.

Greater global interconnectivity driven by international travel and commerce is undoubtedly another key factor. While in the sixteenth century it took several weeks for smallpox, measles, and other Old World pathogens to reach the New World, and even longer for the vectors of diseases like yellow fever to become established in the Americas. Today, international jet travel means that an emerging virus can land in any country or continent on the globe within seventy-two hours. It is not the microbes that are doing this, but our own technology. Wuhan, for instance, is a key domestic and international hub with over one hundred direct flights to more than seventy countries worldwide. Prior to the lockdown, any number of individuals—business people, tourists, foreign language tutors—could have transported the virus beyond China's borders by the simple expedient of boarding a plane. Indeed, tens of millions of us annually make such trips in aircraft for either business or pleasure, and as flights become cheaper and passengers make more and more journeys, the risks are only likely to grow. Herded into airline waiting rooms, then crammed into economy row seats, we resemble nothing more than the captive Amazonian parakeets who introduced psittacosis to Baltimore and other US cities in 1929. The difference is that the parakeets had no choice about their accommodation, whereas we do. As Alfred Crosby put it, international jet travel is like "sitting in the waiting room of an enormous clinic, elbow to elbow with the sick of the world."[2] Yet budget airlines continue to grow in popularity.

Another increasingly important factor is how the growing demand for milk and animal proteins in rapidly industrializing countries, such as China, is putting pressure on previously remote animal habitats where pathogens like coronavirus reside. As an example, for more than three centuries Guangdong, the epicentre of the 2002 SARS outbreak, practised a subsidence farming model, whereby rice-farmers would raise pigs, chickens, and ducks on plots of land adjacent to rice paddies. These backyard farms were ecologically sustainable and provided all the food requirements for farmers and their families. They also produced surpluses that could be sold at market for cash, supplementing farmers' meagre incomes. But with the advent of the Livestock Revolution in the 1980s and the arrival of so-called industrial food production conglomerates this began to change. Heavily capitalized broiler companies began to undercut traditional subsistence farmers, forcing smallholders to look for new sources of protein and income. Many of them turned to farming "wild" animals, such as civet cats and pangolins. As the market for these traditional Chinese delicacies grew and they were rebranded as luxury products, wild animals started to command premium prices at "wet" markets. As the anthropologists Christos Lynteris and Lyle Fearnley explain, one of the advantages of this style of farming is that smallholders are able to transport animals to market without the involvement of large-scale food processing firms and supermarkets.[3] At the same time, however, state-backed enterprises and industrial farms have gobbled up more and more cultivable land, forcing smallholders to look to "uncultivated" plots closer to the edge of rainforests. These areas, of course, are the same zones inhabited by bat populations, a factor that makes the spillover of novel viruses to farmed animals and humans much more likely.

Anthropologists and sociologists, such as Mike Davis, have been warning about the unintended ecological consequences of the Livestock Revolution for years.[4] Unsurprisingly, so have disease ecologist's such as Peter Daszak. Indeed, in 2017 Daszak and his colleagues in the EcoHealth Alliance compared information about emerging infectious diseases "hotspots" with demographic and environmental data, such as climate change and shifts in population density and land-use patterns. They concluded that the risk of disease emergence was "elevated in tropical forest regions, high in mammal biodiversity, and experiencing anthropogenic land use changes related to agricultural practices".[5] In other words, permitting people to farm on the edge of forests that are home to a diverse range of mammalian species, or to penetrate deeper into the same forests in search of timber and bushmeat, presents clear risks for pandemic emergence events.

These insights are valuable, not least because they underline the way in which infectious disease is part of an ecological web that is itself influenced by a constellation of shifting economic, social, and environmental factors. Or, as the Rockefeller researcher René Dubos observed in 1958, "microbial disease is one of the inevitable consequences of life in a world where nothing is stable."[6] That is why Dubos recommended that in a world of rapid environmental, ecological and social change it was incumbent on scientists, to "avoid pride of intellect and guard against any illusion or pretense as to the extent and depth of what he knows". Instead, Dubos advised medical researchers to "develop an alertness to the unexpected, an awareness of the fact that many surprising effects are likely to result from even trivial disturbances of ecological equilibrium".[7]

Dubos was not the only thinker to reject a narrow "germ-eye" view of our interactions with microbes. The social historian of medicine Charles Rosenberg, in an influential essay published in the wake of the AIDS pandemic, also advised against treating germs merely as contagions that needed to be eradicated. Prior to the bacteriological era and the rise of microbe-hunting, disease and health had been viewed in far more holistic terms, he pointed out. In particular, he argued, epidemics were seen as being due to a "unique configuration of circumstances". Contrasting this configuration model with the notion of disease as "contamination", Rosenberg invoked a view of health as a "balanced, integrated, and value-imparting relationship between humankind and its environment".[8]

It was a similar sensibility that towards the end of his career saw Dubos focus increasingly on interactions between man and his environment and to emphasize what he called the "symbiosis of earth and humankind".[9] In Dubos's day, these perspectives found expression in the image of earth as a "spaceship" adrift in a hostile universe, and his call for environmental activists to "think globally, act locally". Today, these ideas find their correlate in the notion of "planetary health" and the call by young activists such as Greta Thunberg to adopt a more holistic and environmentally responsible attitude to our interactions with nature and the lives that depend on it, our own included.[10]

Lurking in the background, informing our response to Covid-19 and whatever other pandemic might be heading our way during the next one hundred years, is the ghost of Spanish flu. If anything has taught scientists the value of caution and the perils of hubris it is the long shadow cast by the 1918-19 influenza pandemic – what the WHO, an organization not known for hyperbole, calls the "most deadly disease event in the history of humanity". Since it became possible to retrieve viral genetic material from the H1N1 pandemic virus using modern molecular pathology techniques, virologists have made huge progress in understanding the factors that made the Spanish flu so virulent. By comparing the 1918 virus to descendent H1N1 strains still in circulation, scientists have also come to a better understanding of its epidemiology and pathophysiology. Moreover, the 1997 outbreak of H5N1 bird flu in Hong Kong, and the subsequent outbreaks of other varieties of bird flu in China and Southeast Asia, have shown that it is not necessary for an avian influenza virus to transit through an intermediary mammalian host first in order for it to be the cause of morbidity and deaths in humans. At the same time, the 2009 scare over the "Mexican" swine flu demonstrated that from time to time different swine and human lineages of H1N1 can recombine to produce new pandemic viruses. However, so far, no bird flu or recombinant swine flu virus has yet managed the trick of wide infectivity and high virulence that was achieved in 1918. Furthermore, while it is known that the H1N1 Spanish flu was infectious to all age groups in 1918-19, scientists are still no closer to solving the riddle of why it proved relatively more deadly to young adults, or why mortality rates were closely associated with the increased incidence of secondary bacterial infections. The result is that despite the tremendous advances in microbiology, immunology, vaccinology, and preventive medicine in the century since 1919, influenza researchers are still no closer to being able to predict when new pandemic strains will emerge or how they will impact human populations. As David Morens and Jeffrey Taubenberger put it: "In recent decades, pandemic influenza has continued to produce numerous unanticipated events that expose fundamental gaps in scientific knowledge . . . These uncertainties make it difficult to predict influenza pandemics and, therefore, to adequately plan to prevent them."[11]

That is why, reviewing the last hundred years of epidemic outbreaks, the only thing that *is* certain is that there will be new plagues and new pandemics. It is not a question of if, but when. Camus was right. Pestilences may be unpredictable, but they *will* recur.

NOTES

PROLOGUE: SHARKS AND OTHER PREDATORS

1. Richard Fernicola, *Twelve Days of Terror: A Definitive Investigation of the 1916 New Jersey Shark Attacks* (Guilford, CT: Globe Pequot Press, 2001), xxiv–xxx.

2. The best narrative account of the New Jersey shark attacks is Michael Capuzzo's *Close to Shore* (London: Headline Publishing, 2001). The attacks also inspired Peter Benchley's best-selling 1974 novel *Jaws*, the basis for the Steven Spielberg film of the same name. In both the book and the film, the shark attacks are transposed to the fictional Long Island resort of Amity.

3. David Oshinsky, *Polio: An American Story* (Oxford: Oxford University Press, 2005), 19–23.

4. John Paul, *A History of Poliomyelitis* (New Haven, CT: Yale University Press, 1971), 148–60; Naomi Rogers, *Dirt and Disease: Polio before FDR*, Health and Medicine in American Society (New Brunswick, NJ: Rutgers University Press, 1992), 2–6.

5. René Dubos, *Mirage of Health: Utopias, Progress and Biological Change* (New Brunswick, NJ: Rutgers University Press, 1996), 266–67.

6. On 12 February 2002, five months after the 9/11 attacks and a year before the invasion of Iraq, the then-US Secretary of Defense Donald Rumsfeld appeared at a Pentagon news conference to field questions about the purported threat posed by the Iraqi dictator Saddam Hussein's secret weapons program. Asked by a journalist what evidence he had that Iraq had supplied or was willing to supply terrorists with weapons of mass destruction, Rumsfeld responded: "Reports that say that something hasn't happened are always interesting to me, because as we know, there are known knowns; there are things we know we know. We also know there are known unknowns; that is to say we know there are some things we do not know. But there are also unknown unknowns—the ones we don't know we don't know."

At the time, Rumsfeld's comments were widely lampooned for their "Alice in Wonderland" quality, but, as many of Rumsfeld's critics subsequently acknowledged, he was drawing on well-known scholarship in the philosophy of knowledge and the social construction of scientific facts. Indeed, much scientific research is based on investigating known unknowns, where scientists develop a hypothesis and then design experiments to test the null hypothesis, or the commonly held view. At the outset the researcher does not know whether or not the results will support the null hypothesis.

However, it is common for the researcher to believe that the result that will be obtained will be within a range of known possibilities. Occasionally, however, the result is completely unexpected, making it an unknown unknown.

Historians of science also routinely apply these ideas to capture the uncertainty surrounding natural events from earthquakes, to climate change, to pandemics, that pose a catastrophic threat to modern societies and where knowledge may be partial and incomplete. However, in addition to the three types of knowledge described by Rumsfeld, they also propose a fourth category—the "unknown known." This captures a situation in which experimenters think they have discovered everything there is to know about a scientific object but are unaware of their ignorance as regards certain important aspects of it (it is sometimes also described as "uncomfortable knowledge"). Pneumonic plague, Psittacosis, Ebola, and Zika belonged to this category. By contrast, Legionnaires' disease, SARS, and HIV were unknown unknowns. To the extent that no one had a way of studying the influenza virus before 1918, Spanish flu could also be considered an unknown unknown, though many researchers had begun to suspect it might be a filter-passer and had become uncomfortable with the state of bacteriological knowledge of the disease. For the background and context of Rumsfeld's remarks, see Errol Morris, "The Certainty of Donald Rumsfeld," *New York Times*, 25 March 2014, accessed 1 September 2017, https://opinionator.blogs.nytimes.com/2014/03/25/the-certainty-of-donald-rumsfeld-part-1/?mcubz=1; for further discussion of Rumsfeld's parsing of the philosophy of knowledge and unknown knowns, see Steve Rayner, "Uncomfortable Knowledge: The Social Construction of Ignorance in Science and Environmental Policy Discourses," *Economy and Society* 41, no. 1 (1 February 2012): 107–25.

7. Thucydides, *History of the Peloponnesian War* (Harmondsworth, UK: Penguin, 1972); David Morens et al., "Epidemiology of the Plague of Athens," *Transactions of the American Philological Association* 122 (1992): 271–304.

1. THE BLUE DEATH

1. Roger Batchelder, *Camp Devens* (Boston: Small Maynard, 1918), 11.

2. Ibid., 94.

3. Carol R. Byerly, "The U.S. Military and the Influenza Pandemic of 1918–1919," *Public Health Reports* 125, suppl. 3 (2010): 82–91.

4. William Osler, Henry A. Christian, and James G. Carr, *The Principles and Practice of Medicine: Designed for the Use of Practitioners and Students of Medicine*, 16th edition (New York and London: D. Appleton-Century, 1947), 41.

5. Victor Vaughan, *A Doctor's Memories* (Indianapolis: Bobbs-Merrill, 1926), 424–25.

6. J. A. B. Hammond et al., "Purulent Bronchitis: a study of cases occurring amongst the British troops at a base in France," *The Lancet* 190, no. 4898 (14 July 1917): 41–46.

7. A. Abrahams et al., "Purulent Bronchitis: its influenzal and pneumococcal bacteriology," *The Lancet* 190, no. 4906 (8 September 1917): 377–82.

8. A. Abrahams et al., "A Further Investigation into Influenzo-pneumococcal and

Influenzo-streptococcal Septicæmia: Epidemic influenzal 'pneumonia' of highly fatal type and its relation to 'purulent bronchitis," *The Lancet* 193, no. 4975 (5 July 1919): 1–11.

9. E. L. Opie et al., "Pneumonia at Camp Funston," *Journal of the American Medical Association* (11 January 1919): 108–16.

10. Byerly, "The U.S. Military and the Influenza Pandemic of 1918–1919," 125.

11. "Letter to Susan Owen, 24 June 1918," in *Wilfred Owen: Collected Letters*, ed. H. Owen and J. Bell (London: Oxford University Press, 1967), 599.

12. This stipulates that in order for a microorganism to be considered the aetiological agent of a disease, the organism must be constantly present in all clinical cases of the disease, and when grown and isolated in pure culture and inoculated into healthy test animals must be able to reproduce the same disease.

13. E. L. Opie et al., "Pneumonia at Camp Funston," *Journal of the American Medical Association* 72, no. 2 (11 January 1919): 108–16.

14. Dorothy A. Petit and Janice Bailie, *A Cruel Wind: Pandemic Flu in America, 1918–1920* (Murfreesboro, TN: Timberlane Books, 2008), 83.

15. Batchelder, *Camp Devens*, 16.

16. Letters and postcards from Pvt. Clifton H. Skillings, *Bangor Daily News*, accessed 6 July 2017: https://bangordailynews.com/2009/05/15/news/letters-postcards-from-pvt-clifton-h-skillings/

17. F. M. Burnet and E. Clark, *Influenza: A Survey of the Last Fifty Years*. Monographs from the Walter and Eliza Hall Institute of Research in Pathology and Medicine, no. 4 (Melbourne: Macmillan, 1942); Anton Erkoreka, "Origins of the Spanish Influenza Pandemic (1918–1920) and Its Relation to the First World War," *Journal of Molecular and Genetic Medicine: An International Journal of Biomedical Research* 3, no. 2 (30 November 2009): 190–94.

18. V. Andreasen et al., "Epidemiologic Characterization of the 1918 Influenza Pandemic Summer Wave in Copenhagen: Implications for Pandemic Control Strategies," *The Journal of Infectious Diseases* 197, no. 2 (2008): 270–78.

19. Petit and Bailie, *A Cruel Wind*, 85.

20. Paul G. Woolley, "The Epidemic of Influenza at Camp Devens, MASS," *Journal of Laboratory and Clinical Medicine* 4, no. 6 (March 1919): 330–43.

21. R. N. Grist, "Pandemic Influenza 1918," *British Medical Journal* 2, no. 6205 (22 December 1979): 1632–33.

22. John M. Barry, *The Great Influenza: The Epic Story of the Deadliest Plague in History* (New York: Viking Penguin, 2004), 187–88.

23. A. Abrahams et al., "A further investigation into influenzo-pneumococcal and influenzo-streptococcal septicaemia," *The Lancet* 193, no. 4975 (5 July 1919): 1–11.

24. Barry D. Silverman, "William Henry Welch (1850–1934): The Road to Johns Hopkins," *Proceedings Baylor University Medical Center* 24, no. 3 (2011): 236–42.

25. "The Four Founding Physicians," Johns Hopkins Medicine, accessed 6 July 2017: http://www.hopkinsmedicine.org/about/history/history5.html

26. Woolley, "The Epidemic of Influenza at Camp Devens, MASS."

27. Vaughan, *A Doctor's Memories*, 383–84.

28. Jim Duffy, "The Blue Death—Flu Epidemic of 1918," *Johns Hopkins School of Public Health*, Fall 2004, accessed 6 July 2017: http://magazine.jhsph.edu/2004/fall/pro-logues/index.html

29. Woolley, "The Epidemic at Camp Devens, MASS."

30. Jeffery K. Taubenberger et al., "The Pathology of Influenza Virus Infections," *Annual Review of Pathology* 3 (2008): 499–522.

31. Barry, *The Great Influenza*, 190–91, 288.

32. Pfeiffer recommended Ziehl-Neelsen's carbol-fuchsin stain. Pickett-Thomson Research Laboratory, ed., *Annals of the Pickett-Thomson Research Laboratory* 9 (London: Bailliere, Tindall & Cox, 1924): 275.

33. Barry, *The Great Influenza*, 289–90.

34. *H. influenzae*—also known as type b (Hib)—can cause many different kinds of infections ranging from mild ear infections, to severe bloodstream infections, to pneumonia. Hib meningitis is a particular danger to unvaccinated children, and even with treatment approximately one in twenty will die.

35. A. Sally Davis et al., "The Use of Nonhuman Primates in Research on Seasonal, Pandemic and Avian Influenza, 1893–2014," *Antiviral Research* 117 (May 2015): 75–98.

36. John M. Eyler, "The State of Science, Microbiology, and Vaccines Circa 1918," *Public Health Reports* 3, no. 125 (2010): 27–36.

37. "Bacteriology of The 'Spanish Influenza' 1," *The Lancet* 192, no. 4954 (10 August 1918), 177.

38. Royal College of Physicians, London, "Prevention and Treatment of Influenza," *British Medical Journal* 2, no. 3020 (16 November 1918): 546.

39. S. W. B. Newson, *Infections and Their Control: A Historical Perspective* (Los Angeles and London: Sage, 2009), 36.

40. Erling Norrby, "Yellow Fever and Max Theiler: The Only Nobel Prize for a Virus Vaccine," *The Journal of Experimental Medicine* 204, no. 12 (26 November 2007): 2779–84.

41. Myron G. Schultz et al., "Charles-Jules-Henri Nicolle," *Emerging Infectious Diseases* 15, no. 9 (September 2009): 1519–22; Ludwik Gross, "How Charles Nicolle of the Pasteur Institute Discovered That Epidemic Typhus Is Transmitted by Lice: Reminiscences from My Years at the Pasteur Institute in Paris," *Proceedings of the National Academy of Sciences* 93, no. 20 (1 October 1996): 10539–40.

42. C. Nicolle et al., "Quelques notions expérimentales sur le virus de la grippe," *Comptes Rendus de l'Académie Sciences* 167 (1918 II): 607–10; C. Nicolle et al., "Recherches expérimentales sur la grippe," *Annales d'Institut Pasteur* 33 (1919): 395.

43. Davis, Taubenberger, and Bray, "The use of nonhuman primates in research on seasonal, pandemic and avian influenza, 1893–2014."

44. The technique was discovered by Ernest Goodpasture at Vanderbilt University, but it was an Australian researcher and future Nobel Prize winner, Frank Macfarlane

Burnet, who first applied the technique to growing influenza virus. F. M. Burnet, *Changing Patterns: An Atypical Biography* (Melbourne: Heinemann, 1968), 41, 90–91.

45. C. R. Byerly, *Fever of War: The Influenza Epidemic in the U.S. Army During World War I* (New York: New York University Press, 2005), 102–3.

46. Nancy K. Bristow, *American Pandemic: The Lost Worlds of the 1918 Influenza Epidemic* (New York and Oxford: Oxford University Press, 2012), 101.

47. "New York prepared for influenza siege," *New York Times*, 19 September 1918, 11.

48. "Vaccine for Influenza," *New York Evening Post* (12 October 1918), 8.

49. Barry, *The Great Influenza*, 279.

50. John M. Eyler, "The State of Science, Microbiology, and Vaccines Circa 1918," *Public Health Reports* 3, no. 125 (2010): 27–36.

51. "Battle Influenza Microbes, Noted Physician Warns," *Chicago Herald Examiner* (6 October 1918), 1.

52. "Spanish Influenza and the Fear of It," *Philadelphia Inquirer* (5 October 1918), 12; "Stop the Senseless Influenza Panic," *Philadelphia Inquirer* (8 October 1918), 12.

53. Herbert French, "The clinical features of the influenza epidemic of 1918–19," UK Ministry of Health, *Report on the Pandemic of Influenza 1918–19* (London: HMSO, 1920), 66–109.

54. Letter from Harry Whellock, Cape Province, South Africa, 10 November 1918. Mullocks sale item.

55. A. E. Baumgardt to Richard Collier, 28 May 1972, Richard Collier Collection, Imperial War Museum. IWM 63/5/1.

56. Albert Camus, *The Plague*, trans. Robin Buss (New York: Penguin Classics, 2002), 31.

57. John F. Bundage et al., "Deaths from Bacterial Pneumonia During 1918–19 Influenza Pandemic," *Emerging Infectious Diseases* 14, no. 8 (August 2008): 1193–99.

58. Jeffery K. Taubenberger et al., "1918 Influenza: The Mother of All Pandemics," *Emerging Infectious Diseases* 12, no. 1 (January 2006): 15–22.

59. T. Tumpey et al., "Characterization of the Reconstructed 1918 Spanish Influenza Pandemic Virus," *Science* 310, no. 5745 (10 July 2005): 77–80; J. K. Taubenberger et al., "Characterization of the 1918 Influenza Virus Polymerase Genes," *Nature* 437, no. 7060 (6 October 2005): 889–93.

60. Ann H. Reid et al., "Evidence of an Absence: The Genetic Origins of the 1918 Pandemic Influenza Virus," *Nature Reviews. Microbiology* 2, no. 11 (November 2004): 909–14.

61. Michael Worobey et al., "Genesis and Pathogenesis of the 1918 Pandemic H1N1 Influenza A Virus," *Proceedings National Academy of Sciences* 111, no. 22 (3 June 2014): 8107–12.

62. The British virologist John Oxford has argued that such a reassortment could have occurred at Étaples in the winter of 1916–17 when hundreds of soldiers at the camp were sickened by "purulent bronchitis." As well as being crowded with troops en route to the Front, Étaples boasted its own piggeries, and many men also kept ducks

and geese as pets, meaning that all the ecological conditions were in place for the direct transfer of an avian flu virus to humans, or its reassortment with a mammalian flu virus first. Similarly, John Barry argues that the ecological conditions for a reassortment with a bird flu virus were in place in Haskell County, Kansas, a sparsely populated farming area three hundred miles to the west of Camp Funston, where people raised poultry and hogs. However, his suggestion that the epidemic at Camp Funston in March 1918 was a precursor of the Spanish flu is undermined by the fact that, unlike during the later autumn wave or the outbreak at Étaples in 1917, there were no reports of heliotrope cyanosis. Even more problematic for Barry's theory is that in the summer of 1918, Copenhagen, and other northern European cites, suffered large flu outbreaks marked by unusual mortality in younger age groups—a hallmark of the later pandemic waves. Moreover, New York saw a similar wave of pre-pandemic flu activity in February–April 1918. According to the authors of the New York study, these findings are "inconsistent with the prevailing hypothesis of a spring 1918 Kansas origin, and … reopen the possibility that the virus had spread from Europe to New York City in the context of troop movement during World War I." John S. Oxford, "The So-Called Great Spanish Influenza Pandemic of 1918 May Have Originated in France in 1916," *Philosophical Transactions of the Royal Society of London, Series B* 356, 1416 (2001): 1857–59; John M. Barry, "The Site of Origin of the 1918 Influenza Pandemic and its Public Health Implications," *Journal of Translational Medicine* 2 (20 January 2004): 3; Viggo Andreasen et al., "Epidemiologic Characterization of the 1918 Influenza Pandemic Summer Wave in Copenhagen: Implications for Pandemic Control Strategies," *The Journal of Infectious Diseases* 197, no. 2 (January 2008): 270–78; Donald R. Olson et al., "Epidemiological Evidence of an Early Wave of the 1918 Influenza Pandemic in New York City," *Proceedings of the National Academy of Sciences of the United States of America* 102, no. 31 (August 2005): 11059–63.

63. Worobey et al., "Genesis and Pathogenesis."

64. Kevin D. Patterson, *Pandemic Influenza, 1700–1900: A Study in Historical Epidemiology* (Totowa, NJ: Rowman and Littlefield, 1986), 49–82.

65. Taubenberger et al., "The Pathology of Influenza Virus Infections."

66. E. W. Goodpasture, "The Significance of Certain Pulmonary Lesions in Relation to the Etiology of Influenza," *American Journal of Medical Science* 158 (1919): 863–70.

67. "Remarks of Dr. William H. Welch, 1926," Chesney Medical Archives, Johns Hopkins University, Baltimore, MD.

68. Terence M. Tumpey et al., "Characterization of the Reconstructed 1918 Spanish Influenza Pandemic Virus," *Science* 310, no. 5745 (2005): 77–80.

69. Worobey et al., "Genesis and Pathogenesis of the 1918 Pandemic H1N1 Influenza A Virus."

70. Susanne L. Linderman et al., "Antibodies with 'Original Antigenic Sin' Properties Are Valuable Components of Secondary Immune Responses to Influenza Viruses," *PLOS Pathogens* 12, no. 8 (2016): e1005806.

71. David M. Morens et al., "The 1918 Influenza Pandemic: Lessons for 2009 and the Future," *Critical Care Medicine* 38, no. 4 suppl. (April 2010): e10–20.

72. Jefferey K. Taubenberger et al., "Influenza: The Once and Future Pandemic," *Public Health Reports* 125, no. 3 (2010): 16–26.

73. F. M. Burnet, *Natural History of Infectious Disease* (Cambridge: Cambridge University Press, 1953).

74. Burnet, *Changing Patterns*.

75. F. M. Burnet, "Influenza Virus 'A' Infections of Cynomolgus Monkeys," *Australian Journal of Experimental Biology and Medicine* 19 (1941): 281–90.

76. F. M. Burnet and E. Clark, *Influenza: A Survey of the Last Fifty Years*. Monographs from the Walter and Eliza Hall Institute of Research in Pathology and Medicine, no. 4 (Melbourne: Macmillan, 1942).

2. PLAGUE IN THE CITY OF ANGELS

1. Walter M. Dickie and California State Board of Health, "Reports on Plague in Los Angeles, 1924–25," 11–30, HM 72874, The Huntington Library, San Marino, CA.

2. Arthur J. Viseltear, "The Pneumonic Plague Epidemic of 1924 in Los Angeles," *Yale Journal of Biology and Experimental Medicine* 1 (1974): 40–54.

3. William Deverell, *Whitewashed Adobe: The Rise of Los Angeles and the Remaking of Its Mexican Past* (Berkeley: University of California Press, 2004), 3.

4. Mark Reisler, *By the Sweat of Their Brow: Mexican Immigrant Labor in the United States, 1900–1940* (Westport, CT: Greenwood, 1976), 180.

5. Dickie, "Reports on Plague in Los Angeles, 1924–25."

6. Emil Bogen, "The Pneumonic Plague in Los Angeles," *California and Western Medicine* (February 1925): 175–76.

7. "The Pneumonic Plague in Los Angeles," 175–76.

8. California State Board of Health, Special Bulletin, no. 46, "Pneumonic Plague, Report of an Outbreak at Los Angeles, California, October–November, 1924," Sacramento: California State Printing Office, 1926.

9. Dickie, "Reports on Plague in Los Angeles, 1924–25."

10. Bogen, "Pneumonic Plague in Los Angeles"; Deverell, *Whitewashed Adobe*, 176–82.

11. Dickie, "Reports on Plague in Los Angeles, 1924–25."

12. Frank Feldinger, *A Slight Epidemic: The Government Cover-Up of Black Plague in Los Angeles* (Silver Lake Publishing Kindle edition, 2008), location 473.

13. "USGS Circular 1372, Plague," accessed 11 May 2016: http://pubs.usgs.gov/circ/1372/

14. Ole Jørgen Benedictow, *The Black Death, 1346–1353: The Complete History* (Suffolk: Boydell Press, 2004), 382.

15. John Kelly, *The Great Mortality* (New York and London: Harper Perennial, 2006), 22.

16. Deverell, *Whitewashed Adobe*, 182.

17. According to the San Francisco–based bacteriologist Karl F. Meyer, the statement was made by Colby. W. E. Carter and Vernon Link, "Unpublished biography of Karl

F. Meyer and related papers, written and compiled by William E. Carter and Vernon B. Link, 1956–1963," Sixth interview, 199, UCSF Library, Archives, and Special Collections, MSS 63–1. Hereafter "Carter MSS."

18. Marilyn Chase, *The Barbary Plague: The Black Death in Victorian San Francisco* (New York: Random House, 2003), 160.

19. In 1898, Paul-Louis Simond, a French researcher based in Karachi, succeeded in transmitting plague from an infected to an uninfected rat by allowing fleas harvested from a cat to feed on the diseased rat, but other experts questioned his methods, casting doubt on his findings. The result was that it was not until 1914, when two British researchers at the Lister Institute repeated Simond's experiment under more rigorous conditions, that flea-rat transmission of plague was unequivocally accepted. Edward A. Crawford, "Paul-Louis Simond and His Work on Plague," *Perspectives in Biology and Medicine* 39, no. 3 (1996): 446–58.

20. The first person to posit the link with marmots was the Russian medical researcher Mikhail Edouardovich Beliavsky. Examining an outbreak in 1894 of bubonic plague at Aksha, on the Russian–Chinese border, Beliavsky argued that the Siberian marmot, or tarbagan, a large rodent hunted by native Mongols and Buryats, might be the carrier of plague, and that the disease spread to humans when they skinned the animal. Four years later, another Russian researcher, Danilo Zabolotny, reached the same conclusion while investigating an outbreak of pneumonic plague in eastern Mongolia. See Christos Lynteris, *Ethnographic Plague: Configuring Disease on the Chinese-Russian Frontier* (London: Palgrave Macmillan, 2016).

21. William B. Wherry, "Plague among the Ground Squirrels of California," *The Journal of Infectious Diseases* 5, no. 5 (1908): 485–506.

22. Chase, *Barbary Plague*, 189. *Citellus beecheyi* has since been renamed *Otospermophilus beecheyi*.

23. In 1914 researchers at the Lister Institute in London demonstrated that plague bacilli multiply and form a block in the proventriculus of *X. cheopis*. This block prevents the ingested blood from reaching the flea's midgut, causing the flea to starve. The resulting increase in the number of feeding attempts by blocked fleas, combined with regurgitation of ingested blood and infectious material from the blockage, makes them dangerous vectors for humans. However, as these blockages can take twelve to sixteen days to form, *X. cheopis* is not thought to be infectious for long enough to be a factor in epizootics. Rebecca J. Eisen et al., "Early-Phase Transmission of Yersinia Pestis by Unblocked Fleas as a Mechanism Explaining Rapidly Spreading Plague Epizootics," *Proceedings of the National Academy of Sciences* 103, no. 42 (2006): 15380–85.

24. McCoy, "Plague Among the Ground Squirrels in America," *Journal of Hygiene* 10, no. 4 (1910–1912): 589–601.

25. Wherry, "Plague Among the Ground Squirrels of California."

26. Meyer, "The Ecology of Plague," *Medicine* 21, no. 2 (May 1941): 143–74 (147).

27. P. C. C. Garnham, "Distribution of Wild-Rodent Plague," *Bulletin of the World Health Organization* 2 (1949): 271–78.

28. W. H. Kellogg, "An Epidemic of Pneumonic Plague," *American Journal of Public Health* 10, no. 7 (July 1920): 599–605.

29. J. N. Hays, *The Burdens of Disease: Epidemics and Human Response in Western History* (New Brunswick, NJ, and London: Rutgers University Press, 2009), 184–85.

30. W. H. Kellogg, "Present Status of Plague, With Historical Review," *American Journal of Public Health* 10, no. 11 (1 November 1920): 835–44; Guenter B. Risse, *Plague, Fear and Politics in San Francisco's Chinatown* (Baltimore: Johns Hopkins University Press, 2012), 156–58, 167–69. The commission was led by Simon Flexner, the head of the Rockefeller Institute for Medical Research in New York, and had the aim of exonerating the Marine Hospital Service.

31. Eli Chernin, "Richard Pearson Strong and the Manchurian Epidemic of Pneumonic Plague, 1910–1911," *Journal of the History of Medicine and the Allied Sciences* 44 (1989): 296–391.

32. Wu Lien-Teh, *A Treatise on Pneumonic Plague* (Geneva: League of Nations Health Organization, 1926).

33. Oscar Teague and M. A. Barber, "Studies on Pneumonic Plague and Plague Immunization, III. Influence of Atmospheric Temperature upon the Spread of Pneumonic Plague," *Philippine Journal of Science* 7B, no. 3 (1912): 157–72.

34. Wu, *Treatise on Pneumonic Plague*.

35. Kellogg, "Epidemic of Pneumonic Plague," 605.

36. Viseltear, "Pneumonic plague epidemic."

37. "Nine Mourners At Wake Dead," *Los Angeles Times* (1 November 1924).

38. Viseltear, "Pneumonic plague epidemic," 41.

39. "Malady outbreak traced," *Los Angeles Times* (5 November 1924), A10.

40. Deverell, *Whitewashed Adobe*, 197.

41. Ibid.

42. Ibid, 185–86.

43. Albert Camus, *The Plague* (New York: Random House, 1948), 35.

44. Emil Bogen, "Pneumonic Plague in Los Angeles: A Review," 1925, MSS Bogen Papers, The Huntington Library, San Marino, CA.

45. Dickie, "Reports on Plague in Los Angeles, 1924–25," 32–34.

46. Deverell, *Whitewashed Adobe*, 197.

47. "Disease Spread Checked," *Los Angeles Times* (6 November 1924), A1.

48. Viseltear, "Pneumonic plague epidemic," 42.

49. Ibid., 43.

50. Feldinger, *A Slight Epidemic*, location 1838.

51. Viseltear, "Pneumonic plague epidemic," 46.

52. Meyer, Carter MSS, Sixth interview, 209.

53. Deverell, *Whitewashed Adobe*, 197–98.

54. Bess Furman, *A Profile of the U.S. Public Health Service 1798–1948* (Bethesda, MD: National Library of Medicine, 1973), 350–51.

55. "Rat War Death Toll Is Heavy," *Los Angeles Times* (30 November 1924), B1.

56. "Malady Outbreak Traced," *Los Angeles Times* (5 November 1924), A10.

57. "Rat War Death Toll Is Heavy."

58. Meyer, Carter MSS, Sixth interview, 211.

59. "Report Hugh Cumming to Secretary of Treasury, 23 June 1925," RG 90 Records of the Public Health Service, General Subject File, 1924–1935, State Boards of Health, California, 0425–70.

60. Meyer, "Ecology of Plague," 148.

61. "Signs of Bubonic Plague in Three American Cities," *New York Times* (8 February 1925); Letter from Cumming to medical officers in charge of U.S. quarantine stations, 22 December 1924, RG 90 General Subject File, 1924–1935, 0452–183 General (Plague).

62. "Quarantine Ordered Against Bubonic Rats," *New York Times* (1 January 1925).

63. Letter from A. G. Arnoll to Robert B. Armstrong, 8 January 1925, RG 90, Records of the Public Health Service, General Subject File, 1924–1935, State Boards of Health, California, 0425–70.

64. "Report Hugh Cumming to Secretary of Treasury, 23 June 1925," RG 90 Records of the Public Health Service, General Subject File, 1924–1935, State Boards of Health, California, 0425–70.

65. Dickie, "Reports on Plague in Los Angeles, 1924–25," 23–24.

66. In 1348, the year the Black Death first visited in Europe, Italian chroniclers recorded symptoms characteristic of both the pneumonic and bubonic forms of the disease. The seventh-century plague outbreaks in Iceland and Norway are also thought to have been largely pneumonic, since in these northerly countries it would have been too cold to maintain rat-flea transmission over the winter and because pneumonic plague is more easily transmitted in cold weather.

67. K. F. Meyer, "Selvatic Plague—Its Present Status in California," *California and Western Medicine* 40, no. 6 (June 1934): 407–10; Mark Honigsbaum, "Tipping the Balance': Karl Friedrich Meyer, latent infections and the birth of modern ideas of disease ecology," *Journal of the History of Biology* 49, no. 2 (April 2016): 261–309.

68. C. R. Eskey et al., *Plague in the Western Part of the United States* (Washington, DC: US Public Health Service, 1940).

69. Meyer, "Selvatic Plague—Its Present Status in California."

70. "Plague Homepage | CDC," accessed 11 May 2016: http://www.cdc.gov/plague/

71. Eisen et al., "Early-Phase Transmission of Yersinia Pestis by Unblocked Fleas as a Mechanism Explaining Rapidly Spreading Plague Epizootics."

72. "Human Plague—United States, 2015," accessed 11 May 2017: http://www.cdc.gov/mmwr/preview/mmwrhtml/mm6433a6.htm?s_cid=mm6433a6_w

73. Wendy Leonard, "Utah Man Dies of Bubonic Plague," DeseretNews.com, 27 August 2015, accessed 11 May 2017: http://www.deseretnews.com/article/865635488/Utah-man-dies-of-bubonic-plague.html?pg=all

74. Kenneth L. Gage and Michael Y. Kosoy, "Natural History of Plague: Perspectives from More than a Century of Research," *Annual Review of Entomology* 50 (2005): 505–

28; "USGS Circular 1372 Plague, Enzootic and Epizootic Cycles, 38–41," accessed 11 May 2016: http://pubs.usgs.gov/circ/1372/

3. THE GREAT PARROT FEVER PANDEMIC

1. V. L. Ellicott and Charles H. Halliday, "The Psittacosis Outbreak in Maryland, December 1929, and January 1930," *Public Health Reports* 46, no. 15 (1931): 843–65; Jill Lepore, "It's Spreading: Outbreaks, Media Scares, and the Parrot Panic of 1930," *New Yorker*, 1 June 2009.
2. "Killed by a Pet Parrot," *American Weekly*, 5 January 1930.
3. Paul de Kruif, *Men Against Death* (London: Jonathan Cape, 1933), 181.
4. Ibid., 182.
5. Ibid., 203.
6. The journal was most likely *La Revista de La Asociación Médica Argentina*. Enrique Barros, "La Psittacosis En La República Argentina," *La Revista de La Asociación Médica Argentina*, Buenos Aires, 1930.
7. "Killed by a Pet Parrot," *American Weekly* (5 January 1930).
8. E. L. Sturdee and W. M. Scott, *A Disease of Parrots Communicable to Man (Psittacosis)*. Reports on Public Health and Medical Subjects, no. 61 (London: H.M.S.O., 1930), 4–10.
9. "30,000 Parrots Here; Amazon Best Talker," *New York Times* (29 January 1930).
10. Katherine C. Grier, *Pets in America: A History* (Chapel Hill: University of North Carolina Press, 2006), 244.
11. Sturdee and Scott, *A Disease of Parrots Communicable to Man*, 10–17.
12. De Kruif, *Men Against Death*, 182.
13. Albin Krebs, "Dr. Paul de Kruif, Popularizer of Medical Exploits, Is Dead," *New York Times* (2 March 1971).
14. Paul de Kruif, "Before You Drink a Glass of Milk," *Ladies Home Journal* (September 1929).
15. Nancy Tomes, "The Making of a Germ Panic, Then and Now," *American Journal of Public Health* 90, no. 2 (February 2000): 191–98.
16. "Topics of the Times: Warning Against Parrots," *New York Times* (11 January 1930).
17. "Vienna Specialist Blames 'Mass Suggestion' for Parrot Fever Scare, Which He Holds Baseless," *New York Times* (16 January 1930).
18. "Stimson's Parrot Is Banished for Cursing," *New York Times* (18 January 1930).
19. Edward. A. Beeman, *Charles Armstrong, M.D.: A Biography* (Bethesda, MD: Office of History, National Institutes of Health, 2007), 45.
20. Jeanette Barry, *Notable Contributions to Medical Research by Public Health Scientists, U. S. Department of Health: A Bibliography to 1940* (Washington, DC: US Department of Health, Education and Welfare, 1960), 5–8.
21. De Kruif, *Men Against Death*, 182, 185.
22. Ibid., 181.
23. Bess Furman, *A Profile of the U.S. Public Health Service 1798–1948* (Bethesda, MD: National Library of Medicine, 1973), 370–73.

24. Beeman, *Charles Armstrong*, 145.

25. "Parrot Fever Kills 2 In This Country," *New York Times* (11 January 1930).

26. "Hunts For Source of 'Parrot Fever,'" *New York Times* (12 January 1930).

27. "Parrot Fever Cases Halted in the City," *New York Times* (19 January 1930).

28. De Kruif, *Men Against Death*, 184.

29. Ibid., 125.

30. Beeman, *Charles Armstrong*, 139.

31. De Kruif, *Men Against Death*, 183–84.

32. "Hoover Bars Out Parrots to Check Disease: Gets Reports of Fatal Psittacosis Cases," *New York Times* (25 January 1930).

33. George W. McCoy, "Accidental Psittacosis Infection Among the Personnel of the Hygienic Laboratory," *Public Health Reports* 45, no. 16 (1930): 843–49.

34. De Kruif, *Men Against Death*, 203.

35. "Parrot Fever Attack Fatal to Dr Stokes," *The Sun* (11 February 1930).

36. Charles Armstrong, "Psittacosis: Epidemiological Considerations with Reference to the 1929–30 Outbreak in the United States," *Public Health Reports* 45, no. 35 (1930): 2013–23.

37. Edward C. Ramsay, "The Psittacosis Outbreak of 1929–1930," *Journal of Avian Medicine and Surgery* 17, no. 4 (2003): 235–37.

38. S. P. Bedson, G. T. Western, and S. Levy Simpson, "Observations on the Ætiology of Psittacosis," *The Lancet* 215, no. 5553 (1 February 1930): 235–36; S. P. Bedson, G. T. Western, and S. Levy Simpson, "Further Observations on the Ætiology of Psittacosis," *The Lancet* 215, no. 5555 (15 February 1930): 345–46.

39. Sturdee and Scott, *A Disease of Parrots Communicable to Man*, 68–74. In Bedson's honour, the organism was named *Bedsoniae*, a nomenclature that stuck until the 1960s.

40. Karl F. Meyer, "The Ecology of Psittacosis and Ornithosis," *Medicine* 21, no. 2 (May 1941): 175–205.

41. Sturdee and Scott, *A Disease of Parrots Communicable to Man*, 88–89.

42. "Deny Parrot Fever Affects Humans," *New York Times* (18 January 1930).

43. Albert B. Sabin, *Karl Friedrich Meyer 1884–1974, A Biographical Memoir* (Washington, DC: National Academy of Sciences, 1980); Mark Honigsbaum, "Tipping the Balance': Karl Friedrich Meyer, Latent Infections and the Birth of Modern Ideas of Disease Ecology," *Journal of the History of Biology* 49, no. 2 (April 2016): 261–309.

44. Karl F. Meyer, *Medical Research and Public Health*. An interview conducted by Edna Tartaul Daniel in 1961 and 1962 (Berkeley: The Regents of the University of California, 1976), 74.

45. Paul de Kruif, "Champion among Microbe Hunters," *Reader's Digest*, June 1950: 35–40.

46. Meyer, *Medical Research and Public Health*, 358.

47. It was on one of these expeditions that they agreed that the lives of these medical men would make "a fantastic story," and Meyer told de Kruif to "forget science and … go into the writing game." De Kruif took Meyer's advice and by 1926 was forging

a new career as a science writer. Indeed, it is said that when Sinclair Lewis was casting around for a real-life disease detective for his novel *Arrowsmith*, de Kruif suggested Meyer as a model for Gustaf Sondelius, Lewis's bombastic Swedish plague-hunter. However, although de Kruif credited Meyer with the inspiration for *Arrowsmith*, he would subsequently claim that Sondelius had "no prototype." Meyer, *Medical Research and Public Health*, 340; de Kruif to Dr Malloch, 16 April 1931. Paul H. de Kruif papers, Rockefeller Institute for Medical Research Scientific Staff, Rockefeller Archive Center, Correspondence, 1919–1940, Box 1, Folder 9.

48. Altogether, some 6,000 horses became diseased during the outbreak and 3,000 died.

49. Technically, equine encephalitis is an arbovirus transmitted from birds to horses by Aedes and other species of mosquitoes. In horses and other animals it frequently attacks the optical nerves and meninges, causing the brain to swell and leading to neurological impairment. The key experiments were conducted in 1941 in the Yakima Valley in Washington, where Meyer's colleagues, Bill Hammon and William Reeves, succeeded in isolating the virus from *Culex* mosquitoes trapped in the wild and from chickens and ducks on which the mosquitoes had been allowed to take a blood meal. Although not definitive proof of mosquito-transmission, the experiments were strong evidence. Subsequent studies demonstrated that chickens were naturally infected with the virus over the winter and that it was only as summer approached and mosquito populations increased and began to feed on chickens that the virus spilled over into horses.

50. Meyer, *Medical Research and Public Health*, 150.

51. Ibid.

52. Karl F. Meyer, "Psittacosis Meeting," Los Angeles, California, 2 March 1932, folio leaves 1–31, 5, Karl Meyer Papers, 1900–1975, Bancroft Library, Berkeley, BANC 76/42 cz, Box 89.

53. W. E. Carter and V. Link, "Unpublished biography of Karl F. Meyer and related papers, written and compiled by William E. Carter and Vernon B. Link, 1956–1963," "Fifth Interview," 157. UCSF Library, Archives and Special Collections. MSS 63–1.

54. Karl F. Meyer, "Psittacosis Meeting," Los Angeles, California, 2 March 1932, folio leaves 1–31, BANC 76/42 cz, Box 89—"Psittacosis study." Aware of the risk of accidental laboratory exposure, Meyer insisted that test animals at the Hooper be kept in a special isolation room and that laboratory workers wear rubber gloves and masks at all times. Unfortunately, the rules were not always observed, and in 1935 it was anonymously reported that a Hooper laboratory worker had been accidentally contaminated with psittacosis during a routine examination of a smear from a mouse spleen. Only years later would it emerge that that worker had been Meyer and that the breach of protocol had occurred when he had removed his rubber gloves to take a phone call.

55. Beeman, *Charles Armstrong*, 142–43.

56. K. F. Meyer and B. Eddie, "Latent Psittacosis Infections in Shell Parakeets," *Proceedings of the Society for Experimental Biology and Medicine* 30 (1933): 484–88.

57. K. F. Meyer, "Psittacosis," *Proceedings of the Twelfth International Veterinary Congress* 4 (1935): 182–205.

58. F. M. Burnet, "Psittacosis amongst Wild Australian Parrots," *The Journal of Hygiene* 35, no. 3 (August 1935): 412–20.

59. Meyer, "The Ecology of Psittacosis and Ornithosis."

60. Julius Schachter and Chandler R. Dawson, *Human Chlamydial Infections* (Littleton, MA: PSG Publishing, 1978), 25–26, 39–41.

61. Frank Macfarlane Burnet, *Natural History of Infectious Disease* (Cambridge: Cambridge University Press, 1953), 23.

4. THE "PHILLY KILLER"

1. "Hyatt at the Bellevue," accessed 6 September 2017: https://philadelphiabellevue.hyatt.com/en/hotel/home.html

2. Gordon Thomas and Max Morgan-Witts, *Trauma, the Search for the Cause of Legionnaires' Disease* (London: Hamish Hamilton, 1981), 68–69, 120.

3. "Statement of Edward T. Hoak," in "Legionnaires' Disease," Hearings before House of Representatives, Subcommittee on Consumer Protection and Finance, 23 and 24 November 1976 (Washington, DC: US Government Printing Office, 1977), 156–57 (hereafter: "House hearings on Legionnaires' Disease"); Thomas and Morgan-Witts, *Trauma*, 101, 120.

4. Thomas and Morgan-Witts, *Trauma*, 103; Robert Sharrar, "Talk—Legionnaires' disease," Legionnaires' disease files and manuscripts, Smithsonian, Box 5.

5. American Thoracic Society, "Top 20 Pneumonia Facts—2015," accessed 1 May 2017: https://www.thoracic.org/patients/patient-resources/fact-sheets-az.php

6. Charles-Edward Amory Winslow, *The Conquest of Epidemic Disease: A Chapter in the History of Ideas* (Madison: University of Wisconsin Press, 1971).

7. David W. Fraser, "The Challenges Were Legion," *The Lancet, Infectious Diseases* 5, no. 4 (April 2005): 237–41.

8. Statement of David J. Sencer, "House hearings on Legionnaires' Disease," 95.

9. Elizabeth W. Etheridge, *Sentinel for Health: A History of the Centers for Disease Control* (Berkeley: University of California Press, 1992), 47–48.

10. In Gaudiosi's defence, Fort Detrick, in Maryland, the site of the US germ warfare program, was just across the state border, and there had been reports that the CIA had been experimenting with hallucinogenic fungi at Toughkenamon, just an hour's drive from Philadelphia. Moreover, the year before, the public had been treated to revelations about MKULTRA, the CIA's clandestine experiments with LSD and other psychotropic drugs in the 1950s that had grown out of the program to counter Soviet efforts to create a "Manchurian candidate." For further discussion, see Thomas and Morgan-Witts, *Trauma*, 179–80; John Marks, *The Search for the Manchurian Candidate* (New York: Norton, 1991), 81.

11. Thomas M. Daniel, *Wade Hampton Frost, Pioneer Epidemiologist, 1880–1938: Up to the Mountain* (Rochester, NY: University of Rochester Press, 2004), xii.

12. Sharrar, "Talk—Legionnaires' disease."

13. "Progress Report Legionnaires Disease Investigation, August 12, 1976," Legionnaires' disease files and manuscripts, Smithsonian, Box 2.

14. Ibid.

15. David Fraser, EPI-2 report on Legionnaires' disease, 21 March 1976, in "Legionnaires' disease: Hearing before the Senate Subcommittee on Health and Scientific Research," 9 November 1977, 85–129.

16. Sharrar, "Talk—Legionnaires' disease," 20.

17. Julius Schachter and Chandler R. Dawson, *Human Chlamydial Infections* (Littleton: PSG Publishing, 1978), 29–32; Karl F. Meyer, "The Ecology of Psittacosis and Ornithosis," *Medicine* 21, no. 2 (May 1941): 175–206.

18. Thomas and Morgan-Witts, *Trauma*, 224–25.

19. Schachter had recently traced an outbreak of psittacosis at UCSF to pigeons roosting on office window sills, a discovery that prompted the university to install antiroost spikes.

20. Gary Lattimer to Theodore Tsai, 20 December 1976, Legionnaires' disease files and manuscripts, Smithsonian, Box 5.

21. Fraser, EPI-2 report, 125.

22. Ibid., 35.

23. The organism is named for Macfarlane Burnet, who did much to elaborate the aetiology of Q Fever following a series of outbreaks in Australia in the 1930s.

24. Joseph McDade, interview with author, 26 May 2016.

25. Ibid.

26. Statements of F. William Sunderman and F. William Sunderman Jr., "House hearings on Legionnaires' disease," 54.

27. Ibid., 51–61.

28. Ibid., 60.

29. "House hearings on Legionnaires' disease," 4–6.

30. Jack Anderson and Les Whitten, "Paranoid Suspect in Legion Deaths," *Washington Post* (28 October 1976), 1.

31. Richard Hofstadter, "The Paranoid Style in American Politics," *Harper's Magazine*, (November 1964).

32. Laurie Garrett, *The Coming Plague: Newly Emerging Diseases in a World out of Balance* (New York: Farrar, Straus and Giroux, 1994), 176.

33. Michael Capuzzo, "Legionnaires Disease," *Philadelphia Inquirer*, 21 July 1986.

34. It would seem Dylan never recorded the song and only played it on one occasion—at a sound check in Detroit on 13 October 1978. By then, of course, the real pathogen had been discovered, so perhaps Dylan lost interest. However, Cross liked the song and recorded it three years later with his Delta Cross Band. Some writers have detected a similarity to the melody of "Hurricane," the song released by Dylan the year before inspired by the wrongful conviction of the Canadian middleweight boxer Rubin "Hurricane" Carter, for a triple homicide in a bar in New Jersey in 1966, a

conviction that was eventually overturned in 1985. "Delta Cross Band Back on the Road Again," accessed 1 May 2017: https://www.discogs.com/Delta-Cross-Band-Back-On-The-Road-Again-Legionaires-Disease/release/2235787

35. "The Philadelphia Killer," *Time* (16 August 1976).

36. After sale to a local developer and extensive renovations, the Bellevue was acquired by San Francisco's Fairmont chain, reopening its doors in 1979 as the Fairmont Philadelphia. Since then, the hotel has changed hands and its name several times.

37. David Fraser, interview with author, 4 February 2015.

38. EPI-2, Second Draft, 15 December 1976, Legionnaires' disease files and manuscripts, Smithsonian, Box 2.

39. Gwyneth Cravens and John S. Karr, "Tracking Down The Epidemic," *New York Times* (12 December 1976), accessed 4 April 2018: https://www.nytimes.com/1976/12/12/archives/tracking-down-the-epidemic-epidemic.html

5. LEGIONNAIRES' REDUX

1. Laurie Garrett, *The Coming Plague: Newly Emerging Diseases in a World out of Balance* (New York: Farrar, Straus and Giroux, 1994), 167.

2. Arthur M. Silverstein, *Pure Politics and Impure Science: The Swine Flu Affair* (Baltimore: Johns Hopkins University Press, 1981), 100–1.

3. Garrett, *Coming Plague*, 175.

4. George Dehner, *Influenza: A Century of Science and Public Health Response* (Pittsburgh: University of Pittsburgh, 2012), 183–84.

5. Ibid., 148.

6. For further discussion, see ibid., 185–88, and Garrett, *Coming Plague*, 180–83.

7. Dehner, *Influenza*, 144.

8. Garrett, *Coming Plague*, 185.

9. The chickens survived, prompting Pasteur to repeat the experiment with both old and new cultures and discover the principle of attenuated vaccines.

10. Joe McDade, interview with author, 26 May 2015.

11. Ibid. Later, CDC researchers would also demonstrate that the organism was present in lung tissue from patients who had died of Legionnaires' disease. Previous attempts to detect the organism had failed, but when researchers used a little-known stain called Dieterle's, the bacteria showed up clearly. Subsequently, researchers also succeeded in growing the bacteria on special agar media and developing a specific reagent to aid diagnosis. "Statement of William H. Foege," in "Follow-up examination of Legionnaires' Disease," US Senate Subcommittee on Health and Scientific Research, 9 November 1977, 42–43.

12. Joseph McDade, interview with author, 26 May 2015.

13. W. C. Winn, "Legionnaires Disease: Historical Perspective," *Clinical Microbiology Reviews* 1, no. 1 (January 1988): 60–81.

14. C. V. Broome et al., "The Vermont Epidemic of Legionnaires' Disease," *Annals of Internal Medicine* 90, no. 4 (April 1979): 573–77.

15. John T. MacFarlane and Michael Worboys, "Showers, Sweating and Suing: Legionnaires' Disease and 'New' infections in Britain, 1977–90," *Medical History* 56, no. 1 (January 2012): 72–93.

16. J. F. Boyd et al., "Pathology of Five Scottish Deaths from Pneumonic Illnesses Acquired in Spain due to Legionnaires' Disease Agent," *Journal of Clinical Pathology* 31, no. 9 (September 1978): 809–16.

17. MacFarlane and Worboys, "Showers, Sweating and Suing: Legionnaires' Disease and 'New' Infections in Britain, 1977–90."

18. Ronald Sullivan, "A Macy's Tower Held Bacteria That Cause Legionnaires' Disease," *New York Times* (12 January 1979), accessed 1 May 2017: http://www.nytimes.com/1979/01/12/archives/a-macys-tower-held-bacteria-that-cause-legionnaires-disease.html

19. G. K. Morris et al., "Isolation of the Legionnaires' Disease Bacterium from Environmental Samples," *Annals of Internal Medicine* 90, no. 4 (April 1979): 664–66.

20. J.P. Euzéby, "Genus *Legionella*," *List of Prokaryotic names with Standing in Nomenclature* (LPSN), accessed 1 May 2017: http://www.bacterio.net/legionella.html

21. R. F. Breiman, "Impact of Technology on the Emergence of Infectious Diseases," *Epidemiologic Reviews* 18, no. 1 (1996): 4–9.

22. Ibid., 6.

23. Alfred S. Evans and Philip S. Brachman, eds., *Bacterial Infections of Humans: Epidemiology and Control* (New York: Springer, 2013), 365.

24. Ibid., 361–63.

25. "Statement of William H. Foege," 43.

26. David Fraser, interview with author, 4 February 2015.

27. H. M. Foy et al., "Pneumococcal Isolations from Patients with Pneumonia and Control Subjects in a Prepaid Medical Care Group," *The American Review of Respiratory Disease* 111, no. 5 (May 1975): 595–603.

28. Willis Haviland Carrier, "The Invention That Changed the World," accessed 1 May 2017: http://www.williscarrier.com/1876–1902.php; Steven Johnson, *How We Got to Now: Six Innovations That Made the Modern World*, reprint edition (New York: Riverhead Books, 2015), 76–83.

29. A. D. Cliff and Matthew Smallman-Raynor, *Infectious Diseases: Emergence and Re-Emergence: A Geographical Analysis* (Oxford and New York: Oxford University Press, 2009), 296.

30. Laurel E. Garrison et al., "Vital Signs: Deficiencies in Environmental Control Identified in Outbreaks of Legionnaires' Disease—North America, 2000–2014," *MMWR. Morbidity and Mortality Weekly Report* 65, no. 22 (10 June 2016): 576–84.

6. AIDS IN AMERICA, AIDS IN AFRICA

1. Ronald Bayer and Gerald M. Oppenheimer, *AIDS Doctors: Voices from the Epidemic* (Oxford and New York: Oxford University Press, 2000), 18.

2. T cells, so-called because they are produced in the thymus, are a type of lymphocyte, or white blood cell. They can be distinguished from other lymphocytes by the presence of a T-cell receptor on their surface.

3. Michael S. Gottlieb, "Discovering AIDS," *Epidemiology* 9, no. 4 (July 1998): 365–67. PCP used to be considered a protozoan infection, but in 1988 it was reclassified as a fungus and renamed *Pneumocystis jirovecii*. However, to avoid confusion, the abbreviation "PCP" was retained. "Pneumocystis pneumonia" CDC, accessed 21 September 2017: https://www.cdc.gov/fungal/diseases/pneumocystis-pneumonia/index.html#5

4. Nelson Vergel, "There When AIDS Began: An Interview With Michael Gottlieb, M.D.," *The Body* (2 June 2011), accessed 10 October 2016: http://www.thebody.com/content/62330/there-when-aids-began-an-interview-with-michael-go.html

5. CMV can be transmitted in saliva, semen, vaginal fluids, urine, blood, even breast milk. Newborns can also contract CMV infections via the placenta or during delivery if their mother's genital tract is infected. Most people contract CMV in childhood and are unaware they carry the virus, but if their immune systems are compromised the infection can be reactivated. Prior to AIDS, CMV was most commonly seen in transplant patients who had received immunosuppressant medication to prevent the rejection of donor organs.

6. Elizabeth Fee and Theodore M. Brown, "Michael S. Gottlieb and the Identification of AIDS," *American Journal of Public Health* 96, no. 6 (June 2006): 982–83.

7. Bayer and Oppenheimer, *AIDS Doctors*, 12–14.

8. Fee and Brown, "Michael S. Gottlieb and the Identification of AIDS."

9. Amyl nitrate reduces blood pressure while increasing heart rate, producing a dizzying "rush" to the head. Poppers were popular at parties, where they were commonly used to break the ice and heighten the pleasure of sex.

10. Garrett, *Coming Plague*, 285.

11. CDC, "Pneumocystis Pneumonia—Los Angeles, 1981," *Morbidity and Mortality Weekly Report* 45, no. 34 (August 1996): 729–33.

12. "The Age of AIDS," *Frontline*, accessed 13 October 2016: http://www.pbs.org/wgbh/frontline/film/aids/

13. "A Timeline of HIV/AIDS," accessed 13 October 2016: https://www.aids.gov/hiv-aids-basics/hiv-aids-101/aids-timeline/; "WHO | HIV/AIDS," *WHO*, accessed 13 October 2016: http://www.who.int/gho/hiv/en/

14. Office of NIH History, "In Their Own Words: NIH Researchers Recall the Early Years of AIDS," interview with Dr Robert Gallo, 25 August 1994, 33, accessed 21 October 2016: https://history.nih.gov/nihinownwords/docs/gallo1_01.html

15. Robert C. Gallo, "HIV—the Cause of AIDS: An Overview on Its Biology, Mechanisms of Disease Induction, and Our Attempts to Control It," *Journal of Acquired Immune Deficiency Syndromes* 1, no. 6 (1988): 521–35.

16. Garrett, *Coming Plague*, 330.

17. Douglas Selvage, "Memetic Engineering: Conspiracies, Viruses and Historical

Agency," *OpenDemocracy*, 21 October 2015, accessed 8 November 2016: https://www.opendemocracy.net/conspiracy/suspect-science/douglas-selvage/memetic-engineering-conspiracies-viruses-and-historical-agency

18. In this stage of the infection, virus levels fall and it becomes harder to pass on HIV via sexual intercourse.

19. The CD4 count of a healthy, uninfected adult generally ranges from 500–1600 cells/mm^3. By contrast, a very low CD4 count (less than 200 cells/mm^3) indicates a compromised immune system.

20. The significance of Mabs to immunology must not be understated. As the historian of medicine Lara Marks puts it, "Before the arrival of Mabs, scientists had as much knowledge of the surface of immune cells as they had of the surface of the moon." Lara V. Marks, *The Lock and Key of Medicine: Monoclonal Antibodies and the Transformation of Healthcare* (New Haven and London: Yale University Press, 2015), 68.

21. Oncoviruses do not always cause tumours. For instance, Epstein-Barr is ubiquitous in infancy, and infections in adolescence usually result in mononucleosis, the so-called "kissing disease." Similarly, while infection with hepatitis B can lead to cirrhosis and liver failure, only a small percentage of people go on to develop hepatocellular carcinomas.

22. Surindar Paracer and Vernon Ahmadjian, *Symbiosis: An Introduction to Biological Associations*, 2nd edition (Oxford and New York: Oxford University Press, 2000), 21. When the human genome was sequenced it revealed some 96,000 retrovirus-like elements. These elements occupied around 8 per cent of the genome, suggesting they might be the remains of ancient virus infections.

23. Mirko D. Grmek, *History of AIDS: Emergence and Origin of a Modern Pandemic* (Princeton, NJ: Princeton University Press, 1990), 56.

24. Bernard J. Poiesz et al., "Detection and Isolation of Type C Retrovirus Particles from Fresh and Cultured Lymphocytes of a Patient with Cutaneous T-Cell Lymphoma," *Proceedings of the National Academy of Sciences* 77, no. 12 (December 1980): 7415–19. Following isolation of the same virus by a Japanese research group, the L in HTLV was changed to "lymphotropic."

25. John M. Coffin, "The Discovery of HTLV-1, the First Pathogenic Human Retrovirus," *Proceedings of the National Academy of Sciences of the United States of America* 112, no. 51 (22 December 2015): 15525–29.

26. Robert C. Gallo, *Virus Hunting: AIDS, Cancer, and the Human Retrovirus: A story of Scientific Discovery* (New York: Basic Books, 1991), 135–36.

27. The Yugoslavian historian of science Mirko Grmek, who made a detailed study of the history of AIDS and the intellectual and technological developments that led to the discovery of HIV, claims that in early 1983 Gallo had dissuaded a researcher at the CDC from pursuing the hypothesis that AIDS was due to a cell-killing virus, insisting "it had to be oncogenic." Grmek, *History of AIDS*, 58.

28. R. C. Gallo et al., "Isolation of Human T-Cell Leukemia Virus in Acquired Immune Deficiency Syndrome (AIDS)," *Science* 220, no. 4599 (20 May 1983): 865–67;

M. Essex et al., "Antibodies to Cell Membrane Antigens Associated with Human T-Cell Leukemia Virus in Patients with AIDS," *Science* 220, no. 4599 (20 May 1983): 859–62.

29. F. Barré-Sinoussi et al., "Isolation of a T-lymphotropic Retrovirus from a Patient at Risk for Acquired Immune Deficiency Syndrome (AIDS)," *Science* 220, no. 4559 (20 May 1983): 868–71.

30. Grmek, *History of AIDS*, 65.

31. Ibid., 60–70; Nikolas Kontaratos, *Dissecting a Discovery: The Real Story of How the Race to Uncover the Cause of AIDS Turned Scientists against Disease, Politics against Science, Nation against Nation* (Xlibris Corp, 2006); Gallo, *Virus Hunting*; Luc Montagnier, *Virus: The Co-Discoverer of HIV Tracks Its Rampage and Charts the Future* (New York and London: Norton, 2000).

32. Jon Cohen, *Shots in the Dark: The Wayward Search for an AIDS Vaccine* (New York: Norton, 2001), 7–10.

33. Kontaratos, *Dissecting a Discovery*, 274–75.

34. Grmek, *History of AIDS*, 63.

35. F. Barré-Sinoussi, "HIV: A Discovery Opening the Road to Novel Scientific Knowledge and Global Health Improvement," *Virology* 397, no. 2 (20 February 2010): 255–59; Patrick Strudwick, "In Conversation With … Françoise Barré-Sinoussi," *Mosaic*, accessed 19 October 2016: https://mosaicscience.com/story/francoise-barre-sinoussi

36. Gallo, *Virus Hunting*, 143.

37. NIH, "In Their Own Words," 4, 31.

38. Grmek, *History of AIDS*, 71.

39. Susan Sontag, *Illness as Metaphor* (New York: Farrar, Straus and Giroux, 1978), 58.

40. Susan Sontag, *AIDS and Its Metaphors* (London: Allen Lane, 1989), 25–26.

41. David France, *How To Survive a Plague: The Story of How Activists and Scientists Tamed AIDS* (London: Picador, 2016), 189.

42. Randy Shilts, *And The Band Played On: Politics, People and the AIDS Epidemic* (New York and London: Penguin Viking, 1988), 302.

43. Anthony S. Fauci, "The Acquired Immune Deficiency Syndrome: The Ever-Broadening Clinical Spectrum," *Journal of the American Medical Association* 249, no. 17 (6 May 1983): 2375–76.

44. Shilts, *And The Band Played On*, 299–302.

45. L. K. Altman, "The Press and AIDS," *Bulletin of the New York Academy of Medicine* 64, no. 6 (1988): 520–28.

46. Evan Thomas, "The New Untouchables," *Time* (23 September 1985).

47. Colin Clews, "1984–85. Media: AIDS and the British Press," *Gay in the 80s* (28 January 2013), accessed 24 October 2016: http://www.gayinthe80s.com/2013/01/1984-85-media-aids-and-the-british-press/

48. John Tierney, "The Big City; In 80's, Fear Spread Faster Than AIDS," *New York Times* (15 June 2001).

49. CDC, "Kaposi's Sarcoma and Pneumocystis Pneumonia among Homosexual Men—New York City and California," *Morbidity and Mortality Weekly Report* 30, no. 25 (3 July 1981): 305–8.

50. Lawrence K. Altman, "Rare Cancer Seen In 41 Homosexuals," *New York Times* (3 July 1981); "*'Gay plague' Baffling Medical Detectives,*" *Philadelphia Daily News* (9 August 1982).

51. CDC, "A Cluster of Kaposi's Sarcoma and Pneumocystis Carinii Pneumonia among Homosexual Male Residents of Los Angeles and Orange Counties, California," *Morbidity and Mortality Weekly Report* 31, no. 23 (18 June 1982): 305–7.

52. Richard A. McKay, "Patient Zero': The Absence of a Patient's View of the Early North American AIDS Epidemic," *Bulletin of the History of Medicine* 88 (2014): 161–94, 178.

53. Gerald M. Oppenheimer, "Causes, Cases, and Cohorts: The Role of Epidemiology in the Historical Construction of AIDS," in Elizabeth Fee and Daniel Fox, *AIDS: The Making of a Chronic Disease* (Berkeley: University of California Press, 1992), 50–83.

54. Garrett, *Coming Plague*, 270–71.

55. Report of the Centers for Disease Control Task Force on Kaposi's Sarcoma and Opportunistic Infections, "Epidemiologic Aspects of the Current Outbreak of Kaposi's Sarcoma and Opportunistic Infections," *New England Journal of Medicine* 306, no. 4 (28 January 1982): 248–52.

56. Michael Marmor et al., "Risk Factors for Kaposi's Sarcoma in Homosexual Men," *The Lancet* 319, no. 8281 (15 May 1982): 1083–87; Henry Masur et al., "An Outbreak of Community-Acquired Pneumocystis Carinii Pneumonia," *New England Journal of Medicine* 305, no. 24 (10 December 1981): 1431–38.

57. D. M. Auerbach et al., "Cluster of Cases of the Acquired Immune Deficiency Syndrome. Patients Linked by Sexual Contact," *American Journal of Medicine* 76, no. 3 (March 1984): 487–92.

58. McKay, "Patient Zero," 172–73.

59. Ibid., 182; France, *How to Survive a Plague*, 87.

60. "Patient Zero," *People*, 28 December 1987.

61. The New York samples were closely related to a strain from Haiti, suggesting that someone arriving from Haiti had introduced AIDS to the United States. Jon Cohen, "Patient Zero' No More," *Science* 351, no. 6277 (4 March 2016): 1013; Michael Worobey et al., "1970s and 'Patient 0' HIV-1 Genomes Illuminate Early HIV/AIDS History in North America," *Nature* 539, no. 7627 (3 November 2016): 98–101.

62. CDC, "AIDS: The Early Years and CDC's Response," Morbidity and Mortality Weekly Report 60, no. 4 (7 October 2011): 64–69.

63. Garrett, *Coming Plague*, 350.

64. Ibid., 352. These were later considered false positives, causing a lot of resentment in Africa.

65. In 1995 Peter Piot became executive director of the United Nations AIDS agency, UNAIDS.

66. Peter Piot et al., "Acquired Immunodeficiency Syndrome in a Heterosexual Population in Zaire," *The Lancet* 324, no. 8394 (July 1984): 65–69.

67. P. Van de Perre et al., "Acquired Immunodeficiency Syndrome in Rwanda," *The Lancet* 2, no. 8394 (14 July 1984): 62–65; T. C. Quinn et al., "AIDS in Africa: An Epidemiologic Paradigm, 1986," *Bulletin of the World Health Organization* 79, no. 12 (2001): 1159–67.

68. Edward Hooper, *The River: A Journey Back to the Source of HIV and AIDS* (London: Penguin, 1999), 95–96.

69. Jacques Pepin, *The Origins of AIDS* (Cambridge: Cambridge University Press, 2011), 6–11.

70. A. J. Nahmias et al., "Evidence for Human Infection with an HTLV III/LAV-like Virus in Central Africa, 1959," *The Lancet* 1, no. 8492 (31 May 1986): 1279–80.

71. Michael Worobey et al., "Direct Evidence of Extensive Diversity of HIV-1 in Kinshasa by 1960," *Nature* 455, no. 7213 (2 October 2008): 661–64.

72. Pepin, *The Origins of AIDS*, 41.

73. "AIDS Origins, Edward Hooper's site on the origins of AIDS," accessed 2 November 2016: http://www.aidsorigins.com/

74. Responding to the study, Duesberg repeated his argument that AIDS is not a specific disease but a battery of previously known and specific diseases and that HIV is merely "a harmless passenger virus." Therefore, Mbeki's decision to withhold AZT did not contribute to the death toll. To prove his point, Crawford reports that at one point, Duesberg even offered to inject himself with AIDS. Dorothy H. Crawford, *Virus Hunt: The Search for the Origin of HIV* (Oxford: Oxford University Press, 2015), 10–12.

75. Celia W. Dugger and Donald G. McNeil Jr., "Rumor, Fear and Fatigue Hinder Final Push to End Polio," *New York Times* (20 March 2006); Stephen Taylor, "In Pursuit of Zero: Polio, Global Health Security and the Politics of Eradication in Peshawar, Pakistan," *Geoforum* 69 (February 2016): 106–16.

76. To date serological evidence of SIV infection has been found in forty species of primates. These viruses appear to be largely non-pathogenic in their natural hosts, despite clustering together with the human and simian AIDS viruses in a single phylogenetic lineage. Paul M. Sharp and Beatrice H. Hahn, "Origins of HIV and the AIDS Pandemic," *Cold Spring Harbor Perspectives in Medicine* 1, no. 1 (September 2011): 1–22.

77. The term "spillover" was popularized by the science writer, David Quammen, and refers to a single event where a pathogen moves from one species to another, typically as a result of contamination with blood or other bodily fluids. However, anthropologists and sociologists have criticized the term as overly simplistic. In particular, they argue that the focus on bushmeat hunting and the consumption of game in spillover events overlooks other types of "contact" between animals and humans in traditional rural settings. Tamara Gilles-Vernick, "A multi-disciplinary study of human beings, great apes, and viral emergence in equatorial Africa (SHAPES)," accessed 21 September 2017: https://research.pasteur.fr/en/project/a-multi-disciplinary-study-of-human-beings-great-apes-and-viral-emergence-in-equatorial-africa-shapes/

78. The simian progenitor virus of HIV-1 is thought to be a hybrid virus consisting of

two monkey viruses that chimpanzees probably acquired from eating other monkeys.

79. Pepin, *The Origin of AIDS*, 50.

80. Ibid., 1–5.

81. Ibid., 110–11.

82. Sharp and Hahn, "Origins of HIV and the AIDS Pandemic."

83. Pepin, *The Origin of AIDS*, 224.

84. Nathan Wolfe, *The Viral Storm: The Dawn of a New Pandemic Age* (London: Allen Lane, 2011), 161–63.

85. Viruses, bacteria, and protozoa are all examples of microparasites. In disease ecology, parasitism designates a non-symbiotic relationship in which one species, the parasite, benefits at the expense of the other, usually referred to as the host.

86. Stephen S. Morse, "Emerging Viruses: Defining the Rules for Viral Traffic," *Perspectives in Biology and Medicine* 34, no. 3 (1991): 387–409.

87. Joshua Lederberg, Robert E. Shope, and S. C. Oaks, eds., *Emerging Infections: Microbial Threats to Health in the United States* (Washington, DC: National Academy Press, 1992), 34–35, 83.

88. Joshua Lederberg, "Infectious Disease as an Evolutionary Paradigm," *Emerging Infectious Diseases* 3, no. 4 (December 1997): 417–23.

89. Garrett, *Coming Plague*, xi.

7. SARS: "SUPER SPREADER"

1. Arthur Starling and Hong Kong Museum of Medical Sciences, eds., *Plague, SARS and the Story of Medicine in Hong Kong* (Hong Kong: Hong Kong University Press, 2006), 2.

2. Stephen Boyden et al., *The Ecology of a City and Its People: The Case of Hong Kong* (Canberra: Australian National University Press, 1988), 1.

3. Tamara Giles-Vernick and Susan Craddock, eds., *Influenza and Public Health: Learning from Past Pandemics* (London and Washington, DC: Earthscan, 2010), 125.

4. Mike Davis, *The Monster at Our Door: The Global Threat of Avian Flu* (New York: The New Press, 2005), 58–60.

5. The initial tests were conducted at the Hong Kong Department of Health. Subsequently, the samples were forwarded to the CDC in Atlanta and laboratories in London and Rotterdam, where they were identified as H5N1. Alan Sipress, *The Fatal Strain: On the Trail of Avian Flu and the Coming Pandemic* (New York and London: Penguin 2010), 53–54; Pete Davis, *The Devil's Flu: The World's Deadliest Influenza Epidemic and the Scientific Hunt for the Virus That Caused It* (New York: Henry Holt, 2000), 8–12.

6. Scientists would subsequently blame the boy's death on the unusual genetic properties of the virus and its effect on white blood cells associated with inflammatory responses. By inducing the release of proinflammatory cytokines, it is thought the H5N1 virus induced an extreme autoimmune reaction known as a "cytokine storm." Robert G. Webster, "H5 Influenza Viruses," in Y. Kawaoka, ed., *Influenza Virology: Current*

Topics (Caister Academic Press, 2006), 281–98; C. Y. Cheung et al., "Induction of Proinflammatory Cytokines in Human Macrophages by Influenza A (H5N1) Viruses: A Mechanism for the Unusual Severity of Human Disease?" *The Lancet* 360, no. 9348 (2002): 1831–37.

7. Davis, *The Devil's Flu*, 46–47.

8. Sipress, *The Fatal Strain*, 57.

9. Mark Honigsbaum, "Robert Webster: 'We Ignore Bird Flu at Our Peril," *The Observer* (17 September 2011), accessed 13 April 2017: https://www.theguardian.com/world/2011/sep/17/bird-flu-swine-flu-warning

10. The statement is by Jeffery Taubenberger, the molecular biologist who in 2005 sequenced all eight genes of the 1918 Spanish flu together with colleagues at the Armed Forces Institute of Pathology at Bethesda, Maryland. Taubenberger is now chief of viral pathogenesis and evolution at the National Institute of Allergy and Infectious Diseases. "The 1918 flu virus is resurrected," *Nature* 437 (6 October 2005): 794–95.

11. K. F. Shortridge et al., "The Next Influenza Pandemic: Lessons from Hong Kong," *Journal of Applied Microbiology* 94 (2003): 70S–79S.

12. Y. Guan et al., "H9N2 Influenza Viruses Possessing H5N1-Like Internal Genomes Continue to Circulate in Poultry in Southeastern China," *Journal of Virology* 74, no. 20 (October 2000): 9372–80.

13. K. S. Li et al., "Characterization of H9 Subtype Influenza Viruses from the Ducks of Southern China: A Candidate for the Next Influenza Pandemic in Humans?," *Journal of Virology* 77, no. 12 (June 2003): 6988–94.

14. Donald G. McNeil and Lawrence K. Altman, "As SARS Outbreak Took Shape Health Agency Took Fast Action," *New York Times* (4 May 2003), accessed 2 October 2017: https://www.nytimes.com/2003/05/04/world/as-sars-outbreak-took-shape-health-agency-took-fast-action.html

15. Thomas Abraham, *Twenty-First Century Plague: The Story of SARS* (Baltimore, MD: Johns Hopkins University Press, 2005), 19.

16. Kung-wai Loh and Civic Exchange, eds., *At the Epicentre: Hong Kong and the SARS Outbreak* (Hong Kong: Hong Kong University Press, 2004), xvi.

17. "Solving the Metropole Mystery," in World Health Organization, *SARS: How A Global Epidemic Was Stopped* (Geneva: World Health Organization, 2006), 141–48; CDC, "Update: Outbreak of Severe Acute Respiratory Syndrome—Worldwide, 2003," *MMWR* 52, no. 12 (28 March 2003): 241–48.

18. Alison P. Galvani and Robert M. May, "Epidemiology: Dimensions of Superspreading," *Nature* 438, no. 7066 (17 November 2005): 293–95.

19. Abraham, *Twenty-First Century Plague*, 64–67; Raymond S. M. Wong and David S. Hui, "Index Patient and SARS Outbreak in Hong Kong," *Emerging Infectious Diseases* 10, no. 2 (February 2004): 339–41.

20. Alexandra A. Seno and Alejandro Reyes, "Unmasking SARS: Voices from the Epicentre," in Loh and Civic Exchange, eds., *At the Epicentre*, 1–15 (10).

21. Abraham, *Twenty-First Century Plague*, 70–75.

22. "Lockdown at Amoy Gardens," in WHO, *SARS*, 155–62.

23. The anthrax mailings, which began one week after 9/11, were the worst biological attacks in US history. In all, five Americans were killed and seventeen were sickened when letters containing anthrax spores arrived at the offices of two congressmen and several news outlets. After a lengthy investigation the FBI concluded the attacks had been perpetrated by a disgruntled microbiologist at the US Army Medical Research Institute for Infectious Diseases at Fort Detrick, Maryland, who had committed suicide shortly before he was due to be arrested. However, the National Academy of Sciences subsequently cast doubt on the agency's findings, accessed 19 February 2017: https://en.wikipedia.org/wiki/2001_anthrax_attacks

24. Abraham, *Twenty-First Century Plague*, 73.

25. David L. Heymann and Guenael Rodier, "SARS: Lessons from a New Disease," in S. Kobler et al., eds., *Learning from SARS: Preparing for the Next Disease Outbreak:Workshop Summary* (Washington, DC: National Academies Press [US], 2004).

26. "How a Deadly Disease Came to Canada," *The Globe and Mail*, accessed 4 February 2017: http://www.theglobeandmail.com/news/national/how-a-deadly-disease-came-to-canada/article1159487/

27. Abraham, *Twenty-First Century Plague*, 111.

28. At that time, a suspect case of SARS was defined as anyone exhibiting fever, cough, or shortness of breath and who had had close contact with a suspect or probable case or who had recently been in an area where transmission had occurred. A probable SARS case had all the features of a suspect case plus X-ray, laboratory, or autopsy findings consistent with the disease.

29. Malik Peiris, interview with author, Hong Kong, 27 March 2017.

30. Ibid.

31. J. S. M. Peiris and Y. Guan, "Confronting SARS: A View from Hong Kong," *Philosophical Transactions of the Royal Society of London Series B, Biological Sciences* 359, no. 1447 (29 July 2004): 1075–79.

32. Peiris, interview with author.

33. J. S. M. Peiris et al., "Coronavirus as a Possible Cause of Severe Acute Respiratory Syndrome," *The Lancet* 361, no. 9366 (19 April 2003): 1319–25.

34. Abraham, *Twenty-First Century Plague*, 118–20.

35. Peiris, interview with author.

36. "Learning from SARS: Renewal of Public Health in Canada," Report of the National Advisory Committee on SARS and Public Health, October 2003, accessed 8 February 2017: http://www.phac-aspc.gc.ca/publicat/sars-sras/naylor/index-eng.php

37. James Young, "My Experience with SARS," in Jacalyn Duffin and Arthur Sweetman, eds., *SARS In Context: Memory, History, Policy* (Montreal: McGill-Queen's University Press, 2006), 19–25.

38. Dick Zoutman, "Remembering SARS and the Ontario SARS Scientific Advisory Committee," in Duffin and Sweetman, eds., *SARS In Context*, 27–40.

39. "How 'Total Recall' Saved Toronto's Film Industry," *Toronto Star* (22 September 2011), accessed 8 February 2017: https://www.thestar.com/news/2011/09/22/how_total_recall_saved_torontos_film_industry.html

40. Christine Loh and Jennifer Welker, "SARS and the Hong Kong Community," in Loh and Civic Exchange, eds., *At the Epicentre*, 218.

41. Keith Bradsher, "A Respiratory Illness: Economic Impact; From Tourism to High Finance, Mysterious Illness Spreads Havoc," *New York Times* (3 April 2003), accessed 2 October 2017: http://www.nytimes.com/2003/04/03/world/respiratory-illness-economic-impact-tourism-high-finance-mysterious-illness.html

42. Sui A Wong, "Economic Impact of SARS: The Case of Hong Kong," *Asian Economic Papers* 3, no. 1 (2004): 62–83.

43. Duncan Jepson, "When the Fear of SARS Went Viral," *New York Times* (14 March 2013), accessed 2 October 2017: http://www.nytimes.com/2013/03/15/opinion/global/when-the-fear-of-SARS-went-viral.html

44. Abraham, *Twenty-First Century Plague*, 70–75.

45. Yi Guan et al., "Isolation and Characterization of Viruses Related to the SARS Coronavirus from Animals in Southern China," *Science* 302, no. 5643 (10 October 2003): 276–78.

46. Wendong Li et al., "Bats Are Natural Reservoirs of SARS-Like Coronaviruses," *Science* 310, no. 5748 (28 October 2005): 676–79.

47. Kai Kupferschmidt, "Bats May Be Carrying the Next SARS Pandemic," *Science* (30 October 2013). To add further confusion, in 2012 another coronavirus, distantly related to SARS, emerged in Saudi Arabia. Serological evidence suggests that the virus, dubbed Middle East Respiratory Syndrome (MERS), had circulated in camels in Africa and the Arabian peninsula for up to twenty years and that camels most likely acquired the virus from a bat native to sub-Saharan Africa. Victor Max Corman et al., "Rooting the Phylogenetic Tree of Middle East Respiratory Syndrome Coronavirus by Characterization of a Conspecific Virus from an African Bat," *Journal of Virology* 88, no. 19 (1 October 2014): 11297–303.

48. Robert G. Webster, "Wet Markets—a Continuing Source of Severe Acute Respiratory Syndrome and Influenza?," *The Lancet* 363, no. 9404 (17 January 2004): 234–36.

49. Gaby Hinsliff et al., "The day the world caught a cold," *The Observer* (27 April 2003), accessed 2 October 2017: https://www.theguardian.com/world/2003/apr/27/sars.johnaglionby

50. Peiris and Guan, "Confronting SARS," 1078.

51. Abraham, *Twenty-First Century Plague*, 42–49.

52. "Panicking Only Makes It Worse: Epidemics damage economies as well as health," *The Economist* (16 August 2014), accessed 2 October 2017: https://www.economist.com/news/international/21612158-epidemics-damage-economies-well-health-panicking-only-makes-it-worse

53. Heymann and Rodier, "SARS: Lessons from a New Disease."

54. Roy M. Anderson et al., "Epidemiology, Transmission Dynamics and Control of

SARS: The 2002–2003 Epidemic," *Philosophical Transactions of the Royal Society B: Biological Sciences* 359, no. 1447 (29 July 2004): 1091–1105.

8. EBOLA AT THE BORDERS

1. Almudena Marí Saéz et al., "Investigating the Zoonotic Origin of the West African Ebola Epidemic," *EMBO Molecular Medicine* (29 December 2014), e201404792

2. Sylvain Baize et al., "Emergence of Zaire Ebola Virus Disease in Guinea," *New England Journal of Medicine* 371, no. 15 (9 October 2014): 1418–25.

3. Paul Richards, *Ebola: How a Peoples' Science Helped End an Epidemic* (London: Zed Books, 2016), 29–31.

4. Baize et al., "Emergence of Zaire Ebola Virus Disease in Guinea."

5. Médecins Sans Frontières (MSF), "Ebola: Pushed to the limit and beyond," 23 March 2015: accessed 29 April 2015: http://www.msf.org/article/ebola-pushed-limit-and-beyond

6. Daniel S. Chertow et al., "Ebola Virus Disease in West Africa—Clinical Manifestations and Management," *New England Journal of Medicine* 371, no. 22 (27 November 2014): 2054–57; Mark G. Kortepeter et al., "Basic Clinical and Laboratory Features of Filoviral Hemorrhagic Fever," *Journal of Infectious Diseases* 204, suppl. 3 (11 January 2011): S810–16.

7. Richard Preston, *The Hot Zone* (London and New York: Doubleday, 1994), 81–83.

8. MSF, "Ebola," 1–21, 5.

9. J. Knobloch et al., "A Serological Survey on Viral Haemorrhagic Fevers in Liberia," *Annales de l'Institut Pasteur / Virologie* 133, no. 2 (1 January 1982): 125–28.

10. "Army Scientist Uses Diagnostic Tools to Track Viruses," US Department of Defense, accessed 7 December 2015: http://www.defense.gov/News-Article-View/Article/603830/army-scientist-uses-diagnostic-tools-to-track-viruses. Later, when the WHO confirmed the outbreak was due to *Zaire ebolavirus*, the journal revised its decision and published Schoepp's paper. Randal J. Schoepp et al., "Undiagnosed Acute Viral Febrile Illnesses, Sierra Leone," *Emerging Infectious Diseases* 20, no. 7 (July 2014): 1176–82.

11. Baize et al., "Emergence of Zaire Ebola Virus Disease in Guinea."

12. WHO, "Ebola Outbreak 2014–15," accessed 6 May 2015: http://www.who.int/csr/disease/ebola/en/

13. Pam Belluck et al., "How Ebola Roared Back," *New York Times*, 29 December 2014, accessed 6 May 2015: http://www.nytimes.com/2014/12/30/health/how-ebola-roared-back.html

14. MSF, "Ebola," 6.

15. In fact, as would subsequently become clear, Ebola had already crossed into Liberia and Sierra Leone and was spreading via several concurrent transmission lines, aided by the passage of the family members incubating the virus across the region's porous borders.

16. Jean-Jacques Muyembe-Tamfum et al., "Ebola Virus Outbreaks in Africa: Past and

Present," *The Onderstepoort Journal of Veterinary Research* 79, no. 2 (2012): 451; David M. Pigott et al., "Mapping the Zoonotic Niche of Ebola Virus Disease in Africa," *eLife*, 8 September 2014, e04395.

17. Neil Carey, "Ebola and Poro: Plague, Ancient Art, and the New Ritual of Death," Poro Studies Association, accessed 16 January 2017: http://www.porostudiesassociation. org/ebola-and-secret-societies/

18. Paul Richards, "Burial/other cultural practices and risk of EVD transmission in the Mano River Region," Briefing note for DFID, 14 October 2014, Ebola Response Anthropology Platform, accessed 16 January 2017: http://www.ebola-anthropology. net/evidence/1269/

19. Mark G. Kortepeter et al., "Basic Clinical and Laboratory Features of Filoviral Hemorrhagic Fever," *Journal of Infectious Diseases* 204, suppl. 3 (1 November 2011): S810–16. doi:10.1093/infdis/jir299.

20. Jean-Jacques Muyembe-Tamfum, interview with author, 29 May 2015.

21. David L. Heymann et al., "Ebola Hemorrhagic Fever: Lessons from Kikwit, Democratic Republic of the Congo," *Journal of Infectious Diseases* 179, suppl. 1 (1 February 1999): S283–86. doi:10.1086/514287.

22. David Heymann, interview with author, 19 March 2015.

23. James Fairhead, "Understanding social resistance to Ebola response in Guinea," Ebola Response Anthropology Platform, April 2015, accessed 16 January 2017: http://www. ebola-anthropology.net/evidence/1269/; Pam Belluck, "Red Cross Faces Attacks at Ebola Victims' Funerals," *New York Times* (12 February 2015), accessed 16 January 2017: https://www.nytimes.com/2015/02/13/world/africa/red-cross-faces-attacks-at-ebola-victims-funerals.html

24. "Ebola and Emerging Infectious Diseases: Measuring the Risk," Chatham House (6 May 2014), accessed 11 November 2015: https://www.chathamhouse.org/events/view/198881

25. Armand Sprecher, "The MSF Response to the West African Ebola Outbreak," The Ebola Epidemic in West Africa, Institute of Medicine, Washington, DC, 25 March 2015.

26. "Outbreak—Transcript," *Frontline*, accessed 5 October 2017: http://www.pbs.org/wgbh/frontline/film/outbreak/transcript/

27. Joshua Hammer, "My Nurses are Dead and I Don't Know If I'm Already Infected—Matter," *Medium* (12 January 2015), accessed 4 February 2015: https://medium.com/matter/did-sierra-leones-hero-doctor-have-to-die-1c1de004941e

28. Oliver Johnson, interview with author, 10 March 2015.

29. "Briefing note to the director-general, June 2014," Associated Press, "Bungling Ebola-Documents," accessed 17 June 2015: http://data.ap.org/projects/2015/who-ebola/

30. "Ebola Outbreak in W. Africa 'totally out of control'—MSF," *RT English*, accessed 30 September 2015: http://www.rt.com/news/167404-ebola-africa-out-of-control/

31. Will Pooley, interview with author, 24 May 2015.

32. Umaru Fofana and Daniel Flynn, "Sierra Leone Hero Doctor's Death Exposes Slow Ebola Response," accessed 12 February 2015: http://in.reuters.com/article/2014/08/24/health-ebola-khan-idINKBN0GO07C20140824

33. Daniel G. Bausch et al., "A Tribute to Sheik Humarr Khan and All the Healthcare Workers in West Africa Who Have Sacrificed in the Fight against Ebola Virus Disease: Mae We Hush," *Antiviral Research* 111 (November 2014): 33–35.

34. Etienne Simon-Loriere et al., "Distinct Lineages of Ebola Virus in Guinea during the 2014 West African Epidemic," *Nature* 524, no. 7563 (6 August 2015): 102–4.

35. Ed Mazza, "Donald Trump Says Ebola Doctors 'Must Suffer the Consequences," *Huffington Post* (4 August 2014), sec. Media, accessed 6 May 2015: https://www.huffingtonpost.com/2014/08/03/donald-trump-ebola-doctors_n_5646424.html

36. Belgium Airways in-flight magazine, March 2015.

37. MSF, "Ebola," 11.

38. Joanne Liu, Global Health Risks Framework, Wellcome Trust workshop, 1–2 September 2015.

39. Preston, *The Hot Zone*, 81–83.

40. Ibid., 289–90.

41. Garrett, *The Coming Plague*, 593–95.

42. Tom Frieden, interview with author, 26 October 2015.

43. "Statement of Joanne Liu at United Nations Special Briefing on Ebola," United Nations, New York (2 September 2014), accessed 27 November 2015: http://association.msf.org/node/162513

44. Martin Meltzer et al., and Centers for Disease Control and Prevention (CDC), "Estimating the Future Number of Cases in the Ebola Epidemic—Liberia and Sierra Leone, 2014–2015," *Morbidity and Mortality Weekly Report. Surveillance Summaries (Washington, DC: 2002)* 63 suppl. 3 (26 September 2014): 1–14.

45. Norimitsu Onishi, "As Ebola Grips Liberia's Capital, a Quarantine Sows Social Chaos," *New York Times* (28 August 2014): http://www.nytimes.com/2014/08/29/world/africa/in-liberias-capital-an-ebola-outbreak-like-no-other.html

46. Breslow, "Was Ebola Outbreak an Exception Or Was It a Precedent?" "Outbreak," *Frontline*, accessed 6 May 2015: http://www.pbs.org/wgbh/pages/frontline/health-science-technology/outbreak/was-ebola-outbreak-an-exception-or-was-it-a-precedent/

47. Mark Honigsbaum, "Ebola: The Road to Zero," *Mosaic*, accessed 5 October 2017: https://mosaicscience.com/story/ebola-road-zero

48. Manny Fernandez and Kevin Sack, "Ebola Patient Sent Home Despite Fever, Records Show," *New York Times* (10 October 2014), accessed 1 October 2016: https://www.nytimes.com/2014/10/11/us/thomas-duncan-had-a-fever-of-103-er-records-show.html

49. Duncan was most likely infected with Ebola in Monrovia on 15 September when he carried his landlord's daughter, who was stricken with Ebola, home from the hospital.

However, he had showed no signs of fever or other symptoms of Ebola when he was screened on 19 September before boarding a flight from Monrovia to Brussels, from where he caught a connecting flight to Washington Dulles, followed by a second to Dallas-Fort Worth. "Retracing the Steps of the Dallas Ebola Patient," *New York Times* (1 October 2014): http://www.nytimes.com/interactive/2014/10/01/us/retracing-the-steps-of-the-dallas-ebola-patient.html

50. MSF, "Ebola," 9.

51. WHO, "Report of the Ebola Interim Assessment Panel—July 2015," *WHO*, Geneva, accessed 6 August 2015: http://www.who.int/csr/resources/publications/ebola/ebola-panel-report/en/

52. Pierre Rollin, interview with author, 26 October 2015.

53. Kevin Belluck et al., "How Ebola Roared Back," *New York Times* (29 December 2014), accessed 1 October 2016: http://www.nytimes.com/2014/12/30/health/how-ebola-roared-back.html

54. Wellcome. "Discussing Global Health at Davos," *Wellcome Trust Blog*, accessed 11 June 2015: http://blog.wellcome.ac.uk/2015/01/21/discussing-global-health-at-davos/. *Black Swan* is the title of a 2010 best-selling book by the Lebanese-American essayist Nassim Nicholas Taleb, and refers to an event for which past experience has not prepared us and which, until it occurs, is widely considered to be an impossibility—the paradigm example being that before the discovery of Australia, people in the Old World were convinced that all swans were white because no one had seen a black one before. According to Taleb, a Black Swan has three key elements: "rarity, extreme impact, and retrospective (though not prospective) predictability."

55. Muyembe-Tamfum, "Ebola Virus Outbreaks in Africa."

56. WHO, "Ebola virus disease, fact sheet 103, updated August 2015. Table: Chronology of previous Ebola virus disease outbreaks," accessed 4 December 2015: http://www.who.int/mediacentre/factsheets/fs103/en/

57. The reasons for this are beyond the scope of this book, save to say that pharmaceutical companies have little commercial incentive to invest in vaccines and drugs for neglected tropical diseases such as Ebola. Having said that, during the outbreak in Guinea an international consortium backed by the WHO were able to demonstrate that an experimental vaccine developed by the Public Health Agency of Canada and the US Defense Threat Reduction Agency that had previously only been tested in monkeys under laboratory conditions conferred 100 per cent protection against Ebola in trial subjects immunized randomly in the field. While questions remain about the safety of the rVSV vaccine and the duration of its protective effect, the prospect is that it could be offered to health workers before they are deployed to the next Ebola outbreak, thereby reducing the incidence of disease and keeping casualties to a minimum. Thomas W. Geisbert, "First Ebola Virus Vaccine to Protect Human Beings?," *The Lancet* 389, no. 10068 (4 February 2017): 479–80.

58. Edward C. Holmes et al., "The Evolution of Ebola Virus: Insights from the 2013–2016 Epidemic," *Nature* 538, no. 7624 (13 October 2016): 193–200.

9. Z IS FOR ZIKA

1. Juliana Barbassa, "Inside the fight against the Zika virus," *Vogue* (5 May 2016), accessed 1 August 2017: https://www.vogue.com/article/zika-virus-doctor-vanessa-van-der-linden

2. Laura Clark Rohrer, "Enigma," *Pitt (University of Pittsburgh)*, Summer 2017, 19–23.

3. Liz Braga, "How a Small Team of Doctors Convinced the World to Stop Ignoring Zika," *Newsweek* (29 February 2016), accessed 1 August 2017: http://www.newsweek.com/2016/03/11/zika-microcephaly-connection-brazil-doctors-431427.html

4. "Chikungunya Fever Guide," accessed 3 August 2017: http://www.chikungunya.in/dengue-chikungunya-differences.shtml

5. Dick Brathwaite et al., "The History of Dengue Outbreaks in the Americas," *The American Journal of Tropical Medicine and Hygiene* 87, no. 4 (3 October 2012): 584–93, doi:10.4269/ajtmh.2012.11–0770.

6. WHO, "Dengue and severe dengue," accessed 3 August 2017: http://www.who.int/mediacentre/factsheets/fs117/en/

7. Carlos Brito, interview with author, 5 January and 24 July 2017.

8. Ibid.

9. Donald McNeil, *Zika: The Emerging Epidemic* (New York: Norton, 2016), 30.

10. "Alexander Haddow and Zika Virus," *Flickr*, accessed 7 August 2017: https://www.flickr.com/photos/uofglibrary/albums/72157668781044525; McNeil, *Zika*, 19–22; G. W. A. Dick, "Zika Virus (II). Pathogenicity and Physical Properties," *Transactions of The Royal Society of Tropical Medicine and Hygiene* 46, no. 5 (1952): 521–34.

11. Mary Kay Kindhauser et al., "Zika: the origin and spread of a mosquito-borne virus," *Bulletin of the World Health Organization* 94 (2016): 675–686C, accessed 7 August 2016: http://www.who.int/bulletin/online_first/16–171082/en/

12. McNeil, *Zika*, 41.

13. Ibid., 43–45.

14. Rachel Becker, "Missing Link: Animal Models to Study Whether Zika Causes Birth Defects," *Nature Medicine* 22, no. 3 (March 2016): 225–27.

15. Rohrer, "Enigma," 19–23.

16. Ernesto Marques, interview with author, 24 July 2017.

17. Braga, "How a Small Team of Doctors Convinced the World to Stop Ignoring Zika."

18. Brito, interview with author, 24 July 2017.

19. G. Calvet et al., "Detection and Sequencing of Zika Virus from Amniotic Fluid of Fetuses with Microcephaly in Brazil: A Case Study," *The Lancet Infectious Diseases* 16, no. 6 (1 June 2016): 653–60.

20. Braga, "How a Small Team of Doctors Convinced the World."

21. "Neurological syndrome, congenital malformations, and Zika virus infection. Implication for public health in the Americas," *PAHO*, Epidemiological Alert, 1 December 2015, accessed 10 August 2017: http://www.paho.org/hq/index.php?option=com_content&view=article&id=11599&Itemid=41691&lang=en

22. David Heymann et al., "Zika Virus and Microcephaly: Why Is This Situation a PHEIC?," *The Lancet* 387, no. 10020 (20 February 2016): 719–21.

23. Margaret Chan, "Zika: we must be ready for the long haul," 1 February 2017, accessed 10 August 2017: http://www.who.int/mediacentre/commentaries/2017/zika-long-haul/en/

24. WHO, "Zika: Then, now and tomorrow," accessed 10 August 2017: http://www.who.int/features/2017/zika-then-now/en/

25. Jonathan Watts, "Rio Olympics Committee Warns Athletes to Take Precautions against Zika Virus," *The Guardian* (2 February 2016), accessed 11 August 2017: https://www.theguardian.com/world/2016/feb/02/zika-virus-rio-2016-olympics-athletes

26. Jonathan Ball, "No One is Safe from Zika: Confirmation that Mosquito-borne Virus Does Shrink Heads of Unborn Babies … and a Chilling Warning," *Daily Mail* (31 January 2016), accessed 11 August 2017: http://www.dailymail.co.uk/news/article-3424776/No-one-safe-Zika-Confirmation-mosquito-borne-virus-does-shrink-heads-unborn-babies-chilling-warning.html

27. Julian Robinson, "Living with 'Zika': Brazilian Parents Pose with Their Children Suffering from Head-shrinking Bug to Highlight Their Plight," *Daily Mail* (25 February 2016), accessed 11 August 2017: http://www.dailymail.co.uk/news/article-3464023/Living-Zika-Brazilian-parents-pose-children-suffering-head-shrinking-bug-highlight-plight.html#ixzz4pR4i82UG

28. Nadia Khomani, "Greg Rutherford Freezes Sperm over Olympics Zika Fears," *The Guardian* (7 June 2016), accessed 11 August 2017: https://www.theguardian.com/sport/2016/jun/07/greg-rutherford-freezes-sperm-over-olympics-zika-fears

29. Andrew Jacobs, "Conspiracy Theories About Zika Spread Through Brazil with the Virus," *New York Times* (16 February 2016), accessed 11 August 2017: https://www.nytimes.com/2016/02/17/world/americas/conspiracy-theories-about-zika-spread-along-with-the-virus.html

30. Sarah Boseley, "Florida Issues Warning after Cluster of New Zika Cases in Miami Neighborhood," *The Guardian* (1 August 2016), accessed 11 August 2017: https://www.theguardian.com/world/2016/aug/01/florida-zika-cases-transmission-neighborhood-miami-dade-county; Jessica Glenza, "Zika Virus Scare is Turning Miami's Hipster Haven into a Ghost Town, *The Guardian* (10 August 2016), accessed 11 August 2017: https://www.theguardian.com/world/2016/aug/10/zika-virus-miami-florida-cases-mosquito-wynwood; Richard Luscombe, "Miami Beach Protests against use of Naled to fight Zika-carrying Mosquitos," *The Guardian* (8 September 2017), accessed 11 August 2017: https://www.theguardian.com/world/2016/sep/08/miami-beach-zika-protests-naled-mosquitos

31. N. R. Faria et al., "Establishment and Cryptic Transmission of Zika Virus in Brazil and the Americas," *Nature* 546, no. 7658 (15 June 2017): 406–10.

32. Celia Turchi, interview with author, 24 July 2017.

33. Ilana Löwy, "Zika and Microcephaly: Can we Learn from History?," *Revista de Saúde Coletiva* 26, no. 1 (2016): 11–21.

34. C. G. Victora et al., "Microcephaly in Brazil: How to Interpret Reported Numbers?," *The Lancet* 387, no. 10019 (13 February 2016): 621–24.

35. W. K. Oliveira et al., "Infection-related Microcephaly after the 2015 and 2016 Zika Virus Outbreaks in Brazil: A Surveillance-based Analysis," *The Lancet* 6736, no. 17 (21 June 2017): 31368–5.

36. W. Kleber de Oliveira et al., "Infection-Related Microcephaly after the 2015 and 2016 Zika Virus Outbreaks in Brazil: A Surveillance-Based Analysis," *The Lancet* (21 June 2017), accessed 19 March 2018: https://doi.org/10.1016/S0140-6736(17)31368–5

37. Stephanie Nolen, "Two Years after Brazil's Zika Virus Crisis, Experts Remain Baffled," *The Globe and Mail* (1 September 2017), accessed 2 September 2017: https://beta.theglobeandmail.com/news/world/zika-crisis-brazil/article36142168/

38. Priscila M. S. Castanha et al., "Dengue Virus–Specific Antibodies Enhance Brazilian Zika Virus Infection," *The Journal of Infectious Diseases* 215, no. 5 (3 January 2017): 781–85.

39. Ewen Callaway, "Rio fights Zika with Biggest Release Yet of Bacteria-infected Mosquitoes," *Nature News* 539, no. 7627 (3 November 2016): 17.

40. Liana Ventura, interview with author, 28 July 2017.

41. "Neglected and Unprotected: The Impact of the Zika Outbreak on Women and Girls in Northeastern Brazil," *Human Rights Watch* (12 July 2017), accessed 24 August 2017: https://www.hrw.org/news/2017/07/12/brazil-zika-epidemic-exposes-rights-problems

42. Rob Sawers, "The beautiful Brazilian beaches plagued by shark attacks," *BBC World News* (27 September 2012), accessed 22 August 2017: http://www.bbc.co.uk/news/world-radio-and-tv-19720455

43. Andrew Spielman and Michael D'Antonio, *Mosquito: The Story of Man's Deadliest Foe* (New York: Hyperion, 2001).

44. "Aedes Albopictus—Factsheet for Experts," *European Centre for Disease Prevention and Control*, accessed 6 October 2017: http://ecdc.europa.eu/en/disease-vectors/facts/mosquito-factsheets/aedes-albopictus

10. DISEASE X

1. Partha Bose and Jilian Mincer, "The Doctor Whose Gut Instinct Beat AI in Spotting the Coronavirus," *Oliver Wyman Forum*, accessed 10 March 2020: https://www.oliverwymanforum.com/city-readiness/2020/mar/the-doctor-whose-gut-instinct-beat-ai-in-spotting-the-coronavirus.html

2. Jeremy Page, Wenxin Fan and Natasha Khan, "How it All Started: China's Early Coronavirus Missteps," *Wall Street Journal*, 6 March 2020, accessed 13 March 2020: https://www.wsj.com/articles/how-it-all-started-chinas-early-coronavirus-missteps-11583508932

3. Wang Lianzhang, "Gone But Not Soon Forgotten: Li Wenliang's Online Legacy," *Sixthtone*, 7 February 2020: https://www.sixthtone.com/news/1005172/gone-but-not-soon-forgotten-li-wenliangs-online-legacy

4. Tian Yang, et al., "Appeal From Chinese Doctors to End Violence," *The Lancet* 382, no. 9906 (23 November 2013): 1703-1704, accessed 13 March 2020: https://www.thelancet.com/journals/lancet/article/PIIS0140-6736(13)62401-0/fulltext

5. Page, "How It All Started: China's Early Coronavirus Missteps."

6. Alexander Boyd, "CCP Report on Death of Dr. Li Wenliang Scapegoats Wuhan Police, Claims Him as Their Own", *Supchina*, 20 March 2020, accessed 24 March 2020: https://supchina.com/2020/03/20/ccp-report-on-death-of-dr-li-wenliang-scapegoats-wuhan-police-claims-him-as-their-own/

7. Page, "How It All Started: China's Early Coronavirus Missteps."

8. Boyd, "CCP Report on Death of Dr. Li Wenliang Scapegoats Wuhan Police, Claims Him as Their Own."

9. Verna Yu, "'Hero Who Told the Truth': Chinese Rage Over Coronavirus Death of Whistleblower Doctor", *Guardian*, 7 February 2020, accessed 29 March 2020: https://www.theguardian.com/global-development/2020/feb/07/coronavirus-chinese-rage-death-whistleblower-doctor-li-wenliang

10. Xu Zhangrun, trans. Geremie R. Barmé, "Viral Alarm: When Fury Overcomes Fear," *China File*, 5 February 5 2020, accessed 29 March 2020: https://www.chinafile.com/reporting-opinion/viewpoint/viral-alarm-when-fury-overcomes-fear

11. Daniel Wrapp, et al., "Cryo-EM Structure of the 2019-nCoV Spike in the Prefusion Conformation", *Science* 367, no. 6483 (13 March 2020): 1260-1263.

12. A recent study in *Nature* found that SARS-CoV-2 is about four times as good at binding to the ACE-2 receptor as classic SARS. The viruses share approximately 80 per cent of the same genes, which makes SARS-CoV-2 a new virus. It is most closely related to strains found in bats and pangolins. This suggests that either SARS-CoV-2 spilled over to humans directly from bats, or from pangolins that had been infected by bats. Before infecting humans, the animal strains picked up key mutations that enabled the virus to spread more easily to humans. Jian Shan et al., "Structural Basis of Receptor Recognition by SARS-CoV-2," *Nature*, 30 March 2020, accessed 31 March 2020: https://www.nature.com/articles/s41586-020-2179-y#Abs1

13. "Mount Sinai Physicians the First in U.S. Analyzing Lung Disease in Coronavirus Patients from China", *Imaging Technology News*, 26 February 2020; Scott Simpson, et al., "Radiological Society of North America Expert Consensus Statement on Reporting Chest CT Findings Related to COVID-19", *Radiology: Cardiothoracic Imaging* 2, no. 2 (25 March 2020): e200152.

14. See for instance, Bill Gates, "Responding to Covid-19—A Once-in-a-Century Pandemic?" *New England Journal of Medicine*, 28 February 2020, accessed 29 March 2020: https://doi.org/10.1056/NEJMp2003762; David Morens, Peter Daszak, and Jeffery Taubenberger, "Escaping Pandora's Box—Another Novel Coronavirus", *New England Journal of Medicine*, 26 February 2020, accessed 29 March 2020: https://doi.org/10.1056/NEJMp2002106

15. Christos Lynteris and Lyle Fearnley, "Why Shutting Down Chinese 'Wet Markets' Could Be a Terrible Mistake", *The Conversation*, 2 March 2020, accessed 22 March 2020: https://

theconversation.com/why-shutting-down-chinese-wet-markets-could-be-a-terrible-mistake-130625

16. H. V. Fineberg, "Pandemic Preparedness and Response—Lessons from the H1N1 Influenza of 2009", *New England Journal of Medicine* 370, no. 14 (3 April 2014): 1335–1342.

17. World Bank, "2014-2015 West Africa Ebola Crisis: Impact Update", 10 May 2016, accessed 25 March 2020: https://www.worldbank.org/en/topic/macroeconomics/publication/2014-2015-west-africa-ebola-crisis-impact-update

18. Kai Kupferschmidt, "Bats May Be Carrying the Next SARS Pandemic", *Science*, 30 October 2013, accessed 6 April 2020: https://www.sciencemag.org/news/2013/10/bats-may-be-carrying-next-sars-pandemic#

19. James Gorman, "How Do Bats Live With So Many Viruses?" *New York Times*, 28 January 2020, accessed 25 March 2020, https://www.nytimes.com/2020/01/28/science/bats-coronavirus-Wuhan.html; Jiazheng Xi, et al., "Dampened STING-Dependent Interferon Activation in Bats", *Cell Host & Microbe* 23, no. 3 (14 March 2018): 2018-03-14.

20. Kevin J. Olival, et al., "Host and Viral Traits Predict Zoonotic Spillover From Mammals", *Nature*, 21 June 2017.

21. Lisa Schnirring, "New SARS-like Virus From Bats Implicated in China Pig Die Off", *CIDRAP*, 5 April 2018: http://www.cidrap.umn.edu/news-perspective/2018/04/new-sars-virus-bats-implicated-china-pig-die

22. Kate E. Jones, et al., "Global Trends in Emerging Infectious diseases", *Nature*, 451, no. 7181 (21 February 2008): 990-993.

23. Bill Gates, "The Next outbreak? We're Not Ready", *TED* 2015, accessed 26 March 2020: https://www.ted.com/talks/bill_gates_the_next_outbreak_we_re_not_ready/transcript?language=en#t-39511

24. WHO, "Blueprint for R&D Preparedness and Response to Public Health Emergencies Due to Highly Infectious Pathogens", 8-9 December 2015, accessed 26 March 2020, https://www.who.int/blueprint/about/en/

25. WHO, "2018 Annual Review of Diseases Prioritized Under the Research and Development Blueprint", 6-7 February 2018, accessed 26 March 2020: http://www.who.int/blueprint/priority-diseases/en/

26. Interview with author, 6 March 2020. The person to whom Daszak is referring is Dr Massinissa Si Mehand, a WHO technical officer whose research interests include "applied mathematics, outbreak preparedness and response, priority setting, decision aid, and risk analysis." Massinissa Si Mehand et. al, "World Health Organization Methodology to Prioritize Emerging Infectious Diseases in Need of Research and Development", *Emerging Infectious Diseases* 24, no. 9 (September 2018), accessed 26 March 2020: https://wwwnc.cdc.gov/eid/article/24/9/17-1427_article

27. Peter Daszak, "We Knew Disease X Was Coming. It's Here Now", *New York Times*, 23 March 2020: https://www.nytimes.com/2020/02/27/opinion/coronavirus-pandemics.html; https://www.globalviromeproject.org/our-history

28. "What is GVP – Fact Sheet", *Global Virome Project*, accessed 26 March 2020: http://www.globalviromeproject.org/fact-sheets

29. CEPI, "Mission", accessed 6 April 2020; Elsevier, "Infographic: Global Research Trends in Infectious Disease," 25 March 2020: https://www.elsevier.com/connect/infographic-global-research-trends-in-infectious-disease

30. World Bank and WHO, "A World at Risk: Annual Report on Global Preparedness for Health Emergencies", *Global Preparedness Monitoring Board*, September 2019.

31. "The Event 201 Scenario", accessed 27 March 2020: http://www.centerforhealthsecurity.org/event201/scenario.html

32. Helen Branswell and Megan Thielking, "Fluctuating Funding and Flagging Interest Hurt Coronavirus Research", *STAT*, 10 February 2020, accessed 27 March 2020; https://www.statnews.com/2020/02/10/fluctuating-funding-and-flagging-interest-hurt-coronavirus-research/

33. Rupert Beale, "Wash Your Hands", *London Review of Books* 42, no. 5 (5 March 2020), accessed 27 March 2020: https://www.lrb.co.uk/the-paper/v42/n06/rupert-beale/short-cuts

34. Angela Giuffrida and Lorenzo Tondo, "'As If a Storm Hit': More Than 40 Italian Health Workers Have Died Since the Crisis Began", *Guardian*, 26 March 2020.

35. Motoko Rich, "'We're in a Petri Dish': How a Coronavirus Ravaged a Cruise Ship", *New York Times,* 22 February 2020, accessed 30 March 2020: https://www.nytimes.com/2020/02/22/world/asia/coronavirus-japan-cruise-ship.html

36. Motoko Rich and Eimi Yamamitsu, "Hundreds Released From Diamond Princess Cruise Ship in Japan", *New York Times*, 19 February 2020.

37. "'Clap for Carers': UK in 'emotional' tribute to NHS and care workers", *BBC News*, 27 March 2020.

38. Robert P. Baird, "What Went Wrong With Coronavirus Testing in the U.S.", *New Yorker*, 16 March 2020.

39. Demetri Sevastopulo and Hannah Kuchler, "Trump's Bluster Fails Crisis Test", *Financial Times*, 27 March 2020.

40. Brad Brooks, "Like the Flu? Trump's Coronavirus Messaging Confuses Public, Pandemic Researchers Say", *Reuters*, 13 March 2020.

41. "Wayne Gretzy: Biography", *Hockey Hall of Fame,* accessed 29 March 2020: https://www.hhof.com/LegendsOfHockey/jsp/LegendsMember.jsp?mem=p199901&type=Player&page=bio&list=ByName

42. Donald G. McNeil Jr., "Inside China's All-Out War on the Coronavirus", *New York Times*, 4 March 2020, accessed 11 March 2020: https://www.nytimes.com/2020/03/04/health/coronavirus-china-aylward.html

43. Stephen Grey and Andrew MacAskill, "Special Report: Johnson listened to his scientists about coronavirus - but they were slow to sound the alarm", *Reuters*, 7 April 2020, accessed 9 April 2020, https://www.reuters.com/article/us-health-coronavirus-britain-path-speci-idUSKBN21P1VF

44. Emily Shapiro, "Read Gov. Cuomo's Moving Speech About Defeating the Novel

Coronavirus", *ABC News*, 27 March 2020, accessed 29 March 2020: https://abc news.go.com/US/read-gov-cuomos-moving-speech-defeating-coronavirus/story?id= 69839370

45. Kenya Evelyn, "Trump On Urgent Requests For Ventilators: 'I Don't Believe You Need 30,000'", *Guardian*, 27 March 2020, accessed on 29 March 2020: https://www.the guardian.com/us-news/2020/mar/27/trump-ventilators-coronavirus-cuomo-new-york

46. Ebony Bowden, Carl Campanie and Bruce Golding, "Worker at NYC Hospital Where Nurses Wear Trash Bags as Protection Dies from Coronavirus", *New York Post*, 25 March 2020.

47. Alfred W. Crosby, *America's Forgotten Pandemic: The Influenza of 1918* (Cambridge: Cambridge University Press, 2003), 322.

48. Mark Honigsbaum, *Living With Enza: The Forgotten Story of Britain and the Great Flu Pandemic of 1918* (London: Macmillan, 2009), 83-84.

49. Thomas Friedman, "Our New Historical Divide: B.C. and A.C.—the World Before Corona and the World After", *New York Times*, 17 March 2020.

50. Robert Verity, et al., "Estimates of the Severity of Coronavirus Disease 2019: A Model-Based Analysis", *The Lancet Infectious Diseases*, 30 March 2020, accessed 1 April 2020: https://www.thelancet.com/journals/laninf/article/PIIS1473-3099(20)30243-7/ abstract

51. The Spanish flu killed an estimated 50 million to 100 million people worldwide. Adjusting for world population growth that is equivalent to between 140 million to 425 million deaths today. John Barry, "The 1918 Influenza Pandemic in its Time –Will We Learn For the Future?' *Nature Research Microbiology Community*, accessed 10 October 2018: https:// naturemicrobiologycommunity.nature.com/users/79120-john-barry/posts/29254-the-1918-influenza-pandemic-in-its-time-will-we-learn-for-the-future

52. Arundhati Roy, "The Pandemic is a Portal", *Financial Times*, 3 April 2020.

53. Samanth Subramanian, "It's a Razor's Edge We're Walking: Inside the Race to Develop a Coronavirus Vaccine", *Guardian*, 27 March 2020.

EPILOGUE: THE PANDEMIC CENTURY

1. Commission on a Global Health Risk Framework for the Future, and National Academy of Medicine, Secretariat, *The Neglected Dimension of Global Security: A Framework to Counter Infectious Disease Crises* (Washington, D.C.: National Academies Press, 2016), accessed 26 September 2017: http://www.nap.edu/catalog/21891

2. Crosby, *America's Forgotten Pandemic*, xiii.

3. Christos Lynteris and Lyle Fearnley, "Why Shutting Down Chinese 'Wet Markets' Could be a Terrible Mistake", *The Conversation*, 2 March 2020, accessed 22 March 2020: https:// theconversation.com/why-shutting-down-chinese-wet-markets-could-be-a-terrible-mistake-130625

4. Mike Davis, *The Monster at Our Door: The Global Threat of Avian Flu* (New York and London: The New Press, 2005), especially Chapter 7: "The Triangle of Doom", pp. 97-115.

5. Toph Allen, et al., "Global Hotspots and Correlates of Emerging Zoonotic Diseases", *Nature Communications* 8, no. 1 (October 24, 2017): 1-10, accessed 22 March 2020: https://www.nature.com/articles/s41467-017-00923-8

6. René Dubos, "Infection into Disease", *Perspectives in Biology and Medicine* 1, no. 4 (Summer 1958): 425–35.

7. René Dubos, *Mirage of Health* (New Jersey: Rutgers University Press, 1988), 271.

8. Charles E. Rosenberg, *Explaining Epidemics and Other Studies in the History of Medicine* (Cambridge: Cambridge University Press, 1992), 295.

9. René Jules Dubos, "Symbiosis of Earth and Humankind", lecture at American University, Washington D.C., 6 May 1978, RU450 D851, Box 119, Folder 5, René Jules Dubos papers, Rockefeller Archive Center.

10. Samuel Myers and Howard Frumkin (eds), *Planetary Health: Protecting Nature to Protect Ourselves* (Washington; London: Island Press, 2020).

11. David M. Morens and Jeffery K. Taubenberger, "Pandemic Influenza: Certain Uncertainties", *Reviews in Medical Virology* 21, no. 5 (September 2011): 262–84.

ABBREVIATIONS

AFRO	Africa Regional Office
AIDS	Acquired Immune Deficiency Syndrome
ARDS	Acute Respiratory Distress Syndrome
CDC	Centres for Disease Control and Prevention
CMV	Cytomegalovirus
CSF	Cerebrospinal Fluid
CZS	Congenital Zika Syndrome
DRC	Democratic Republic of the Congo
EID	Emerging Infectious Disease
EIS	Epidemic Intelligence Service
ELISA	Enzyme-Linked Immunosorbent Assay
ELWA	Eternal Love Winning Africa
ETU	Ebola Treatment Unit
GOARN	Global Outreach and Response Network
GPHIN	Global Public Health Intelligence Network
GRID	Gay-Related Immune Deficiency
HIV	Human Immunodeficiency Virus
HTLV	Human T-cell Leukaemia Virus
IAM	Instituto Aggeu Magalhães
KS	Kaposi's Sarcoma
LAV	Lymphadenopathy Virus
LCL	Levinthal-Coles-Lillie
MSF	Médecins Sans Frontières
NGO	Nongovernmental Organization
NIAID	National Institute of Allergy and Infectious Diseases
NIH	National Institutes of Health
PAHO	Pan American Health Organization
PCP	*Pneumocystis carinii pneumonia*
PCR	Polymerase Chain Reaction
PHS	Public Health Service

ABBREVIATIONS

ProMED	Program for Monitoring Emerging Diseases
RT-PCR	Reverse Transcriptase Polymerase Chain Reaction
SIV	Simian Immune-Deficiency Virus
UNMEER	United Nations Mission for Ebola Emergency Response
USAMRIID	U.S. Army Medical Research Institute of Infectious Diseases
WHO	World Health Organization

ACKNOWLEDGMENTS

This book is the product of over a decade of research and thinking about infectious disease. My interest in epidemics and pandemics began in 2005 when I went to speak to John Oxford, then Professor of Virology at Queen Mary and Westfield School of Medicine in East London, about avian influenza. A few months earlier a strain of the H5N1 bird flu virus had sparked a spate of deaths in Vietnam, and I had asked John to give me a tutorial on the ecology and virology of influenza before heading to Hanoi to write a feature article for *The Observer*. Very quickly our conversation turned to other notable outbreaks of infectious disease, including the 1918–19 Spanish influenza pandemic. It was the beginning of an obsession with influenza that has led, by way of a PhD and a research fellowship, to a deeper engagement with the history of bacteriology and disease ecology. That research has been generously supported by the Wellcome Trust, allowing me to visit archives in the United States and Australia, where I was able to consult primary documents on the Spanish flu as well as several of the other epidemics canvassed in this book. In 2015, the Wellcome Trust also funded my travel to Sierra Leone to document the impressions of patients, clinicians, and research scientists swept up in the Ebola epidemic, and in Chapter 8 I have drawn on several of these interviews.

Since 1918 there has been a huge change in the scientific understanding of infectious disease and of virology in particular, and I am acutely aware of the scope for error in seeking to summarize this shifting scientific knowledge in relation to such a wide range of infectious pathogens. I have been fortunate in being able to consult some of the leading experts in their fields to help me avoid more obvious errors and summarize past and current scientific knowledge of these pathogens accurately (any errors that remain are my own). In particular, I would like to thank the following for their comments on specific chapters and passages: Wendy Barclay, Kevin De Cock, David Fraser, David Heymann, Michael Kosoy, Ernesto Marques, Joe McDade, David Morens, Malik Peiris, Celina Turchi and Liana Ventura.

ACKNOWLEDGMENTS

I would also like to thank the librarians and archivists who helped me locate key documents and who directed my attention to collections that I might otherwise have missed. In particular: Diane Wendt, Curator of Medicine and Science at the National Museum of American History; Louise E. Shaw, Curator of the David J. Sencer CDC Museum; and Polina E. Ilieva, the Head of Archives and Special Collections at the University of California San Francisco. My thanks also to the staff at the Wellcome Library in London, the National Library of Medicine and National Archives in Bethesda, Maryland, and the librarian in the Library of Congress's newspaper room, who helped me locate the January 1930 report in Hearst's *American Weekly* about the outbreak of parrot fever in the theatrical troupe in Buenos Aires.

Writing a book—especially one of this size—is not a task to be undertaken lightly, and for urging me on and encouraging me that my initial proposal would find an enthusiastic editor, I would like to thank my agent, Patrick Walsh. I would also like to thank Anne Bogart for her knowledge of Los Angeles and her comments on the pneumonic plague chapter, and my wife, Jeanette, who perhaps missed her vocation as a copy editor but has more than made up for it since. No one has read more drafts than she has, and I cannot thank her enough for her intellectual and emotional support. Finally, I am very pleased that the editors who "got" this book and wanted to publish it were John Glusman, whom I had previously worked with at Farrar, Straus and Giroux, and Jon de Peyer at Hurst.

INDEX

327

INDEX